ETHNIC
RHINOPLASTY

Springer Science+Business Media, LLC

ETHNIC RHINOPLASTY

STEVEN M. HOEFFLIN, M.D., F.A.C.S
Department of Surgery, Division of Plastic Surgery
UCLA School of Medicine
Los Angeles, California

With 264 Figures, 65 in Color

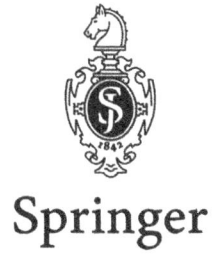

Springer

Steven M. Hoefflin, M.D., F.A.C.S.
Associate Clinical Professor
Department of Surgery, Division of Plastic Surgery
UCLA School of Medicine
Los Angeles, CA 90025
USA

Cover illustration by Hermine Kavanau

Library of Congress Cataloging-in-Publication Data
Hoefflin, Steven M.
   Ethnic rhinoplasty / Steven M. Hoefflin.
     p. cm.
   Includes bibliographical references and index.
   ISBN 978-0-387-94691-7   ISBN 978-1-4612-1646-9 (eBook)
   DOI 10.1007/978-1-4612-1646-9
   I. Rhinoplasty. 2. Black race—Surgery. 3. Mongoloid race—
Surgery. 4. Latin Americans—Surgery. I. Title.
   [DNLM: 1. Rhinoplasty. 2. Nose—anatomy & histology. 3. Ethnic
Groups. WV 312 H693e 1997]
RD119.5.N67H64 1997
617.5'230592—dc21   97-7621

Printed on acid-free paper.

© 1998 Springer Science+Business Media New York
Originally published by Springer-Verlag New York, Inc. in 1998

Production coordinated by University Graphics and managed by Terry Kornak; Manufacturing super-
vised by Jacqui Ashri.
Typeset by University Graphics, York, PA.

9 8 7 6 5 4 3 2 1

ISBN 978-0-387-94691-7

This book is dedicated to my parents, David and Gloria Hoefflin, my wife, Pamela, and my two sons, Jeff and Brady Hoefflin, whose love, encouragement, and inspiration have been so important in my life.

Foreword

When Dr. Hoefflin asked me to write the foreword to his new text, I was apprehensive about introducing yet another book on rhinoplasty until I looked over the manuscript. Dr. Hoefflin has focused his attention on a very special area of rhinoplasty: the ethnic nose. More specifically, he has selected a narrow segment of ethnic rhinoplasty and has included only three groups: black, Asian, and Hispanic. There is a logic in this selection, since they share many common anatomic similarities. And after all, anatomic variation is part of the new approach to rhinoplasty that is so important to the success of the operation. He also includes his personal approach to patient education, preoperative work-up, anesthesia, and postoperative care, which emphasizes the fact that there is more to rhinoplasty than just the surgical essentials.

The publication of a work as significant as a book reflects a high level of dedication and commitment to the specialty that has given so much to all of us. Dr. Hoefflin has had a special interest in the surgical management of the black, Asian, and Hispanic nose and his willingness to share his ideas and experiences will benefit anyone who undertakes this challenging surgery. I am pleased and proud to write this foreword to a work that will add to the ever growing body of information on rhinoplasty.

Jack H. Sheen, M.D.

Acknowledgments

It would be impossible to acknowledge all those who have made contributions, suggested changes, or provided assistance in the creation of this book.

I especially want to acknowledge and thank Ted O. Mills, Peter S. Nicholas, Steven A. Teitelbaum, M.D., and Edward Sorourian, M.A., who actively helped in the organization and editing of the manuscript. The excellent artwork by Hermine Kavanau makes a wonderful contribution, for which I am deeply thankful.

I have tremendous respect for and sincerely thank my mentor Jack H. Sheen, M.D., whose vision, example, and direction have been so important to me over these many years.

Steven M. Hoefflin, M.D., F.A.C.S.

Contents

5 Postoperative Nasal Packing and Dressings 94

6 Postoperative Patient Instructions 99

7 Risks, Complications, and Revisions 104

8 The Ten Commandments of Ethnic Rhinoplasty 121

Introduction

My interest in ethnic (or non-Caucasian) rhinoplasty spans more than 20 years. Historically, the ethnic nose has presented some difficult anatomical challenges. Because of the difficult anatomy of the nose, many patients of various ethnic backgrounds were formerly denied the benefits of rhinoplasty. The main difficulty in noses of Asian, black, and Hispanic ancestry is the discordance between the thick nasal skin and the relative lack of cartilaginous-bony support. The varying balances of these two, as well as soft-tissue volume, offer widely divergent but solvable challenges to the rhinoplastic surgeon. During my early plastic surgical training, conventional reduction rhinoplasty was the standard procedure used on non-Caucasian patients, often yielding unsatisfactory results. However, improved surgical techniques have allowed rhinoplastic surgeons to better address the ethnic nose, with more satisfactory and predictable results.

I believe it important to share with other surgeons experiences and techniques gained and modified over the years. Rhinoplastic surgery requires an ongoing assessment of the surgical plan and technical challenges during surgery, as well as the surgical results and inevitable changes occurring during the healing process. Although the biological healing process is somewhat predictable, different body types and different ethnicities can exhibit very different healing processes, times, and results—keeping even the experienced surgeon humble.

The wide ethnic variety of our patients with their many racial and individual differences tests the surgeon's aesthetic perception, skill, and technical abilities. Just as the talents of sculptors throughout the centuries have shown great variation, we surgeons possess dissimilar aesthetic perceptions, preferences, and skills. While the importance of communicating and sharing ideas and perspectives relating to anatomy, physiology, and techniques is generally recognized, there has historically been much less discussion and sharing of aesthetics and technical aesthetic abilities. Rather than be pessimistic about our abilities, we should maintain our optimistic eagerness to learn more about aesthetics and technical innovations for the betterment of our patients and our students.

There are few areas in plastic surgery where improved results are more self-evident than in nasal surgery. Rhinoplasty has long been one of the most popular and frequently requested aesthetic surgical procedures in the United States. It was the technique of combined reduction-augmentation rhinoplasty as popularized by Sheen and others that served as a stimulus for my current surgical technique.

This is not an "all-inclusive" rhinoplasty publication, but just one link in the chain of accumulated experience and learning on which new techniques are built in order to attain the "perfect" rhinoplasty—a goal that all of us would like to meet, but realize is the challenge that forever keeps us learning.

Although one of the most commonly performed plastic surgical procedures, rhinoplasty has only recently gained widespread popularity and acceptance among non-Caucasians. Improvements in technique, public education, economic parity, and successful results among highly visible individuals have created a growing demand for the procedure. With population and affluence rapidly increasing, it seems unlikely that this demand will diminish in the near future.

There are many distinctively attractive features found in each and every race, and while no two noses are exactly alike, even within an ethnic group, each of these groups presents several characteristics which commonly stimulate requests for rhinoplastic changes and require the implementation of new techniques. These special techniques, which I have developed over the last 20 years, will be our focus. I have chosen to concentrate on the black nasal configuration because it is the most different from the Caucasian. Understanding black rhinoplasties translates into knowledge of most non-Caucasian rhinoplasties.

Historically, black African ethnicity has often involved the use of spectacular body painting and other kinds of decoration. Scarification has often been thought of as a beautification process among native tribes and cultures. Indeed, attention to looking attractive has a long and beautiful history among people of all races and ethnicities. Naturally, each and every race possesses unique, beautiful features. However, it appears that the appeal of one nasal shape predominates. There does, though, appear to be a mixed, heterogeneous blending of the "ideal" of one culture's nose with another among many patients. Worldwide communications medias have served to spread and popularize the "Western look" as a world standard of beauty. This Western "ideal" nose is moderately thin, tapered, angular, and subtly projecting. These features have recently become highly sought after by many cultures and races.

Although the aesthetic goal is a common one, techniques for achieving it are not. Standard reduction techniques, which generally work for the thin, architecturally prominent Caucasian nose, are usually not effective on the thick, nonsupportive, non-Caucasian nose. Ethnic noses tend to have a modest osteocartilaginous framework, thick skin, and flimsy alar cartilages that mandate an altered surgical approach. This includes a combination of judicious soft-tissue reduction and osteocartilaginous augmentation. While cephalometric studies may be helpful in determining a successful result, the most important factor is the shared artistic vision of the surgeon and his or her patient. This is where the art of rhinoplasty is separated from the science.

One can get a good sense of the significant nasal variances in the world's different ethnicities by spending an evening in a large, well-stocked, quality bookstore looking through books containing photographs of faces from various regions of the world, specifically, Africa, Asia, Europe, Central and South America, and the South Seas. The histological difference in dermal thickness and sebaceous gland activity provides an important hint to the difficulty of sculpturing the thick sebaceous tip. It appears that in areas with historical extremes in temperature (near either pole or equator) thick nasal skin provides protection from temperature extremes. The very thick, firm sebaceous nasal tip skin found in certain South Seas tribal members is at one end of a spectrum, while the very thin skin of certain European peoples is at the other end.

Thick, bulky nasal soft tissue is predponderant in much of the darker-skinned population, with only a relatively few having significant osteocartilaginous support. This has proven to be a significant challenge for the plastic surgeon. Conservative rhinoplasties, while yielding a high safety margin, have often resulted in dissatisfied patients and surgeons alike. More radical surgery using standard techniques has unfortunately caused a higher-than-acceptable rate of complications as well as poor surgical results. Consequently, Asian, black, and Hispanic patients were often told that they were poor candidates for aesthetic rhinoplasty. My initial surgical attempts only served to confirm this. Reducing an already deficient tip support structure often resulted in a more flattened, bulbous appearance, while reducing soft tissue produced a distorted look. These frustrations led me (as many historical surgical challenges have led others) to an intense quest for improvement.

Following their basic surgical training, most rhinoplastic surgeons gain proficiency and expertise, and refine or develop favored techniques. The collegial sharing of experience, knowledge, and these techniques is critical to further the profession and increase the quality of patient care. Although the importance of sharing with one another our awareness of anatomy, physiology, and surgical techniques is generally recognized, the importance of identifying, developing, and sharing aesthetic issues and abilities has been less well recognized. This book is only one link in that chain of aesthetic experience ultimately geared toward the "perfect rhinoplasty," a goal we would like to meet, but a challenge, again, that forever keeps us searching.

We should also recognize the challenge patients face in matching their physiology and aesthetic goals to the reality of an individual surgeon's technical abilities and aesthetic sensitivity. As much as sculptors have differed in technical ability and artistic sensibilities through the centuries, so too do the technical competencies and artistic skills of today's surgeons.

After performing several hundred non-Caucasian rhinoplasties over the last 20 years, I have found that a combination of supplementing skeletal support with specialized contoured autogenous grafts and soft-tissue reduction with advanced, technically sound techniques provides the most satisfactory results. Reductive and/or augmentative techniques alone often fail to give acceptable results, while a judicious combination of both enables the surgeon to create a more balanced nose with greater aesthetic appeal.

There are literally hundreds of different ethnic groups located on Earth and modern changes in transportation and visual communication may ultimately blend everyone's nose (or at least the "ideal" nose) into a more uniform shape, size, and structure in future centuries. In the meantime, wide ethnic variations exist, while the size and shape of the "ideal" nose narrows and shrinks. With much of the world's population being non-Caucasian, reshaping ethnic noses into the new universal ideal is growing in popularity.

In addition to surgical skill and knowledge, a surgeon must possess the ability to clearly communicate with his or her patients. With an aesthetic procedure, it is paramount that the patient's psychological desires are understood and met. This can only be achieved through effective communication. Any misunderstanding or assumption that allows the patient's and physician's goals to be at odds will only breed dissatisfaction. I find that most patients desire a tip with greater projection, less dorsal augmentation, and an overall thinner-appearing nose than I might have envisioned at the start of my specialization in ethnic noses.

I have established the personal guidelines and special techniques discussed in this book in the hope of encouraging and assisting the rhinoplastic surgeon in his or her work with the non-Caucasian nose. The greatest benefit of these improved techniques is, of course, a more satisfied and happy patient—our common goal.

Steven M. Hoefflin, M.D., F.A.C.S.

1

Asian, Black, and Hispanic Anatomy

While a complete anatomical/ethnographical nasal study of all the different races with every possible variation within the groups might be interesting, I have limited myself to three non-Caucasian groups who commonly request rhinoplasty: Asians, blacks, and Hispanics, with a special emphasis on the black nose. Again, understanding black nasal anatomy is the key to attaining facile comprehension and good surgical technique for most ethnic rhinoplasties.

The Asian Nose

Throughout the world, the Asian sense of aesthetics has been appreciated for centuries. One need only examine a mother-of-pearl inlay or carved jade figurine to appreciate the intricate fine detail. Exquisite attention to style in clothing, jewelry, makeup, and furnishings gives testimony to the "fine eye" of Asian design, art, and aesthetics.

Although the ability to provide Asian noses with fine tapering, detail, definition, and a sculptured appearance is widely sought, attainable surgical results are somewhat dependent on the actual thickness of the draping tissues. The experienced rhinoplastic surgeon is well aware of this potential conflict between the Asian aesthetic nasal ideal and the frequently presented thick nasal skin of an actual Asian nose.

In the author's opinion, even the rigorous Asian aesthetic challenge can be met through use of tip sculpturing, the "pea-pod" tip graft, and internal and inferior alar reductions which result in a more defined and "thinner" nose. Even thick tip skin visually presents some progressive thinness when a "pea-pod" tip graft is used. Autologous cartilage and soft-tissue bolstering (placing a small plug of postauricular fascia over the tip of the cartilage) can also be utilized and has never (in the author's experience) resulted in extrusion. Thick *alae* have usually been successfully improved only with internal and inferior alar wall thinning. External scars not at the alar crease line have especially limited aesthetic acceptance in ethnic patients.

Asian tip skin may often be thicker and more fibrous than black or Hispanic skin. But a thinness in Asian nasion and dorsal skin is often contrastingly different from the thicker tip and alar skin. A more substantially augmented nasion and dorsum may help to balance that dichotomy. One must be very cautious to not overreduce tip skin or alar cartilage in the Asian patient, as both are normally already quite small and flimsy. Instead,

1

implanting the "pea-pod" tip graft adds definition and reduces the impact of thicker tip and alar skin.

Within the three ethnic/racial types considered here (Asian, black, and Hispanic), the Asian nose lies somewhere between the black and Caucasian nose. But a wide variation in nasal and facial contour exists among Asians. The Chinese characteristically exhibit a round, flat face with minimal nasal projection, while Koreans exhibit more prominent, angular features, such as higher cheekbones and greater nasal projection. The Koreans also have a higher incidence of maxillary retrusion. The Japanese face is even more accented and angular, with greater nasal osteocartilaginous definition. East Asians generally have proportionally smaller noses and shorter septums than their West Asian, Indian, and Arabic counterparts, whose noses are long and often ptotic, with acute nasolabial angles. Southeast Asians possess broader, flatter noses, with prominent supraorbital ridges.

Asians also tend to have small or "weak" chins, a fact that must be considered by the surgeon when planning the surgery. Another factor to consider is the Asian patient's propensity for keloid and hypertrophic scar formation. As with the black patient, it is essential to have surgical goals that treat "facial units" with no suture lines or incision sites extending past the boundaries of these established units. The osteocartilaginous framework is generally very small and flat, in some cases even appearing hypoplastic. Other principal characteristics of the Asian nose (Fig. 1-1a, 1-1b) are:

A. The *radix* tends to be flat and depressed. It is slightly narrower than the black & Hispanic radix and much deeper than the Caucasian radix.

Figure 1-1a, 1-1b
This Asian female had somewhat atypical findings for an Asian nose. Although she had a deep-set nasion, she had a very prominent bony-cartilaginous hump. Her nose had moderate thinness, but she was primarily concerned about the shape and size of her bridge. The alar cartilages were not significantly enlarged, but the tip prominence was low and dependent. The nasal spine was hypoplastic, as was the maxilla.

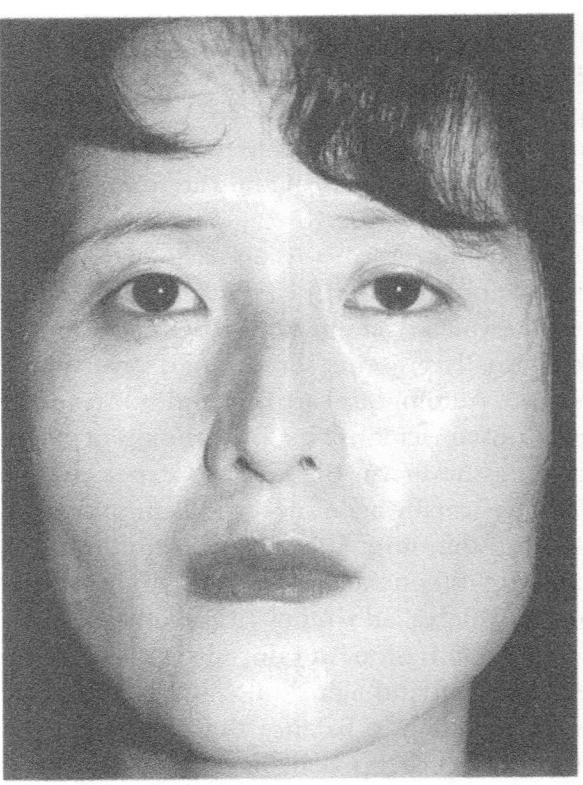

a

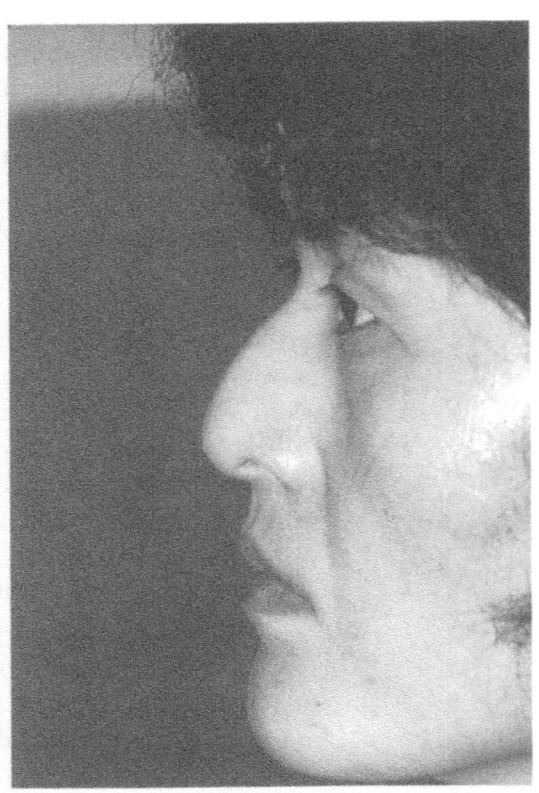

b

B. The *bridge* is usually low, wide, and flat. There is often a deficiency of osteocartilaginous support. The average bridge width is 2.3 cm. The average nasion-to-tip length is 4.5 cm. Depending on a more Northern influence, the Asian bridge may be fuller and more prominent than expected.
C. The *dorsum* is thin and flat and projects even less than the black dorsum.
D. The *tip* is usually thick-skinned, with an abundance of fibrofatty tissue. It is often ptotic, with a slight-to-moderate projection deficit. It is usually more defined than the black tip. The average tip height is 2.2 cm. The average tip width is 2.6 cm.
E. The *base* is usually wide and flaring, but narrower than that of the black nose. The nostrils are oblique in shape, as opposed to the more horizontal configuration of the black nostril, and can range in size from small slits to large openings. The average base width is 3.4 cm.
F. The *columella* is usually short and is recessed 2 to 3 mm.
G. The *nasolabial junction* is characterized by a nasolabial angle of 90 degrees or more.
H. The *maxilla* is usually retrusive and/or has a lack of septal support. The dental arch may be prominent.
I. The *skin* is thick, heavy, and sebaceous, but less so than the skin of the black nose.

The Black Nose

The black nose must be carefully evaluated preoperatively. Any aesthetic imbalance may be accentuated by hyperplastic superior orbital ridges and/or frontal bone, a hypoplastic maxilla, large lips, and/or a retrusive chin. These features require conjoined assessment and may also need treatment to achieve the optimal aesthetic result. Principal characteristics of the black nose (Fig. 1-2a, 1-2b) are:

A. The *radix* is usually low, deep and inferiorly-set, with an obtuse nasofrontal angle averaging 130 degrees to 140 degrees. The lack of radix projection may be further accentuated by a wide intercanthal distance.
B. The *bridge* is usually wide and flat with short nasal bones. The average bridge width is 2.5 cm. There is often a deficiency in osteocartilaginous support, which is particularly striking in relation to the full tip. Due to the inferiorly set radix, the nose is quite short, averaging 5.0 cm from nasion to tip.
C. The *dorsum* is often flat or depressed, lacking anterior height.
D. The nasal *tip* is usually thick-skinned, round, and slightly-to-moderately underprojecting, with the apex lying below the dorsal line. The domes are broad, and there is abundant subcutaneous tissue. Because of the fullness, there is minimal definition and a lack of landmarks and sculpting. The average tip height is 2.4 cm. The average tip width is 2.8 cm.
E. The *base* is wide with thickened alar side walls. The nostrils are usually more horizontal than vertical, causing a flattened appearance. The alar walls usually project beyond the intercanthal line. The nostrils are flaring with a wide interalar distance. The average base width is 3.8 cm.
F. The *columella* is usually short and recessed with hypoplastic medial

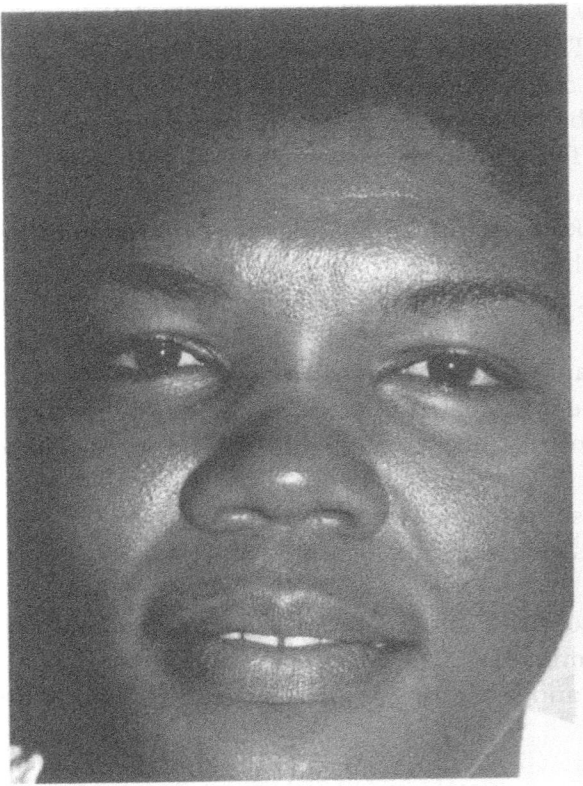
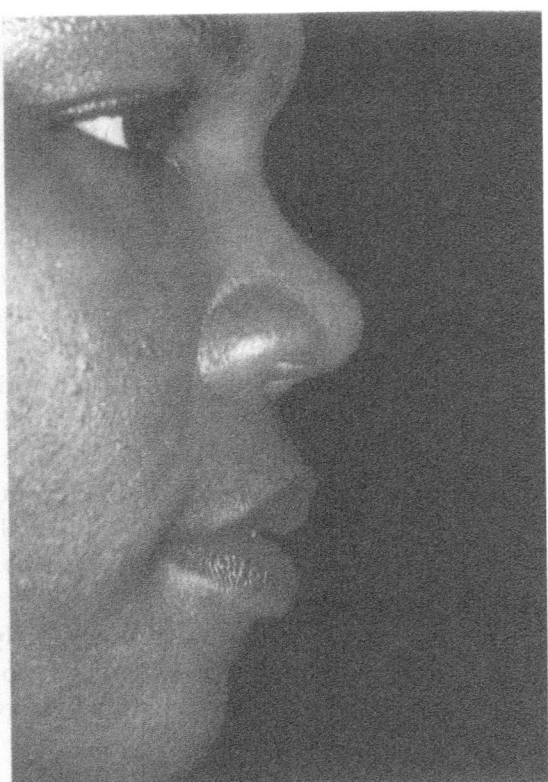

Figure 1-2a, 1-2b
This black female shows the very obvious discrepancy of full, thick, bulky nasal tip with thick, flaring alae, versus the hypoplastic appearance of the nasal bridge. She has a slightly reduced nasion, but a low hyperplastic nasal bridge with widely placed nasal bones. The tip and alae soft tissue is thick and glabrous, and the alae are prominent, but the columella and nasal spine are retracted. The upper alar ridge is retrusive.

crura. There is an alar-columellar disproportion resulting in little or no columellar show.

G. The *nasolabial junction* is usually retracted. The nasal spine is underdeveloped and the maxilla is retrusive. The nasolabial angle is usually less than 90 degrees.

H. The *maxilla* is usually hypoplastic.

I. The *skin* is generally thick and bulky, containing vast amounts of fibrofatty tissue and sebaceous glands.

The Hispanic Nose

Within the three ethnic/racial groups, the Hispanic nose bears the closest anatomical resemblance to the Caucasian nose, probably due to a strong European genetic influence. Hispanic nasal shapes, such as those found in the peoples of Mexico and Central and South America, represent a strong mixture of American Indian, African, and European traits, but the Hispanic nose itself is a unique entity. The Hispanic face is generally wide and somewhat short. Other principal characteristics of the Hispanic nose (Fig. 1-3a, 1-3b) are:

A. The concavity of the *radix* is usually less than that of the black radix and is considered to be within normal bounds when compared to the Caucasian.

B. The *bridge* is usually wide, although slightly less so than the black bridge, and averages 2.4 cm in width. The average nasion-to-tip length is 5.0 cm.

C. The *dorsum* is slightly convex and occasionally has a small osteocartilaginous hump. The osteocartilaginous vault is small and lacks anterior projection, yet expands rapidly in width from the bridge to the tip.

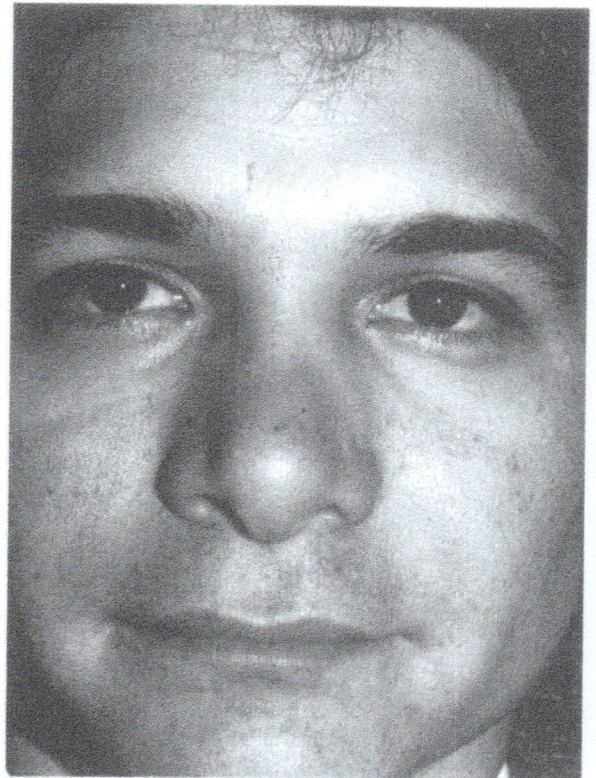
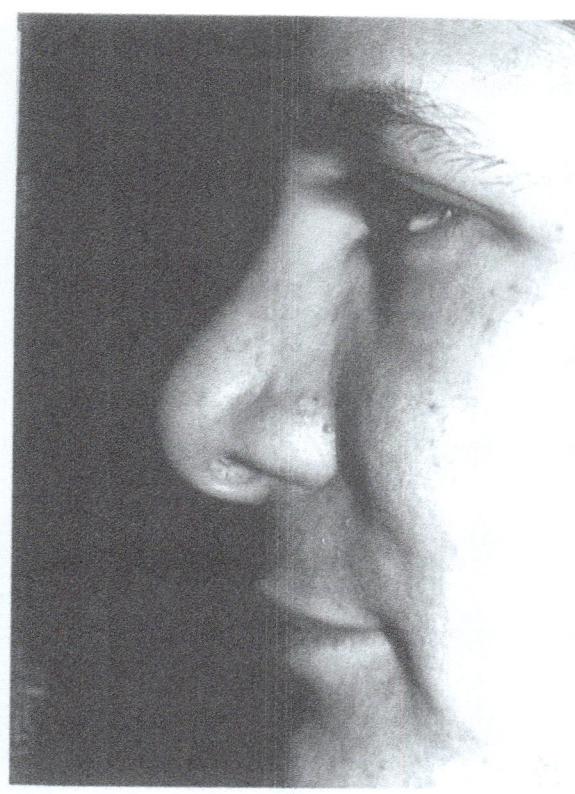

a   b

Figure 1-3a, 1-3b
This Latino male had four previous rhinoplastic attempts at soft tissue and bony-cartilaginous skeletal reduction, resulting in a bulbous, unbalanced globular appearance to the nose. The nasion appeared to be normal. The nasal dorsum was overresected. The nasal tip was bulbous and ill defined, and the columella was hanging and nonsupported. The alar were slightly full. The spine and intermaxillary and alveolar structures were retrusive. Previous osteotomies were high, leaving a wide base.

D. The nasal *tip*, with its wide domes, is generally broad and depressed, lacking both definition and projection. The average tip height is 2.5 cm. The average tip width is 2.4 cm.

E. The *base* tends to be wide, with moderately thick alar walls. The alae have a propensity to flare and the nostrils tend to be horizontal in shape due to a short columella and wide base. The base is wider than in the Asian nose, but less so than in the black nose. The average base width is 3.6 cm.

F. The *columella* tends to be short, contributing to inadequate tip projection. However, when compared to the black or Asian nose, the Hispanic tip possesses relatively good projection, though not enough to meet current aesthetic preferences.

G. The *nasolabial junction* is characterized by an acute nasolabial angle, averaging 70 to 75 degrees, due to the short columella and the prominent dental arches.

H. The *maxilla* tends to fall within normal bounds.

I. The *skin* itself has abundant sebaceous glands, resulting in an oily appearance, with a moderately thick layer of subcutaneous fat.

J. The *radix* may be low.

Desired Rhinoplastic Changes

What is the "ideal" nasal shape?

For whatever reason—be it the influence of advertising and the predominance of Western media, or a desire to "fit in"—the currently accepted standard of beauty for the nose is most often represented by the Western (Caucasian) nasal shape. But for all patients the nasal contour must be in

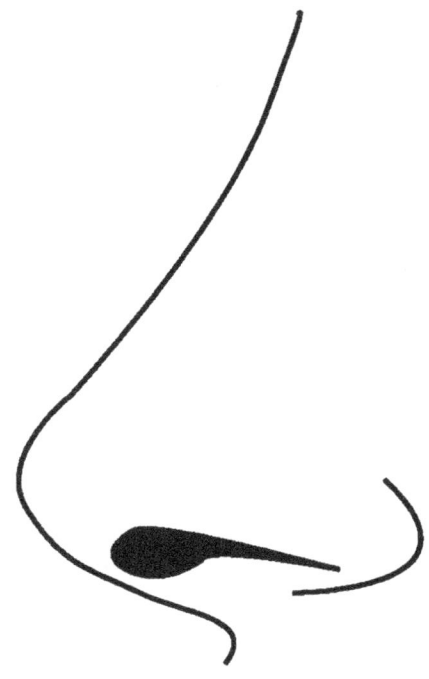

harmony and balance with the patient's ethnicity, gender, age, as well as facial and overall body proportions. The nasal contour must be in line with the patient's desires and goals and within the bounds of aesthetic acceptability and surgical possibility. The Caucasian "standard nose" comprises the following characteristics (Fig. 1-4):

1. A slightly convex frontal bone, with a moderate nasofrontal angle
2. A strong, straight, or slightly concave dorsum
3. A narrow bridge of uniform width along its entire length
4. A tip of moderate thickness and projection
5. Vertical-oblique nostrils with thin alae
6. An open nasolabial angle
7. Skin of thin-to-moderate thickness

Most ethnic rhinoplasty patients wish to trade their nose, which is usually thick and poorly defined, for one that is thinner, more angular, and better defined. At the same time, most patients also wish to retain some of their ethnicity. Again, the "proper" shape is dictated by an aesthetic balance of ethnicity, gender, age, and facial and body proportions. While the desires and expectations of all individuals differ, most of my non-Caucasian rhinoplasty patients have exhibited most or all of the following anatomical characteristics (Fig. 1-5a, 1-5b):

1. The *radix* usually lacks significant anterior projection.
   Desired: A subtle concavity that is in harmony with the supraorbital ridge.

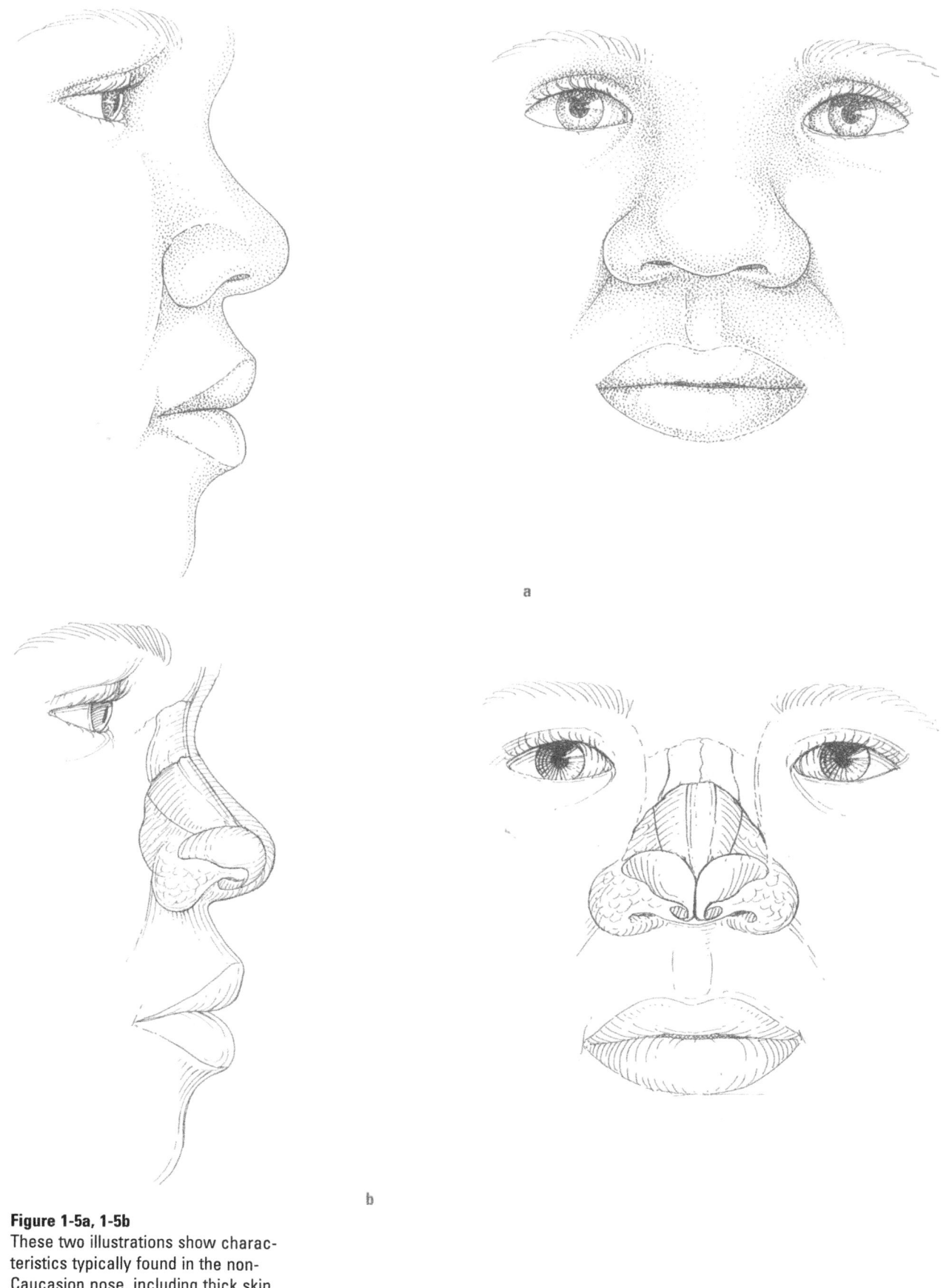

a

b

Figure 1-5a, 1-5b
These two illustrations show characteristics typically found in the non-Caucasion nose, including thick skin and a flat, bulbous nasal tip.

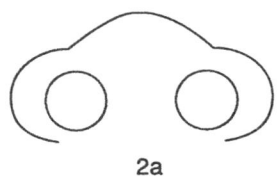

2a

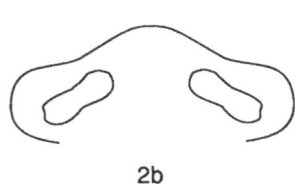

2b

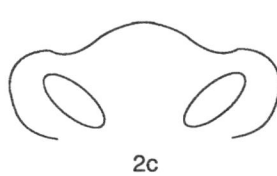

2c

Figure 1-6
Patients nostrils tend to fall into one of these three shapes, central-round being the most common.

2. The *bridge* is usually wide and flat.

Desired: A bridge that is neither too prominent nor too thin but is of uniform and moderate width from the nasion down to the alar groove. The supraorbital ridge should flow and blend in with the bridge.

3. The *dorsum* is wide and flat and may be significantly depressed.

Desired: A straight or slightly concave dorsum. Most patients initially want to limit the size of the dorsal graft, fearing that their nose will appear too large.

4. The *tip* is flat, bulbous, poorly projecting, and ill defined.

Desired: A shapely tip with a contoured projection above the dorsal line. The desired degree of thinness, definition, and sharpness varies from individual to individual. Many non-Caucasian patients want more nasal tip projection than one might initially anticipate.

5. The *base* is broad, tending to accentuate the lack of tip projection. Overhanging alae often hide the columella in profile. The alar rims are thick due to excess fibrofatty tissue. The nostrils tend to be flared and usually fall into one of three categories: (1) central-round, (2) medial horizontal-oblique, or (3) lateral horizontal-oblique (Fig. 1-6).

Desired: Vertical-oblique nostrils that are neither flaring nor pinched. The alar sidewalls should be of thin-to-moderate thickness. The nasal base should be triangular in shape and should fit within the intercanthal-distance dimensions.

6. The *columella* is short, lacks structural support, and is often hidden.

Desired: A columella of adequate length that projects slightly below the alar margin. A desirable columellar "show" is 3 to 5 mm. The nasal spine-columellar junction should be neither too retrusive nor too full.

7. The *nasolabial junction* is usually retracted with an acute angle.

Desired: A slightly obtuse (greater than 90 degrees) nasolabial angle.

8. The *maxilla* is usually retrusive.

Desired: A maxilla that provides good support to the nasal base.

9. The *skin* is thick, bulky, and inelastic, often containing vast amounts of subcutaneous tissue and excess sebaceous glands.

Desired: Skin of thin-to-moderate thickness that provides good tip definition.

2

Preoperative Nasal Evaluation and Surgical Planning

To obtain a satisfactory surgical result in the eyes of both the surgeon and the patient, one needs a broad base of knowledge. My goal is to provide some basics that apply to standard rhinoplasties as well as to the more difficult ethnic nose.

In many ways, a successful rhinoplasty is like a successful work of architecture. Both are constructed with aesthetic balance and function in mind, and both require detailed planning before construction begins. Just as a successful architect will first evaluate the land and its foundation before erecting a building, a good rhinoplastic surgeon will thoroughly evaluate a patient's general physical makeup, psychology, facial contour, and nasal structure prior to surgery. The rhinoplastic surgeon determines not only what is excessive, deficient, or in need of modification but also what is sound and physically possible. A detailed preoperative evaluation and organized surgical plan are as important to the surgeon as preliminary studies and blueprints are to the architect.

Ethnic noses characteristically provide the challenge of managing thick skin. The bulky, thick nasal covering, particularly at the tip, provides the highest number of complaints, the most formidable surgical challenge, and the greatest difficulty in managing secondaries.

Patients presenting themselves for nasal changes usually have a very specific desire in mind. They usually communicate the goal in general terms, and the evaluating surgeon must then press for specifics. Not infrequently they simply comment that their nose is "too large." Specifics of shape, balance, width, and projection of the nose should then be evaluated. Twenty years ago rhinoplastic training of the time discouraged showing pre- or postoperative photographs to patients. I find, however, that in addition to its aid in conversation, the practice is actually extremely helpful in discouraging unrealistic expectations.

I make a practice of showing patients basic slides, including both intra- and extranasal anatomy, diagrammatic techniques, and "before and after" photographs of average results. At the end of the slide carousel are photos of specifically "good" results, as well as complications for when patients wish to see them. After a thorough discussion of the procedure, anesthesia, recovery period, risks, and, specifically, limitations, I will thoroughly examine the patient. I will sit the patient down in front of a three-view mirror and spend an ample amount of time showing the patient those areas I feel I can improve and those that have certain limitations. This examination provides both the patient and surgeon with a realistic appraisal of the type of results that can be obtained. I also make diagrammatic notes of this discussion. Just before surgery, the same appraisal is given in front of a mirror as markings are made.

In my experience, the order of importance for most of my ethnic patients is the following:

1. A thinner, more shapely tip
2. A narrow nasal base
3. Augmentation or reduction of the dorsum
4. Reduction of the bony pyramid

Despite many wonderful tip graft techniques developed by other authors, I feel the more durable "pea-pod" graft has been an important addition to my armamentarium. When elevating and "tenting" the thickened nasal tip skin to increase projection and definition this has been the most reliable graft in my hands. I found that mere "add-on" grafts without "tenting" effect from the base of the columella to the nasal tip usually added bulk, and not projection, to the tip.

Advancement techniques with nasal alar base reduction allow one to excise more alar soft tissue. Previous to the "pea-pod" tip graft, larger nasal base excisions resulted in a triangular spreading and flattening of the nose. When cheek skin is advanced medially, a more acute angle is developed and the normal curvature of the nostril is maintained.

The combination of "pea-pod" tip graft and alar base excision techniques has assisted tremendously in solving the problem of the thickened nasal tip, which normally cannot be removed without significant scarring. It is beneficial to excise the alar base to provide a semblance of nasal thinness.

The desired degree of augmentation in my patients has not been significant unless there is an imbalance between the dorsum and nasal tip. As years have gone by, more patients now desire a very slight convexity, instead of a perfectly straight nose. I mention to my patients that there are no straight lines in the human body and that slight curves, particularly in the facial area, are normal. While I am not in favor of "ski-slope" noses, one must be cautious when creating a large nose with a large tip—even if "balanced," as such patients are frequently dissatisfied. Erring on the side of a smaller nose with a more concave dorsum typically results in greater patient satisfaction. Taking a convex bridge and narrowing the pyramid a moderate, but not substantial, degree provides more balance. This is particularly true when there is a significant width to the bony pyramid.

When dealing with difficult anatomical challenges we all learn both from our patients' preferences and surgical experience. I find it most rewarding to sit in the consultation room and present a mirror to my patients while sitting across from them and to ask them what bothers them about their nose.

On a frontal view, patients usually discuss tip fullness, tip ptosis, width of the nasal base, flaring nostrils, width prominence, or deficiency of bridge projection. It is true that most patients who view their noses do so head-on.

This view can give a somewhat magnified impression of the tip, particularly with mirrors, which I bring to their attention. In addition, photographs bring to patients' attention the width and size of their nose, particularly when they are smiling. I caution patients not to judge their nose when smiling, as everybody's nose does spread and depress during the smiling movement. Muscles such as the depressor nasi can sometimes be interrupted to decrease tip ptosis.

The major complaint to come from patients is the full tip and wide base. If the skin is quite thick, again a formidable challenge is present. It is not possible to remove thickened skin, although it is possible to reduce the entire distal envelope by alar base reduction. The technique by alar base incision and advancement of base skin medially allows one to excise more alae soft tissue and rotate the alae inferiorly and medially, giving a normal convexity and curvature to the alar wall.

The "pea-pod" tip graft has been the most significant step that I have used to obtain improvements in nasal appearance in difficult thick, bulky, wide nasal tips. Other types of tip grafts merely add cartilage and do not provide a significant degree of support from the columellar base to the tip, and therefore do not provide the "tenting" effect that is necessary to provide a semblance of tip thinness.

The combination of a substantial "pea-pod" tip graft, alar base excisions, and remodeling the rest of the nose for balance has given results that were above my initial expectations, based on earlier utilized techniques. Shortly before surgery I will again sit patients in front of a mirror and discuss with them what their desires are and the limitations in improving their appearance. A thick nasal envelope requires discussing with the patient the limited degree of improvement and balance that can be obtained unless the enlarged nasal tip is addressed. A balanced nose with a more defined nasal envelope is more attractive than a small, bulky nose without definition. I use the analogy of the thick glove with a finger in it. If I were to reduce the finger by pulling it back, the thick glove would become ptotic and not retain its shape. I tell my patients that it is important, because we cannot reduce the glove itself, that sometimes adding skeletal support will sometimes give the semblance of a thinner-appearing glove without reducing the glove fabric itself.

One extremely important point is the realistic degree of swelling—often quite prolonged—that occurs postoperatively with thick skin. The development of a postoperative pressure-taping technique has been very well accepted by patients. The patient and doctor work together to reduce postoperative swelling. Although shunned in earlier training, use of triamcinolone acetonide suspension 10 mg/ml (Kenalog) further diluted shows a significant improvement in edema resolution. If necessary, the first Kenalog injection is timed 4 to 6 weeks postoperatively. A maximum of three injections are timed 4 to 6 weeks apart, and are done in conjunction with a postinjection taping program (see Ch. V, Dressing Technique and Postop. Care). Kenalog and taping has shown significant improvement with very few complications, particularly in the first 6 to 12 months when a nose might swell unexpectedly due to sun or heat exposure or increased salt ingestion, etc.

Infrequently, hyperpigmentation can be a problem at the tip and alar reduction sites, especially in darker skin patients. Very porous skin may also be a problem. I prepare patients preoperatively with a combination of Retin-A and hydroquinone, having them apply each once or twice daily for 2 to 4 weeks preoperatively. This tends to cause a slight decrease in glandular activity and significantly decreases any pigmentary changes, particularly if the patient goes on a progressive taping program postoperatively (but taping CAN irritate the skin and cause hyperpigmentation).

The number of requested revisions, I feel, is almost inversely proportional to the amount of time the surgeon spends discussing limitations with the patient. Some patients continue to have unrealistic expectations as to the thinness of the nose, even after these discussions. A good amount of time discussing representative photographs of noses like theirs, with slides or textbooks, may provide a more realistic surgical goal and likely result.

I do not use computerized imaging. In the early years when I tried imaging, it appeared to take a significant period of time and did not give a true representation of the likely results. I find it much more beneficial to show slides projected on a drawing board, and to make changes at that point. As the technology improves I am sure that the units will become much more user-friendly and will be applicable to both a surgeon's time constraints and a patient's desire for an honest prediction of results.

Nasal Evaluation

The key to a successful preoperative evaluation is good communication between the physician and patient. From the patient's point of view, a surgeon's communication skills are nearly as important as his or her surgical skills. In addition to carefully analyzing a patient's anatomy and basic physiological profile, it is paramount that the physician understand the patient's emotional goals and motivation. No matter how remarkable the rhinoplastic surgery, it is unsuccessful if the patient's expectations were different than the outcome. Therefore, it is essential that the surgeon and the patient communicate thoroughly and realistically concerning the aesthetic goals before entering the operating room.

Asian, black, and, frequently, Hispanic patients nearly consistently relate to me that their perceptions of nasal beauty and their desire for a thinner, more tapered nose are based on their years growing up. My Asian patients commonly complain of a concave dorsum and thick nasal tip, which explains the decades-old attempts at dorsal augmentation using prosthetic materials. My black patients frequently desire reduction in the size and width of the nasal tip, particularly when there is a wide base and significant alar flaring. In reference to width, Hispanic patients fall in between the Asian and black noses, depending on individual shape and size.

This is an area in which the surgeon's experience, judgment, aesthetic eye, and well-tuned ear are critical to understanding the patient's concerns and needs and correctly assessing the patient's facial balance and surgical possibilities. In the author's experience, many patients with large thick noses desire a nose that might be thinner and more tapered than a surgeon would normally recommend given the patient's facial balance. It is important that the rhinoplastic surgeon develop the ability to palpate the soft tissues of the nose, specifically noting differences from the nasion to the tip. The principal postoperative ethnic nasal complaint concerns the nasal tip.

While maintaining an open, friendly, and empathetic conversation with the patient, the surgeon must use expert communication skills to provide ethnic nasal patients with a complete understanding of the actual procedures and timeframes necessary to arrive at a realistic surgical goal.

The Consultation

The use of diagrams, photographs, and slide presentations during the consultation can assist the surgeon and patient in sorting the desirable from the undesirable and the obtainable from the unobtainable. During the consultation, the surgeon should make every effort to place him or herself behind the eyes of the patient and visualize the results that can be expected. *The final measure of success in aesthetic surgery is the attainment of the patient's desires, with guidance from the surgeon.* In other words, patients frequently feel they are right; but they may not always be practical. A patient's misguided goals, based only on a wish, have to be properly channeled by an experienced surgeon to avoid dissatisfaction, multiple revisions, etc. This is where an honest assessment of what can be achieved surgically is crucial. A complete and honest prognosis is very important. If the patient's expectations are unrealistic, the physician must moderate them. If they are too ambiguous, he or she must help define them. A lack of communication in which the two are at odds can only provide a breeding ground for patient dissatisfaction, whereas an honest, clearly communicated and understood appraisal can only be beneficial. The surgeon's role is to provide insight into the balance, aesthetics, and possibilities of nasal surgery and to help guide the patient toward realistic expectations. Enough information should be provided so the patient may make a proper informed consent. Another important factor is to not totally disregard function over aesthetics. Functional and anatomical aspects of the procedure, alternatives, risks and possible complications, and the possibility of secondary procedures should all be discussed during the consultation. During the consultation, patients are given informational handouts on their particular procedure(s) and a general handout on homeopathic therapies.

While miscommunication between patient and surgeon is a concern when contemplating any aesthetic procedure, ethnic rhinoplasty introduces unique problems. For example, most of my non-Caucasian patients with thick-skinned noses request a "smaller nose." It is actually more beneficial, however, to maintain or even increase the size of the nose to achieve greater definition and tip projection. The difficulty is in convincing patients that *adding* something to their nose will actually *improve* their appearance. Once this has been properly communicated, however, often with the aid of photographic examples, most patients not only accept, but prefer, a slight increase in nasal projection.

Surgical Planning

Modifying the form and function of a nose requires experience, skill, and detailed planning. Difficult procedures often require the surgeon to draw heavily upon his or her reconstructive surgical background. When planning a non-Caucasian rhinoplasty, even though specifics vary with each individual, proper preparation and a few general principles will assist in forming an appropriate surgical plan.

Nasion

Does the nasion (root of the nose) or frontal bone need to be grafted or reduced?

Bridge and Dorsum

Are both bridge and dorsum flat and depressed, lacking anterior height?
Is there a hump that requires removal, or a low root that needs augmenting?
Does the dorsum need to be straightened or to be made slightly concave?
Do osteotomies need to be performed?

Tip

Does the tip lack adequate projection and require grafting?
Does the nasal tip require narrowing through alar cartilage reduction or tip grafting?
Can altering thin alar cartilages influence a thick tip?

Base

What type and size of alar reduction will be required?
Should the width of the alar bases be changed?
Should the shape of the nostrils be changed?
Should the patient have a Sheen Type I or Type II alar reduction?

Septum and Turbinates

What amount and type of septal and turbinate surgery is indicated?
Does the septum require straightening?
Do the turbinates require trimming or is injection sufficient?

EXAMPLE: The non-Caucasian nose usually requires both dorsal and tip grafting. With grafting indicated, the following questions should be satisfactorily answered by the surgeon preoperatively:

1. *From which source will the graft be taken?*
2. *What is the required size of the graft?*

3. *Is there enough graft material available at the appropriate donor site?*
4. *What about possible backup grafts?*
5. *Will the graft need to be wrapped in mastoid or temporalis fascia?*

In the author's opinion, conchal cartilage is ideal construction material for the special type of tip graft required for these types of noses. The modification of thick nasal tips may require a special type of tip graft that is capable of yielding a great deal of support and projection. Usually one ear is sufficient for both dorsal and tip grafting. However, both ears may be needed and should be discussed preoperatively with the patient. While the Caucasian dorsum is commonly elevated with septal cartilage, this is not always the case with non-Caucasians. Lacking in osteocartilaginous support, the non-Caucasian nose may not house as much septal cartilage as the Caucasian and, therefore, may require alternative graft donor sites. Excised cartilage from a deflected septum may also be used as dorsal graft material if it is not too irregular or insufficient.

A general preoperative checklist which helps obtain a patient history, perform a complete nasal examination, assess the aesthetic goals of each patient, and organize an efficient surgical plan is useful (Fig. 2-1). It is very helpful to complete a detailed diagrammatic plan before surgery. Thorough planning makes intraoperative surprises remarkably rare. A complete physical examination should also be performed.

PREOPERATIVE NASAL EVALUATION AND CHECKLIST

I use a checklist when preoperatively assessing patients. It assists me in obtaining a history, assessing the aesthetic goals of the patient, and performing a complete nasal examination. In addition, a complete medical history and physical examination should be performed prior to surgery.

NASAL CHECKLIST

Name:_____ Date:_____

Previous History Of:

Childhood or adulthood injuries?   Yes_____ No_____ If yes, explain:_____

Nasal Surgery?   Yes_____ No_____
  Date and Specifics?   _____
  X-Rays?   Yes_____ No_____

_____Nasal Airway Obstruction: Left_____ Right_____ Both_____ Consistent_____
                                                                                   Intermittent_____

_____Sinus Infections: Yes_____ No_____ When:_____

_____Nasal Allergy Symptoms: Yes_____ No_____
                              _____Stuffiness   _____Sneezing   _____Postnasal Drip

_____Nasal Spray Use: Yes_____ No_____
                              Type:_____ Frequency:_____

_____Nasal Bleeding: Yes_____ No_____

_____Smoking: Yes_____ No_____ How much_____PPD

_____Aspirin or Aspirin-like Medication Use:_____

_____Hypertension: Yes_____ No_____

_____Previous History of Troublesome Scarring: Yes_____ No_____
                              Where_____ Specifics_____

Additional Comments: _____

                                           _____

Figure 2-1
Preoperative Nasal Evaluation and Checklist.

Nasal Examination:

A basic general physical examination should be performed.

I. Skin:
    ___Normal   ___Medium   ___Thick   ___Hypopigmented
    ___Sebaceous   ___Normal Pigment
    ___Scars   ___Hyperpigmented

II. Septum:
    ___Straight   ___Deviated   ___Left   ___Right
                     ___% Obstruction   ___Left   ___Right
    ___Sufficient For Use As Graft   ___Yes   ___No

III. Vomer:
    ___Straight
    ___Deflected: ___Left   ___Right
    ___Spurred: ___Left   ___Right

IV. Nasal Valve:
    ___Open
    ___Narrow
    ___Compromised

V. Turbinates:
    ___Small   ___Right   ___Left   ___Both
    ___Deep   ___Normal   ___Right   ___Left   ___Both
    ___Flat   ___Enlarged   ___Right   ___Left   ___Both

VI. Nasion: Angle: _____

VII. Dorsum/Bridge:
    ___Convex   ___Straight   ___Concave
    ___Narrow   ___Wide   ___Normal Width
    ___Regular   ___Irregular

VIII. Upper Lateral Cartilage: ___Narrow   ___Medium   ___Wide

IV. Tip: ___Narrow   ___Normal   ___Wide
    ___Adequate Projection
    ___Insufficient Projection

X. Columella: ___Normal   ___Retracted   ___Hanging
    ___Angle: _____   ___Narrow   ___Wide

XI. Nasal Spine: ___Small   ___Normal   ___Large

XII. Alar Base: ___Normal   ___Moderate Width   ___Excessive Width

Patient's Aesthetic Goals:

I. Dorsum/Bridge
    ___Retain Convexity
    ___Retain Width
    ___Reduce Bridge Width
    ___Reduce Dorsum To:
        ___Straight   ___Slight Concavity
        ___Moderate Concavity
    ___Graft Dorsum   ___Graft Nasion   ___Graft Frontal Bone
    ___Other: _____

II. Tip
    ___No Change
    ___Reduce Width
    ___More Tip Projection
    ___No Angle Change
    ___Elevate Angle To _____

III. Alar Base
    ___No Change
    ___Narrow
    ___Graft Nasal Base

Additional Comments/Procedures: _____
_____
_____

Surgical Plan:

Grafting To Be Performed: ___Yes ___No

Source Of Graft: ___Cranial Bone
___Auricular
___Septum
___Other: _____

I. Nasion
___No Change
___Ostectomy
___Graft

II. Septum
___Septectomy
___Septoplasty
___Vomer Spur Ostectomy
___Packing ___Yes ___No — Left ___ Right ___ Both ___

III. Turbinates
___Inject Left ___ Right ___ Both ___
___Cauterization Left ___ Right ___ Both ___
___Clamping/Excis. Left ___ Right ___ Both ___
___S.M. Resections Left ___ Right ___ Both ___

IV. Dorsum/Bridge
___Ostectomies
___Narrow
___Osteotomy
___Graft
___Septum
___Auricular
___Cranial
___Other

V. Columella
___No Change
___Raise To___ Angle

Additional Comments/Procedures: _____

_____

_____

Surgical Plan: (continued)

VI. Tip
    ____No Change
    ____Reduce Alar Cartilages
        Approach: ____Cartilage Splitting Incisions
                       ____Rim Incisions
                       ____Open Technique

    ____Tip Grafting: Yes ____   No ____
        ____Septum
        ____Auricular
        ____Other:_____

VII. Base
    ____No Change
    ____Reduce Spine
    ____Augment Spine
    ____Augment Maxilla

VIII. Alae
    ____No Change
    ____Reduce
        ____Small
        ____Medium
        ____Large

Additional Comments/Procedures: _____

_____

_____

3

Approaching the Perfect Anesthetic Experience

Providing a pleasant, safe, and comfortable anesthetic experience is the goal of both the plastic surgeon and the anesthesia professional. As plastic surgeons, we are in the unique position of caring for patients who are for the most part healthy and desirous of elective procedures. Those patients expect good results both aesthetically and *anesthetically*. Patients will often volunteer information about the pleasant and the not-so-pleasant aspects of their anesthetic experience. Because I have administered intravenous sedation or observed the administration of general anesthesia on more than 20 thousand patients, I have received a lot of feedback. Using that feedback, we have prepared a checklist that helps us provide a high degree of patient satisfaction.

Assessing and trying to assuage a patient's fears, before and after a procedure, are more important than administering the perfect anesthetic. No matter how perfect the anesthetic, many patients experience anxiety at the loss of control or the fear of the unknown and cannot be made comfortable until those fears have been addressed. Your patients need to feel that you and the anesthesiologist understand their fears and that you will both watch over them as carefully as you would a member of your own family.

By following a few simple steps before, during, and after surgery you can help make the experience a pleasant one for your patient. Success begins by extending every possible courtesy to the patient and by clearly explaining each procedure. The majority of the author's patients are concerned, demanding, and perfectionistic—welcomed qualities that provide author and staff with a constant challenge to be better. Our goal is to ensure that each patient is a happy patient.

The following checklist of steps, techniques, and ideas is currently used in our outpatient facility for *all* types of surgery, not just nasal procedures. The anesthesiologists, nurses, and technicians with whom the author works have all contributed to this program. I believe these techniques can help you to provide a positive experience for your patients. Obviously, you may wish to modify this program, depending on the patient and your own personal experience and judgment.

Patient Care Kit

The following list of suggested items can be purchased by nursing personnel and made available for the patient's care and comfort.

Mentholatum or Vicks (for coating lips)

Lorann oils (for masks)

Walkman type stereo with headphones and musical or hypnosis tapes (to occupy the patient during the preoperative wait)

Heating pad

Warm blankets

Plastic bags (to cover the extremities for retention of body heat)

Breath spray

Preanesthesia Checklist

1. The patient is called by a member of the nursing staff several days prior to elective anesthesia to review the patient's medical history and answer any questions the patient may have.

2. The patient is called the evening before surgery by the anesthesiologist to provide additional assurance and to answer any further questions.

3. Consider bedtime sedation the night before surgery. Patients often find that 50 mg of over-the-counter diphenhydramine (Benadryl) provides good, safe sedation.

4. After the patient arrives, the nursing staff checks the patient into the facility and asks the patient pertinent questions in an unrushed manner.

5. Make sure the patient has a warm blanket and booties or socks. The patient should be calm. Background music can have a calming effect. The patient can use portable stereo earphones, if desired.

6. All patients who receive preoperative medications must be kept warm. Blankets, caps, booties, etc. are used to prevent heat loss. This is especially true if the patient will encounter any kind of wait in the preoperative holding area.

7. Consider a fluid warmer for cases over 2 hours. Intravenous fluids may also be warmed.

8. Always use a local anesthetic before insertion of the IV.

9. Antecubital space or forearm IVs are often more comfortable than those inserted in the hand or wrist. If time permits, a small dose of oral Valium can be given to provide sedation and amnesia prior to starting the IV.

10. Intravenous fluids containing high amounts of sodium should be avoided, unless fluid and electrolyte replacement is necessary.

11. Preoperatively, the surgeon should see and talk with the patient outside the operating room.

12. Make sure the operating room table is warmed with blankets or a heating pad.

13. Give the patient breath spray prior to mask application (patients often worry about their breath following surgery).

14. Cast padding should be used under automatic blood pressure cuffs to avoid ecchymosis of the skin during prolonged procedures.

15. Place the pulse oximeter on the arm opposite the blood pressure cuff.

16. Apply a drop of flavored Lorann oil inside mask.
17. Patients usually like to hold their own mask for a few seconds.
18. Use in-line humidification.
19. Keep noise and/or talk in the operating room to a minimum until the patient is completely asleep.
20. Give the patient a small stereo headphone set playing Baroque-type music, if desired.
21. Always tell the patient exactly what you are doing before induction.
22. Use a RAE tube for nasal or facial cases.
23. Apply a thin layer of 2% Xylocaine jelly to the tube prior to insertion.
24. Consider giving 1.5–2.0 mg/kg of lidocaine hydrochloride intravenously, prior to intubation, to decrease light bucking, especially if a difficult intubation is anticipated.
25. Use soft cuff, tube, and Laryngeal Trachea Anesthesia (LTA) kits. Administer Xylocaine 200 mg intratracheally, and mask for 1 to 2 minutes prior to intubation.
26. Use depolarizing agents for intubation, such as vecuronium bromide (Norcuron). Always protect the central incisors by placing a guard or a piece of adhesive tape over them. Disposable plastic laryngoscope blades are less likely to damage teeth.
27. Consider the use of a saline-soaked, pharyngeal and oral packing to keep the oral mucosa moist and to stabilize the tube. This packing can decrease the dryness, sore throat, and discomfort that some patients experience postoperatively. Some of the packing can be placed between the molars to prevent the patient from biting on the tube.
28. Always protect the eyes with ointment and paper tape. The corneas of contact lens wearers will be more sensitive to dryness after lens removal. Be careful also of patients who may be wearing false eyelashes. Alternatively, the surgeon can suture the eyelids closed with 6-0 nylon.
29. As much as 90% of patient heat loss during surgery can be eliminated by covering the arms (to the elbows), legs (to the knees), and head with plastic bags.
30. Apply petroleum jelly such as Vaseline, Mentholatum, or Vicks to the lips. Watch for excessive tube pressure on the lips. Always secure the tube with paper—not adhesive—tape. It may be helpful to secure the tube to the teeth with dental floss.
31. Since the tube cuff will expand during the procedure as the room air is replaced by nitrous oxide, either fill the cuff with anesthetic or remove gas from the cuff periodically, as required.
32. Consider placing small rolls under the neck, lumbar, and knee areas during lengthy procedures.
33. Consider placing ace wraps around the legs if the procedure takes more than 2 hours.
34. Pad any bony areas, especially if the patient is thin. Heels and sacrum are areas that are often overlooked.
35. Consider placing a Foley catheter and/or minimizing intravenous fluids for operations expected to last over 3 hours to prevent a full bladder postoperatively.

36. Securely restrain the patient's arms without using tape on the skin. Place the arms in a comfortable position with ulnar padding.

37. When patients have long hair, wrap the hair carefully in a cap and secure the cap with paper tape.

38. With most facial cases, the surgeon will inject a local anesthetic with epinephrine. Transient tachycardia may be seen. PVCs should be treated as indicated. Xylocaine 50 mg IV may be necessary. A beta-blocker, such as labetalol hydrochloride (Labetalol) or propanolol hydrochloride (Inderal) may be indicated.

39. During long cases, the nursing staff should flex and extend the patient's ankles every 15 minutes. The bony prominences should be checked throughout the procedure. The heels should be elevated off the bed and padded.

40. To decrease swelling, the following triad of medications can be administered after the patient is asleep:
    a. Decadron phosphate (Decadron) 10 mg IV slowly
    b. Diphenhydramine hydrochloride (Benadryl) 50 mg IV
    c. Cefazolin sodium (Ancef or Kefzol) 1 g IV

41. If the patient is allergic to penicillin, and a prosthesis or graft is planned, then vancomycin hydrochloride 500 mg can be given IV, slowly. Otherwise, use erythromycin 250 mg IV, slowly. The patient will receive an additional dose in the recovery room.

42. If indicated, use preoperative clonidine hydrochloride 0.1 mg to minimize anesthetic requirements and to avoid hypertension.

43. When significant blood loss is expected, the surgeon should regularly gauge the blood loss him or herself every 15 to 30 minutes. The surgeon may be better able to do this than the anesthesiologist.

44. Repeat prophylactic antibodies every 2 to 4 hours during a long case.

Before Extubation Checklist

For a smooth extubation phase:

1. The anesthesia specialist should ask the surgeon for a 30-minute warning before extubation.

2. Small amounts of 0.25% marcaine hydrochloride (Marcaine) with epinephrine can be sprayed into the wound to markedly decrease or eliminate postoperative pain.

3. Thirty minutes before extubation, the anesthetist should slowly start to lighten the anesthesia for a smoother emergence.

4. Twenty minutes before extubation, slowly give droperidol 0.25–0.5 cc IV, to decrease postoperative nausea.

5. Have the operating room nurses prepare warm solutions for washing the patient and warm blankets for the bed.

6. Consider administering physostigmine salicylate 1.0 mg IV 10 minutes before extubation, to control postoperative hyperactivity, especially in active young males.

7. Ten minutes before extubation, turn off the nitrous oxide to get a higher oxygen concentration.

8. One and one-half to 3 minutes before extubation, give lidocaine hydrochloride (Xylocaine) 0.5–1.0 mg/kg IV to decrease "bucking."
9. Remove the pharyngeal pack.
10. Suction the oropharynx early to avoid excessive stimulation—be gentle.
11. Use a peripheral nerve stimulator to assess any residual neuromuscular block. Never allow the patient to know that he or she is intubated. Never allow bucking. A small dose of midazolam hydrochloride (Versed) may help to decrease recall in cases where the patient wakes up too early.
12. If the patient is to sit up for the dressing application, do it while the patient is either fully anesthetized or after extubation, in order to avoid bucking. Do *not* sit the patient up while he or she is "light" because this can cause bucking.
13. Wash the patient off with water or saline that has been warmed.
14. In refractory cases, those patients who are very prone to nausea can benefit from dronabinol (Marinol) 5 mg sublingually, 20 minutes before extubation. The capsule can be punctured with an 18 g needle and the contents squirted under the tongue. This dose appears to decrease nausea without giving a "high."

After Extubation Checklist

1. Warm the patient immediately, and keep him or her warm in the recovery room. Use electric blankets (if safe) or warmed blankets. Plastic bags can be left in place on arms and legs.
2. Do not use tight masks after nasal cases. An oxygen tube can be taped neatly at the mouth or nose to provide supplemental oxygen.
3. For shivering: Fentanyl citrate 0.5 cc (25 mg) IV or meperidine hydrochloride (Demerol) 25 mg IV, slowly.
4. Remove sticky EKG leads from the back area so the patient will not lie on them.
5. Consider placing stereo earphones on the patient prior to leaving the operating room, especially if the recovery area is noisy.
6. Follow-up by the anesthetist, either in person or by phone, is appreciated by the patient.

A Standard Nasal Technique

1. A saline-moistened pack is placed in the oral pharynx covering the tongue to keep the oral mucosa moist.
2. After specular evaluation, place petroleum jelly ribbon gauze deep within the nose.
3. 0.5% Bupivacaine hydrochloride (Marcaine) with epinephrine is injected at the supraconchlear, infraorbital, and palatine nerves to block sensory nerves. Infiltration with local anesthetic is started at the piriform aperture and the lateral nasal bridge, alar base, and base of the columella. The ear or septum are infiltrated if grafting is planned. Using a burnt needle decreases ecchymosis.
4. The rim incision, intercartilaginous incision sites, and tip are next anesthetized, and 5 mg/cc Kenalog (triamcinolone acetonide sus-

pension 10 mg/ml) is then injected into the tip, columella, and turbinates.

5. Approximately 10 minutes should elapse before starting the operative procedure. Very detailed intranasal prepping is performed.

6. Intercartilaginous incisions are made and the dorsum is freed. A careful subperiosteal dissection is carried out. If a dorsal implant is planned, then the dissection will only go just barely beyond the dimensions of the implant. The periosteum is left attached to the nasal-maxillary suture. This supports the nasal bones during infracturing.

7. The membranous septum is released and dissection is carried down to the nasal spine, if augmentation or reduction is anticipated.

8. The alar bases are usually incised and freed for better nasal exposure. The incisions are made just a fraction of a millimeter above the alar crease and the entire alar structure is released. The quantity of resection can be previously marked and initial conservative resection planned. The "bucket handle" rim incisions are then carried out and the alar cartilages then delivered. A subdermal dissection is carried out so that all fibrofatty tissue is left on the cartilages. Once the cartilage is delivered, the fibrous soft tissue is dissected off. The superior three-fifths of the alar cartilage is then excised. All soft tissue and cartilaginous specimens are saved. They may be used for future grafting.

9. The author uses an open approach with tip revisions. If a tip graft is planned, the auricular conchal cartilage site would be initially infiltrated with the nose. Approximately 0.5 cc or 0.5% bupivacaine hydrochloride (Marcaine) with epinephrine is utilized to first block the great auricular nerve, then the postauricular site, and then anteriorally. A pea of petroleum jelly pack is placed in the ear canal prior to injection.

10. A curvilinear incision is made postauricularly. A supraperichondrial dissection is carried out. The ear is retracted forward and a postauricular incision through the cartilage is made. Anterior dissection is carried out with a Freer subperiosteal dissector. A large ellipse of conchal cartilage is then taken and placed on a saline sponge.

11. A saline-moistened sponge is then packed into the ear defect. The ear is usually left open until the end of the procedure because additional cartilage harvesting may be necessary. Bleeding points are then controlled with a Bovie coagulator. 0.25% Bupivacaine hydrochloride (Marcaine) with 1:200,000 epinephrine and 5 mg/cc Kenalog are sprayed into the wound.

12. The alar rim incision is carried down just anterior to the medial crus, 3 mm behind the columellar edge. The entire area is dissected so that the surgical plane just above the level of the alar cartilage is all the way down to the medial crus. Anterior to this incised dissection plane all alar cartilage and soft tissue are freed. This is the same dissection plan as the open procedure, only the columellar incision is not made. Attention then turns to construction of the "pea-pod" graft.

13. The tip of a curved clamp is placed on the tip of the nose and measurement performed from the desired elevation of the tip to the nasal spine. This measurement is used for the length of the "pea-pod" graft.

Elliptical excisions of cartilage are then performed. The dimensions are at least 3 cm × 2.5 cm. The cartilaginous segment is then split. An approximation together of the concave cartilage segments is then performed. These are suture-secured in place utilizing 5.0 Dexon. Sutures are placed at both base and apex of the tips and then wrapped around and press sutured together to give a very stiff tip graft. The sutures are left long at the tip and base, with the needles attached for stabilization pull-out suturing through the skin. The turbinate or septal work is then carried out. If necessary, dorsal union grafting is carried out.

14. Turbinate procedures usually consist of cross-clamping, excision, and cauterization. Turbinate resection is performed only where there is significant obstruction (more than 85%). The alar base resection is then performed. The excision is made in a conservative fashion. The alae are then temporarily approximated to the base and appraisal of the degree of resection made. At this point, the "pea-pod" tip graft is then placed into the tip (usually through the right side). The opposite side or left columellar skin and soft tissue are left intact for a buttress. The base of the graft is placed first. Usually a clamp is placed into the base of the defect, spread, and a needle holder supported suture placed through the base of the columella for stabilization. Double hoods are utilized to elevate skin and expose the tip defect. This site is usually both laterally and centrally viewed to have the optimal tip-projection site. A loose French knot is positioned and later paper taped into place to stabilize the grafts.

15. When osteotomies are planned, a subperiosteal dissection is carried out at the junction of the nasal and maxillary bones laterally (nasal pyramidal base). Osteotomies are performed with a 2-mm osteotome and digital approximation performed. The osteotome is introduced through the piriform aperture and "walked" up the nose. Afterwards, pressure is applied for AT LEAST 5 minutes to ensure minimal bruising and swelling.

16. The rim incisions are then closed with 5-0 plain catgut. 5-0 PDS sutures are utilized to approximate the base of the bare alae to the piriform periosteum in order to obtain a narrower base. A suture is placed through the alae, which are then curvilinearly approximated to the base in a medial fashion utilizing one single base approximation suture of 5-0 PDS. The wound is then closed with 6-0 nylon, and Xeroform dressing is placed at the base. Benzoin tape dressings are then applied.

17. The "pea-pod's" apex suture is pulled up and tape is utilized to secure the tip. Two layers of tape are bent around the suture. A form-fitting aluminum splint is then used to compress the area. Further supportive taping is performed. If significant septal work is performed, Merocel sponges are gently placed in the nasal area and soaked with topical anesthetic (4% lidocaine hydrochloride [Xylocaine]). Reinjecting the facial or nasal sensory nerves is then performed and the operative procedure completed.

Personal Ethnic Rhinoplasty Technique

Overview of Personal Ethnic Rhinoplasty Approach

Even the primary ethnic rhinoplasty provides challenges and demands an arsenal of grafting and reduction techniques rivaling the most difficult of secondary nonethnic cases. Having tried a variety of these techniques over the years, I came to the following conclusions:

Rib or conchal cartilage grafts generally lead to postoperative bending or curling, particularly in the dorsum. This postoperative curling is well confirmed in laboratory and clinical settings by measuring the cartilage's internal stresses. Septal cartilage, on the other hand, has proven ideal for dorsal grafts because of its ability to retain its inherent shape and straightness (unless otherwise cut, scored, or torsioned). Bone grafts are ideal as a **second** source for dorsal grafting.

Although conchal cartilage tends to distort more frequently than septal cartilage (because of natural ear curvature), it has been the author's experience that suturing concave-to-concave shapes of conchal cartilage together into "pea-pod" grafts is highly successful. Circumferential and intermittent mattress suturing of the "pea-pod" decreases distortion, and leaving the perichondrium intact increases suture stabilization. Conchal cartilage does not react to crushing as well as septal cartilage. Ear cartilage fragments more easily, especially if the perichondrium has been removed. Incorporating temporalis fascia around grafts, especially when crushing has resulted in fragmentation, can help save a graft and often provides a smoother result. Nowhere does suture stabilization appear more important than when using auricular cartilage in a tip graft.

Using the "pea-pod" graft to provide a semblance of thinness, sculpturing, and definition in the ethnic nose requires "tenting" force at the tip. Such tension can easily result in distortion, particularly if the basic cartilaginous forces are not equalized. While utilizing one piece of acceptably straight cartilage can be satisfactory, more frequently, two or even three pieces of somewhat-curved auricular cartilage are placed concave-to-concave with mattress sutures equalizing opposing forces into a more durable graft. The author not infrequently finds that interposing a small piece of straight ethmoid between the layers of auricular cartilage adds further support and straightness to the tip.

When this small bone graft is under stress, total resorption is not expected. "Pea-pod" grafts are not only placed under a certain degree of stress but are certainly in a well-vascularized bed. The avascular nature of both septal and auricular cartilage decreases its susceptibility to necrosis as long as the graft is covered with vascular soft tissue.

Tight closures have sometimes resulted in some intranasal exposure of both dorsal and tip grafts. A limited excision of the exposed part and further closure or use of antibiotic ointment for 7 to 10 days usually results in reepithelialization and cartilage coverage. This has not been the case where either nonautologous or allographic material has been used.

Stabilization pull-out sutures, particularly 5-0 Dexon, are not only very helpful with graft positioning but, with gentle tightening and taping, result in the cartilage's closer placement against the vascular subdermal plexus. This placement decreases local dead space where vascularization within 48 hours is necessary to decrease graft resorption. Even where positioning grafts is otherwise quite easy, the author has found that pull-out sutures taped to the skin under a very small amount of tension have assisted in maintaining positioning during the swelling period and have not resulted in any discernible problem. Dexon is utilized because its delayed resorption eliminates the possibility of long-term presence of foreign bodies and its rough surface allows easier placement without slippage. Pull-out sutures are usually clipped at the skin's edge. The sutures are retaped after a period of 48 to 72 hours.

When the nasal dressing is removed a few days postoperatively, if graft malpositioning is noted, it remains easy enough to then pull on the proximal and distal sutures to reposition and retape the graft, usually for only an additional 24 to 48 hours.

Cartilage Pearls of Wisdom

1. Grafts should be harvested LARGER than the estimated size needed. Returning to a donor site to remove a larger graft may be problematic, particularly if the septum and auricular areas have been previously salvaged.

2. The ear provides a very abundant amount of cartilage for grafting, and harvesting leaves little, if any, donor deformity—particularly if the antehelical cartilaginous fold is left intact. Cartilage can be excised all the way down to the osteocartilaginous junction of the ear canal without disturbing the canal itself.

3. When salvaging septocartilage, a small piece of ethmoid should be taken to potentially assist in grafting. If harvesting additional cartilage may become necessary, the ear should be packed with a saline-soaked, very dilute Betadine sponge and left open until the end of the case. The ear can be returned-to if further cartilage grafting is necessary.

4. The postauricular mastoid area has abundant fascia and soft tissue for grafting. A thin layer of fascia is usually taken in anticipation of needing soft tissue to "fill" the nose or cover a graft.

5. In major revisions or reconstructions, it is a good idea to prep both ears and have them draped within the surgical site, in case the opposite ear is needed.

6. A 0.5% bupivacaine hydrochloride (Marcaine) with epinephrine auricular nerve block administered prior to awakening is very beneficial to decrease patient discomfort. In the author's experience, next-day patient complaints about pain are alleviated by readministration of local nerve block. The author has very little experience with cadaver or irradiated grafts, but a very large experience with primary and revision nasal surgery spanning more than 20 years. During that time there has been no more than limited necessity to turn to other sources of allogeneic material.

7. There are areas where grafts do not need to be under tension, but are solely used for "fill." Postauricular or temporalis fascia is a good source of graft fill material. If the site is relatively unscarred and easily expandable when using local anesthesia, long-term taking of this soft-tissue graft material has been the author's preference.

8. Estimating the exact volume of required small graft fill is made easier by initially correcting the defect under local anesthesia and then determining the exact volume of needed soft-tissue graft material. The required volume can be closely estimated by placing the graft into saline in a small syringe and measuring the displacement in 0.1-cc increments.

9. Cartilage diced or minced into very small fragments and injected through a 14- or 16-gauge needle has been utilized on several occasions. The results have been satisfactory for the correction of deeper defects where this material can be injected over bone or cartilage having a fairly thick soft-tissue covering. It is necessary to undermine and create a small defect which can incorporate the cartilage fragment fill under minimal but acceptable tension.

10. In revision dorsal and tip grafts, particularly where Silastic grafts have been used and a scar capsule is present, it is important to remove or scrape away as much of the capsule as possible to provide a vascular bed for the autologous graft material. When completely excising the graft is not possible, such as with a very thin soft-tissue covering, scalpel scoring the capsule in a criss-cross fashion may be of benefit to improve vascular regularity.

11. Diagrammatic measurements of planned cartilage grafts are very helpful in determining the availability of graft material. Unless previous graft salvaging has taken place, utilizing septal cartilage for the dorsum and auricular cartilage from the conchal area for the "pea-pod" is preferred. Appropriate measurement and clinical evaluation of the quantity of available graft material needed and available are very important to avoid intraoperative surprises and multiple graft sites. One technique to ascertain the degree of septum present is the use of the "double-light/Q-Tip" trick: a headlight is utilized along with a speculum to look through one nostril and with an opposing light on the opposite side. This allows one to see light penetrating through part/s of the septum lacking cartilage. In addition, a cotton-tip applicator can be used to examine for the presence of cartilaginous and bony septum. It is not rare to find the regeneration of septal, and to some degree, even auricular cartilage where the perichondrium was left intact.

This material appears to be more fibrous than cartilaginous and does not work as well as grafting material.

12. There are some applications in which form-fitting an aluminum splint over distorted nasal graft cartilage can be used. Experience in pediatric plastic surgery has shown that form-fitting a mold over deformed ears can actually result in a reformed cartilage framework. In patients who have early dorsal cartilage twisting, the regular nighttime wearing of a splint for up to 6 weeks may produce some improvement. This is particularly true if there is some cartilage mobility. Suture repositioning under local anesthetic with dorsal taping and splinting for a short period of time may also be effective.

Caucasian vs. Non-Caucasian Techniques

The differences between the non-Caucasian and Caucasian nasal anatomy require some modifications in surgical technique. After many years of altering and combining techniques to obtain a series of good results, I have established a personal operative plan.

The Caucasian nasal anatomy can be characterized as follows: (1) the bony vault is large, if not excessive, and may contain humps in the bridge or dorsum; (2) the middle vault is also large, and may contain a deviated septum; (3) the alar cartilages are usually full and thick with sidewalls of average thickness; (4) the nasolabial angle is neutral or acute; and (5) the nasal spine is usually normal or prominent.

Standard reduction techniques often provide satisfactory results in the Caucasian rhinoplasty patient. Greater definition and thinness are achieved by simply narrowing or reducing the wide or enlarged area. Balancing reduction and augmentation techniques is much more common in ethnic than in Caucasian rhinoplasties. Should the tip require augmentation, standard onlay or shield grafting techniques usually suffice.

However, that is not the case for most ethnic noses. The anatomical construction of the ethnic nose necessitates new approaches. Several key characteristics provide the impetus for innovation:

1. A small to normal bony vault accompanied by significant concavity, particularly in Asians and blacks
2. A bridge of normal width, or wide and splayed, as seen in many Asians and Hispanics
3. Flimsy and relatively unsupportive alar cartilages
4. Horizontally oriented nostrils
5. Thick, bulky nasal skin and soft tissue
6. A drooping, ptotic tip

The ethnic nose's distinct combination of thick, bulky nasal soft tissue with a relatively small quantity of osteocartilaginous support poses the most challenging problem to the rhinoplastic surgeon. Reduction rhinoplasty techniques alone were historically used for ethnic noses, often with disappointing results. Reducing an already deficient osteocartilaginous framework led to a more flattened, bulbous appearance, while reducing the soft-tissue cover resulted in a distorted, unattractive tip. Standard onlay grafting techniques have likewise proven inadequate. Those techniques simply do not achieve the projection, support, and contour required for improving the ethnic nose.

I have found that definition is best achieved in these types of noses by creating the illusion of thinness rather than by actually reducing the size of the nose. This illusion is created by combining a limited amount of selective soft-tissue reduction and incorporating a more supportive tip graft which is capable of a great deal of projection. Indeed, adequate tip projection is crucial for a successful result. When tip projection and a precisely elevated dorsum are correctly balanced, the illusion of a narrower bridge is created and osteotomies sometimes become unnecessary (Fig. 4-1). While reduction techniques are still valuable, most of the "thinning" of the nose actually comes from augmentation techniques. Dorsal grafting supports the small, concave bony vault, while a prominent "pea-pod" graft helps to support the flimsy alar cartilage. This "pea-pod" graft, along with limited tip defatting, provides greater definition to the bulky nasal tip.

A smaller nose can be achieved by reducing osteocartilaginous support and soft-tissue coverage, but usually only at the expense of definition. It is more effective to create definition by increasing—rather than decreasing—the dorsal and tip osteocartilaginous support. It should also be noted that most ethnic patients do prefer this increase in nasal projection because of the significant increase in definition it can provide.

Preoperative Surgical Preparation

I use the following techniques to obtain the best results:

1. I prefer general anesthesia. These procedures often can last 2 to 3 hours, and even the well-blocked, heavily sedated patient may be restless and uncomfortable. Maintaining blood pressure in the range of 85 to 90 psi with the use of safe hypotensive anesthetic techniques significantly helps to decrease bleeding, swelling, and bruising.

2. The "BASICS" also markedly decrease postoperative swelling and bruising and are administered preoperatively:

   Benadryl, 50 mg intravenously

   Antibiotics: Intravenous cefazolin sodium (Ancef) 1 g, or erythromycin 250 mg, or vancomycin hydrochloride 500 mg in the penicillin-allergic patient

   Steroids: Intravenous dexamethasone phosphate (Decadron) 6 to 10 mg

   Ice

   Compression after injection of local anesthetic

   Standard intra- and extranasal preparation with dilute povidone-iodine cleanser (Betadine)

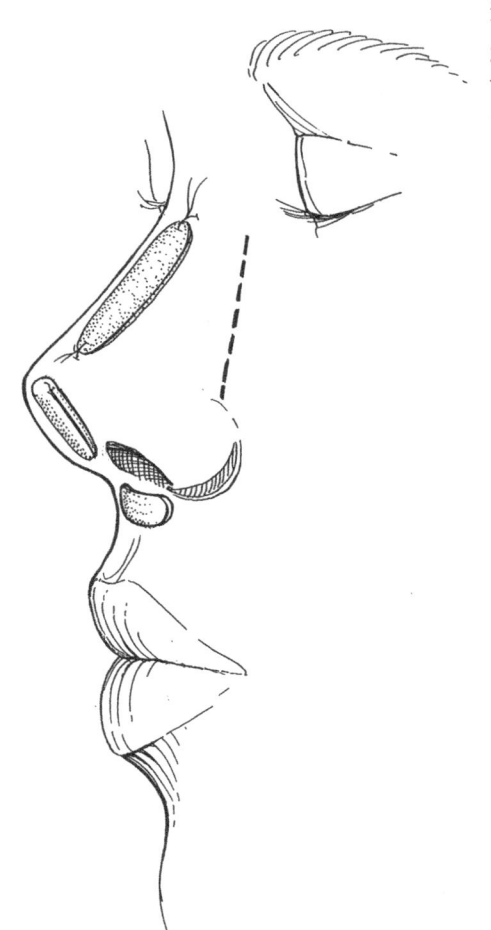

Figure 4-1
Several steps may be required to obtain a satisfactory result in the non-Caucasian nose: (1) dorsal bone or cartilage grafting, (2) thinning of the bridge through osteotomies, (3) alar wedge resectioning, (4) maxillary or nasal base grafting, and (5) nasal tip grafting.

3. Saline-moistened deep pharyngeal packs are always placed during long procedures. Dried blood in the pharynx can cause substantial irritation and postoperative coughing and gagging. These packs also help stabilize the endotracheal tube, thus decreasing the incidence of sore throats.

4. Before injecting the local anesthetic, cotton pledgets (or Vaseline gauze) moistened with topical 4% lidocaine hydrochloride (Xylocaine) are placed deep within the nasal vault. This prevents any local anesthetic from spilling onto the pharyngeal wall and causing numbness and postoperative swallowing difficulties.

5. The local anesthetic used is bupivacaine hydrochloride (Marcaine) 0.5% with epinephrine 1:100,000. It is freshly mixed as 50 cc of bupivacaine hydrochloride (Marcaine) 0.5%, with 0.5 cc of epinephrine 1:1000, along with 750 units of hyaluronidase (Wydase). This mixture is injected into the external and internal nasal structures. Approximately 5 to 10 cc are used for complete infiltration.

6. The tips of the inferior turbinates are *slowly* injected with the steroid of choice. I use 2.5 to 5.0 mg/cc dilute Kenalog (triamcinolone acetonide suspension 10 mg/ml) or dexamethasone phosphate (Decadron) 4 mg/cc. Care should be taken to draw back on the syringe prior to injection to avoid intravascular delivery of steroid solution. Dilute Kenalog is also injected into the nasal tip and the maxillary junction at the osteotomy sites. An ice bag is held over the injection sites for approximately 5 minutes. The ice helps to decrease the amount of reactive turbinate swelling than can occur. Later, gentle outfracturing is performed as needed.

7. The external and intranasal areas are prepped completely, along with the ear(s) and temporalis areas if these are to be utilized. If the ear is designated as the cartilage donor site, the following is performed: (1) the entire external ear is prepped with povidone-iodine cleanser (Betadine); (2) the ear canals are cleaned thoroughly and then packed with povidone-iodine-cleanser (Betadine)–soaked cotton pledgets or ear plugs; (3) an otoscopic examination of the ear is first done to ensure that the tympanic membrane is intact. The surgeon then scrubs and allows several minutes for the epinephrine to take effect. Nasal vibrissae are trimmed when necessary with a small scissors coated with bacitracin zinc.

Standard Ethnic Rhinoplasty Operative Sequence

The following procedures are performed in the order listed, but obviously not every patient requires every procedure.

1. Harvesting of Grafts

The initial procedure is harvesting septal or ear cartilage, cranial bone, or temporalis fascial grafts. Autologous conchal cartilage is the preferred choice for most ethnic rhinoplasties.

2. Septoplasty and Turbinectomy

Appropriate corrective septal and turbinate procedures are then carried out as indicated. The standard turbinate reduction involves cross-clamping and excision distal to the clamp. The turbinates are then outfractured.

3. Compression via Vaseline Packing

The previously placed cotton pledgets are removed and firm-fitting Vaseline packing is packed bilaterally into the posterior nasal cavity to help control swelling and prevent blood from entering the oropharynx. If postoperative packing is to be retained, the Vaseline is replaced with Merocel tampons prior to the end of the surgery.

4. Incisions and Skeletonization

Intercartilaginous incisions are made and a conservative skeletonization of the nasal bones performed. A transfixion incision is also made, if indicated. Light ice compression is applied to the nose at this time. If a dorsal or radix graft is planned, the dissection should be made only slightly larger than the planned graft so as to avoid subsequent graft mobility.

5. Dorsal Rasping or Osteotomies

Scissors are inserted through the intercartilaginous incision and the tissues overlying the dorsum are freed in a subperiosteal plane. Rasping or osteotomies of the dorsum is then performed.

6. Osteotomies

Medial canthal and/or piriform periosteal incisions are made and osteotomies performed.

7. Ice Compression and Carving of Grafts

Three to 5 minutes of intraoperative ice compression is applied to the osteotomy sites and nasal dorsum to decrease the likelihood of subsequent ecchymosis and edema. During this time, the surgeon is free to carve the previously harvested grafts.

8. Alar Rim Incisions

Alar rim incisions are then made and a wide dissection is performed. A "bucket handle" approach is performed and the lower lateral cartilages are delivered.

9. Alar Cartilage Reduction

Limited tip defatting and reduction of alar cartilage is performed. With proper dissection, fat can be left on the alar cartilage and trimmed later. The cephalic three-fifths of the cartilages are trimmed as needed, taking care to curve up at the lateral extent of the excision. As much soft tissue as possible is delivered with the cartilages for subsequent removal.

10. Caudal Septal Excision and Rim Incision

Any necessary caudal septal excision or recontouring is done at this point. A rim incision is made bilaterally and carried down to the midcolumella on the right side for future placement of the nasal tip strut.

11. Nasal Spine and Carving of Smaller Grafts

The anterior nasal spine is reduced or augmented, and maxillary grafts are carved, as indicated.

12. Alar Wedge Excision

After the base has been meticulously measured for tissue excision, a curvilinear incision is made a millimeter above the alar crease. A wedge excision is performed. Take care to excise more skin than mucosa in most situations, though in the occasional ethnic situation with disproportionately wide bases and small nostrils, lobular excision alone (Type I) excisions should be considered.

13. Undermining at the Alar Base

Skin is undermined for a few millimeters on the cheek to allow for medial displacement after closure is accomplished.

14. Placement of Merocel Packing

At this juncture, if indicated, the intranasal Vaseline packing is removed, and Merocel tubular tampons, after being coated with an antibiotic ointment, are placed. All packing should be placed prior to the placement of grafts, since forceful packing can displace grafts.

15. Placement of Grafts

Radix, dorsal, and/or tip grafts are then placed and inserted with Dexon pull-out skin-stabilization sutures. Maxillary, nasal spine, or nasal base grafts may also be inserted at this time.

16. Alar Closure

Intranasal mucosal closure is performed.

Alar wedge excision sites are advanced and closed in a layered fashion, using deep anchoring sutures to the periosteum of the maxilla near the piriform aperture, followed by mucosal closure.

Cartilage Graft Harvesting

The natural size and contour of septal cartilage provides ideal graft material for augmenting and elevating a low dorsum. One can frequently "kill two birds with one stone" when excising a deflected septum by using the excised cartilage as graft material. Unfortunately, most ethnic noses do not usually contain as much septal cartilage as Caucasian noses. It is very important to predetermine if the septum will be an adequate donor site. If the amount of septal cartilage appears inadequate, the ears should be prepped in anticipation of harvesting conchal cartilage (any need for rib and/or cranium grafts should also be anticipated). It should also be noted that turbinate tissue (bony contents) has been found to be poor graft material. Mucosal remnants can be accidentally incorporated into the graft, often leading to later mucous cyst formation.

When given a choice, I prefer using conchal cartilage to construct nasal grafts, especially for more complicated grafts and nasal tip grafts. The convex shape of the concha more closely simulates the normal curvature of the nasal tip cartilages. The straight septum, when layered and placed into the nasal tip, may give a too straight and sharp appearance. While this problem may be alleviated by crushing or placing additional cartilage grafts to soften the straightness of the septal grafts, the consistency and curves of the concha make it the ideal donor site. I prefer a postauricular approach to obtain a conchal cartilage graft, which is the superior method in patients prone to increased pigmentation and scarring or whenever a very large segment of cartilage must be removed. Patients who have a history of problematic scarring or keloid formation (caused by trauma or ear piercing) should be forewarned about potential problems.

A large cartilage donor site may frequently be needed for both dorsal and tip grafting (Fig. 4-2, on page 37). Not infrequently, both ears may be used, contingent upon the desired degree of projection and the size of the ears. I recommend starting with a graft of at least 3.0 cm × 0.75 cm. The final tip graft size may be as large as 3.25 cm × 1.0 cm, but is usually smaller. A constructed tip graft that fails to provide sufficient projection, due to its limited size, may force a larger, second graft to be taken from the opposite ear. Obtaining a sufficient length of graft material during the first excision is therefore of the utmost importance. Attempting to lengthen a short tip graft by adding smaller lengths of cartilage will only result in decreased strength and support, and is not recommended. When salvaging the auricular graft, 25% of additional length should be added as a future corrective margin. Grafts are easily reduced by trimming but very difficult to ex-

Figure 4-2
One ear usually provides sufficient cartilage for both a small-to-medium-sized "pea-pod" tip graft as well as dorsal grafts. However, larger graft requirements may necessitate the use of both ears. Starting with a graft that measures at least 3 cm .75 cm is recommended. A larger graft is rarely necessary.

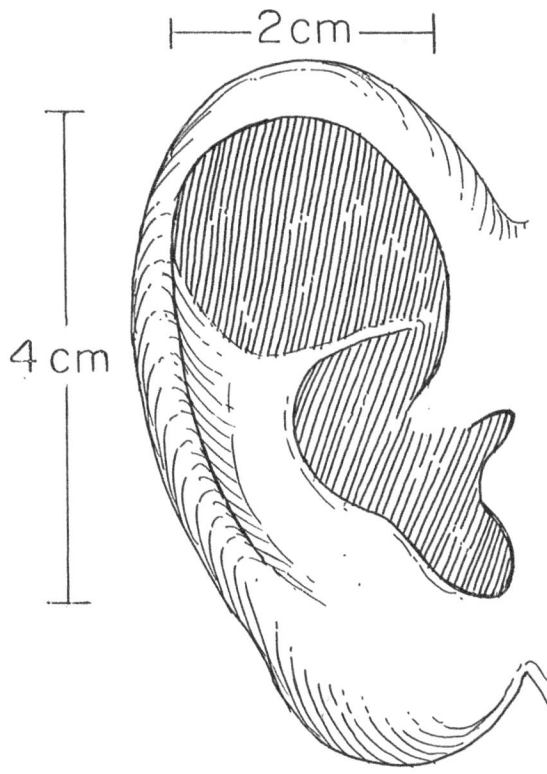

tend. Remember that if a graft is too small, the opposite ear must be used to obtain a complete single length graft.

A wavy, curvilinear incision is made 0.5 cm above the postauricular sulcus (Fig. 4-3a, 4-3b, on page 38). There are numerous advantages to this approach. First, the curvilinear-postauricular approach allows for easier conchal cartilage excision. Second, the postauricular approach gives wide exposure, allowing mastoid fascia and soft tissue to be harvested at the same time, if indicated (Fig. 4-4a, 4-4b, on page 39). Incorporating mastoid fascia and soft tissue onto the graft assists whenever tip skin is thin or extra soft-tissue fill is needed. This padding decreases tip sharpness, reduces the need for additional trimming, and helps to increase projection without causing an undue amount of "pointing." And, again, it has been the author's experience that closing a straight-line incision along the curved postauricular skin has resulted in more hypertrophic scars than when a curved incision is used.

After the postauricular incision is made, a supraperichondrial plane is dissected posteriorly and a subperichondrial plane anteriorly (Fig. 4-5a, 4-5b, on page 40). Typically, a supraperichondrial dissection is performed only if additional soft mastoid tissue is needed to be included with the graft. Great care must be taken when incising the superficial aspect of the cartilage that the anterior auricular skin is not violated. Usually, a large portion of the concha is excised. If possible, the medial aspect of the horizontal, helical bar should be avoided because of the support and contour it provides. The lateral portion of the bar can be removed in continuity for a

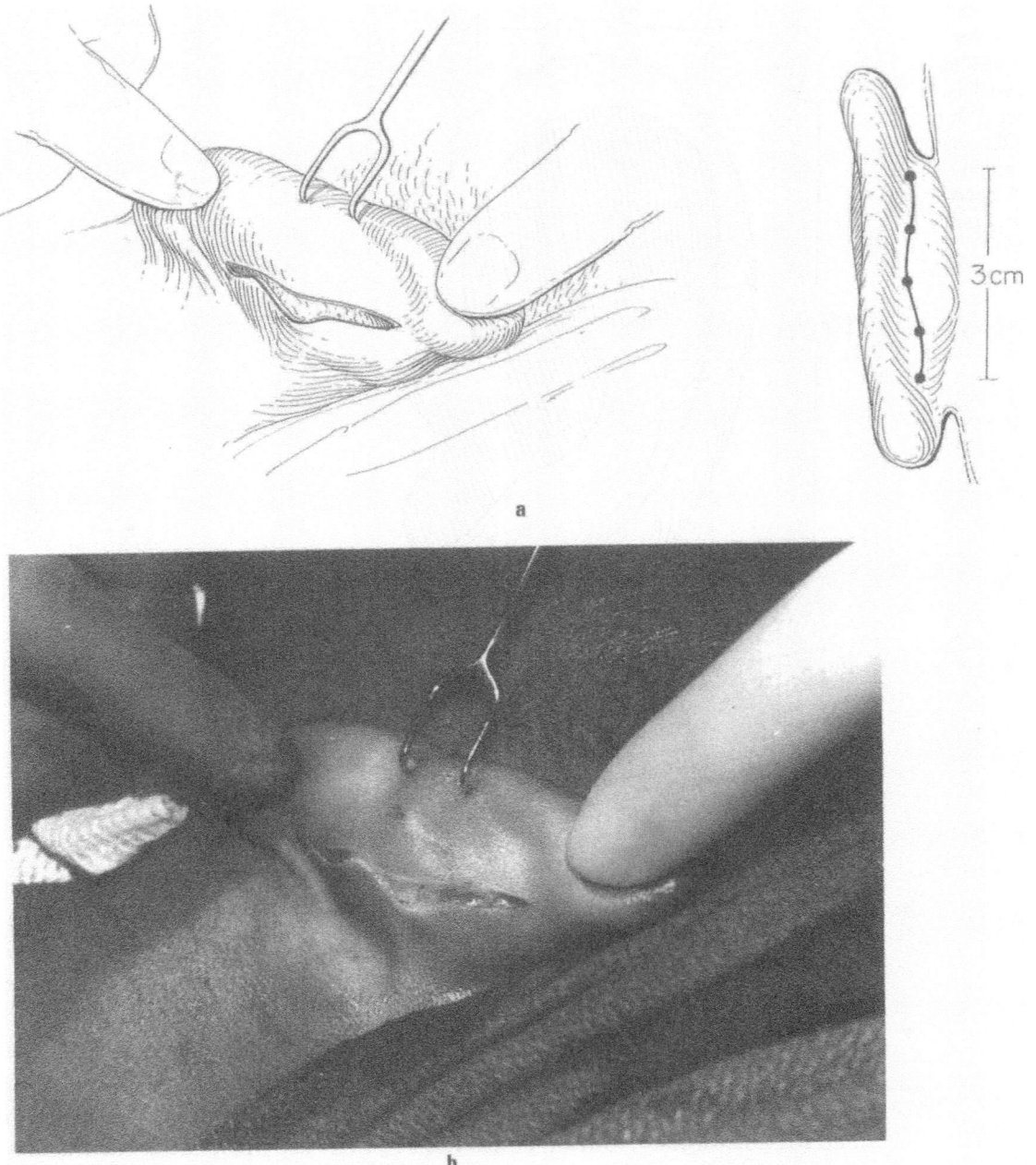

Figure 4-3a, 4-3b
A curvilinear incision is made approximately 0.5 cm above the postauricular sulcus. Here, the skin is thinner and less prone to hypertrophic scarring, and the closure is easier.

longer graft. A significant amount of cartilage can be removed from the concha without ear distortion (Fig. 4-6a, 4-6b, on page 41).

After removal of sufficient conchal cartilage and mastoid fascia, the postauricular incision is irrigated with dilute povidone-iodine cleanser (Betadine) and saline. The area is then sprayed with 0.5% bupivacaine hydrochloride (Marcaine) with epinephrine, and a greater auricular nerve block is performed for prolonged anesthesia. A small suction or Penrose drain is placed. The incision is then closed with 4-0 Dexon and 5-0 nylon sutures (Fig. 4-7a, 4-7b, on page 42). (For postoperative dressings, see chapter 5: "Postoperative Nasal Packing and Dressings".)

Figure 4-4a, 4-4b
This curvilinear-postauricular incision provides excellent access to the conchal cartilage. Required graft measurements can at this time be transferred to the conchal cartilage by use of a marking pen. The premeasured and marked cartilage can then be excised.

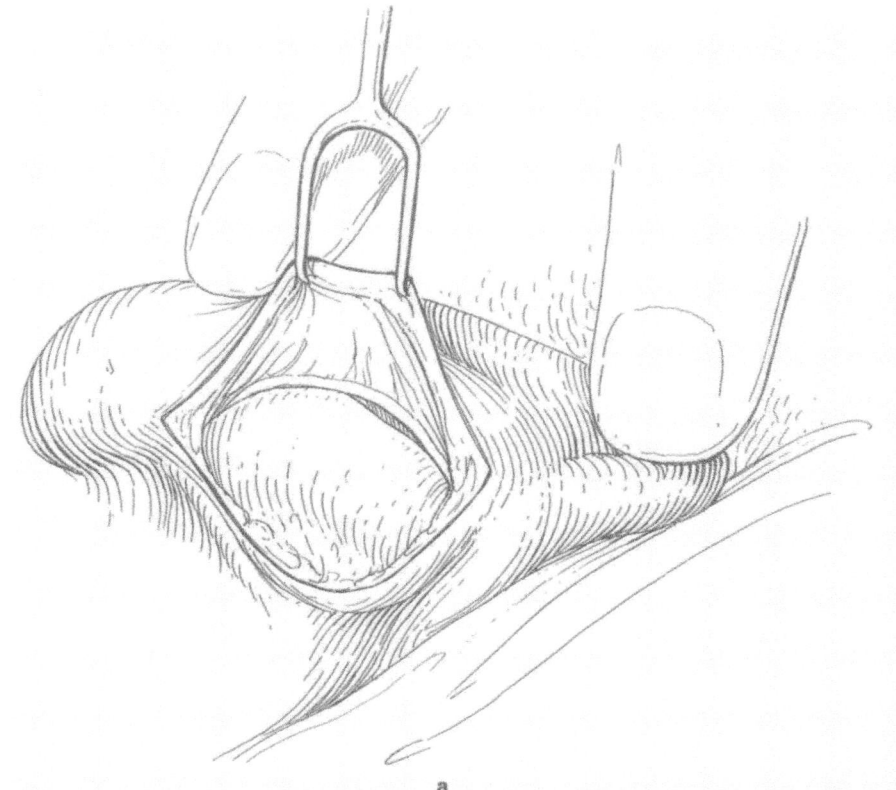

a

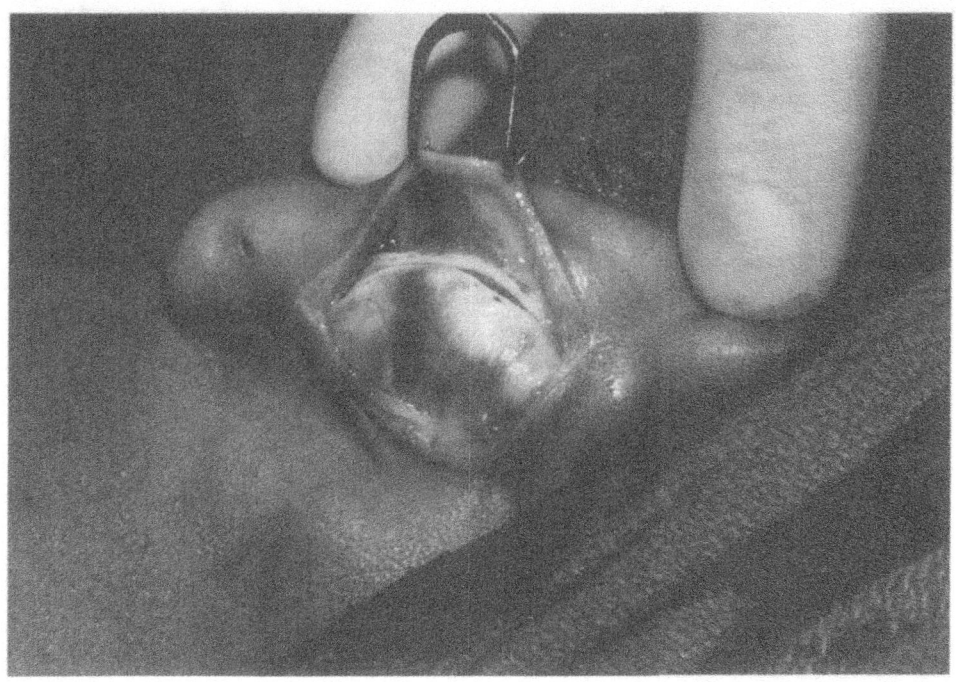

b

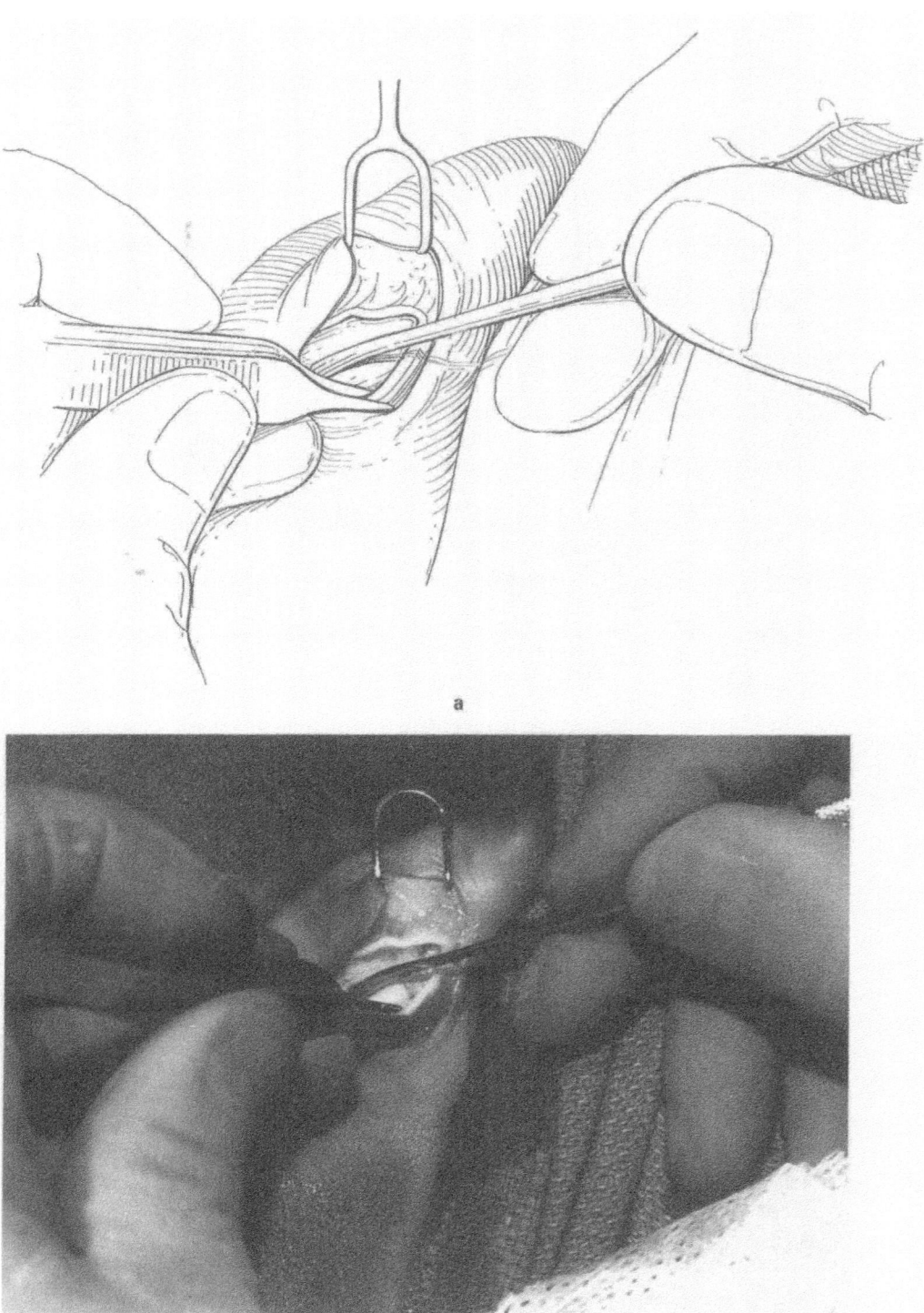

Figure 4-5a, 4-5b
A large segment of conchal cartilage is excised using a #15 blade and a Freer elevator. When additional mastoid soft tissue is not needed for fill or graft padding, a subperichondrial dissection is performed.

Exposure and Incisions

Despite the current popularity and increased exposure allowed by open transcolumellar techniques, I do not recommend them for primary ethnic rhinoplasties, particularly where a highly supportive tip graft has been placed and large alar resections and tip defatting have been performed. There are two reasons for this: safety and graft positioning.

Figure 4-6a, 4-6b
Much of the conchal cartilage can be removed without causing a deformity. The anterior portion of the horizontal bar, however, should be preserved, while the posterior portion of the bar can be removed in continuity with the graft.

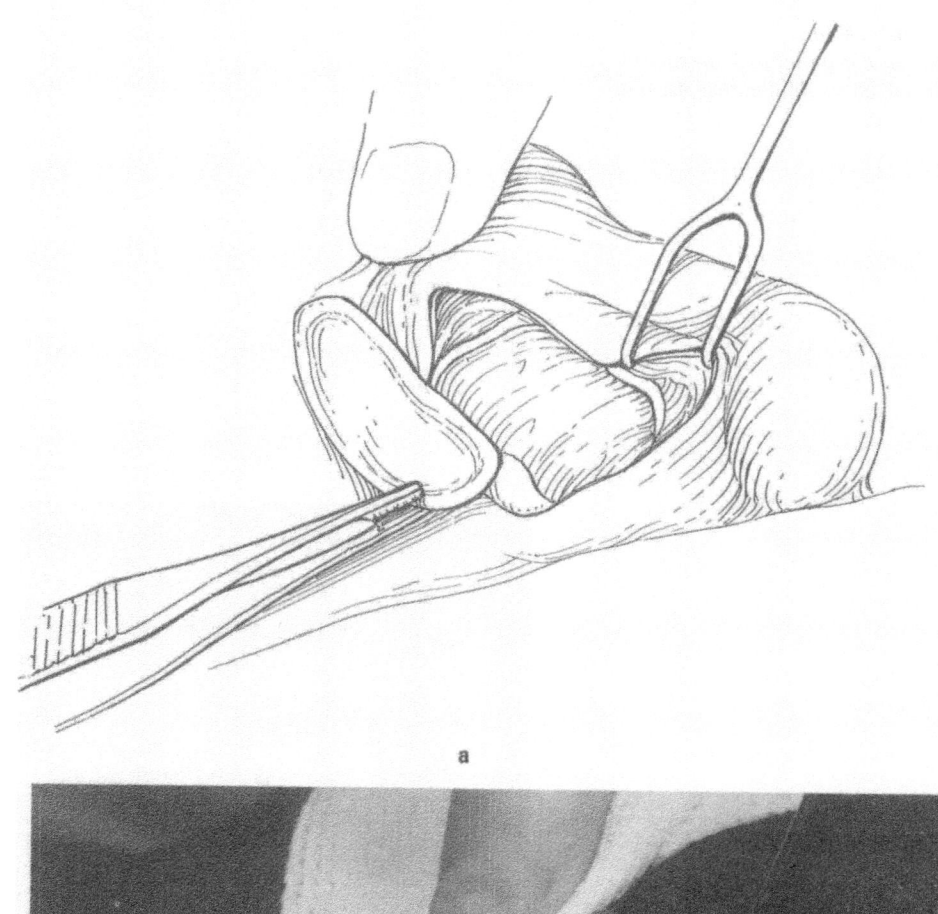

a

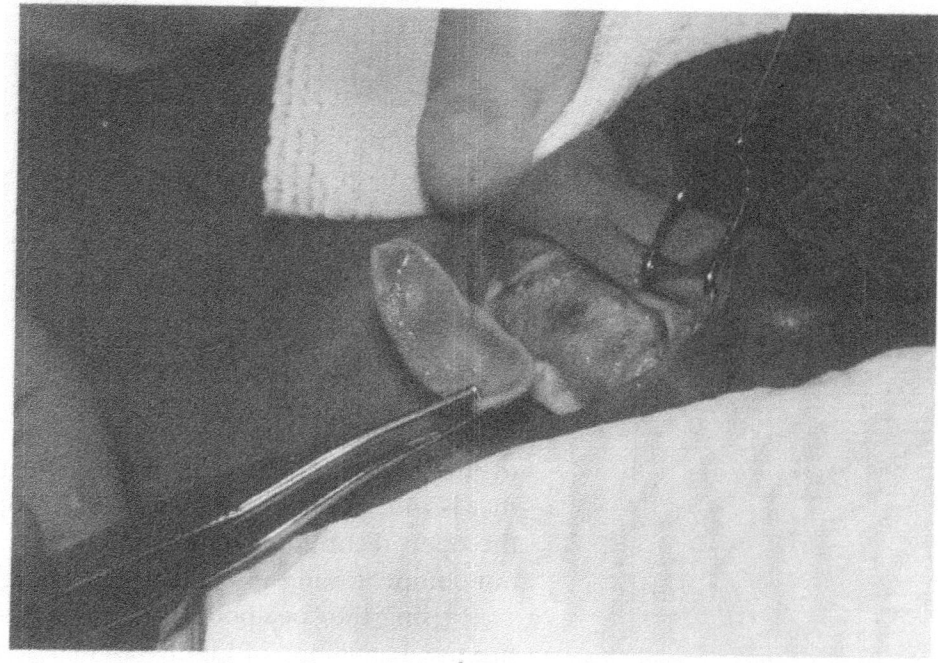

b

First, whenever multiple incisions and grafting have been performed, tip vascularity is already challenged, and a transcolumellar incision could push it beyond the margin of safety. Second, open tip approaches do not accommodate proper graft positioning. When properly placed, the "pea-pod" graft should lie under the columellar skin, over and inferior to the alar cartilages from the dome down to the medial crus. With the open rhinoplasty approach, the skin is elevated but the cartilage from the alar dome

Figure 4-7a, 4-7b
Hemostasis is performed, the incision is closed, and a .25" Penrose drain is brought out.

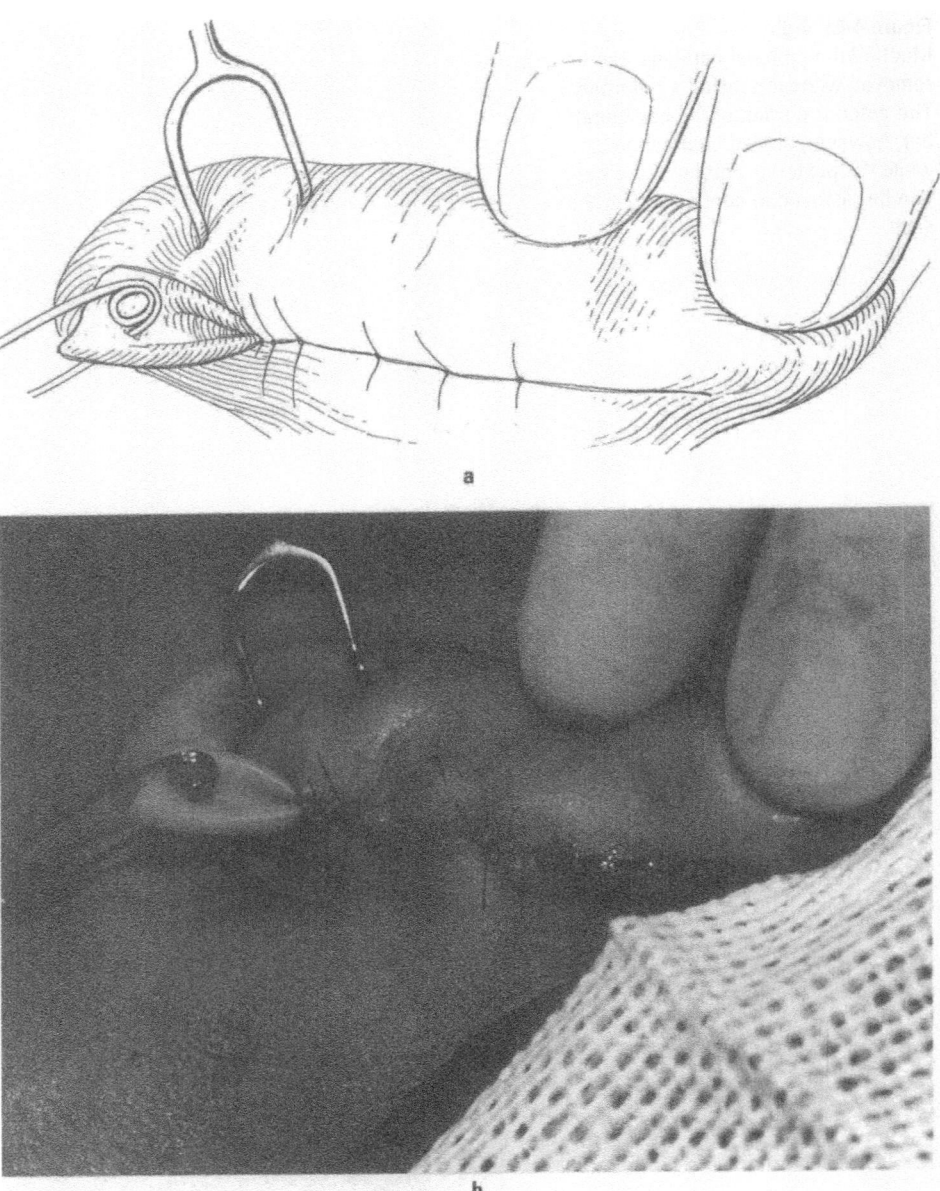

to the medial crus remains intact, creating a bed for the "pea-pod" graft that is too small to afford sufficient projection. In revision cases, however, the open technique is quite efficacious. It provides superb exposure without compromising vascularity or healing.

Using the "pea-pod" graft (see "Pea-Pod" section) and leaving the entire nasal envelope of highly vascularized soft tissue intact (except for right columellar incision) project graft vascularity. Placing the tensioned graft in a more stable base helps assure proper placement and prevent graft resorption. An "open" technique would minimize the continuous soft-tissue envelope, possibly increasing resorption and vascularization. Open techniques have been most beneficial in secondaries when a patient can accept an initially hypopigmented scar to be later improved with tattooing.

Exposure of the nasal tip begins with a standard marginal rim incision in the right ala, which is carried down to the midlateral columella. It is usually 2 to 3 mm behind the edge of the columella but in front of the medial

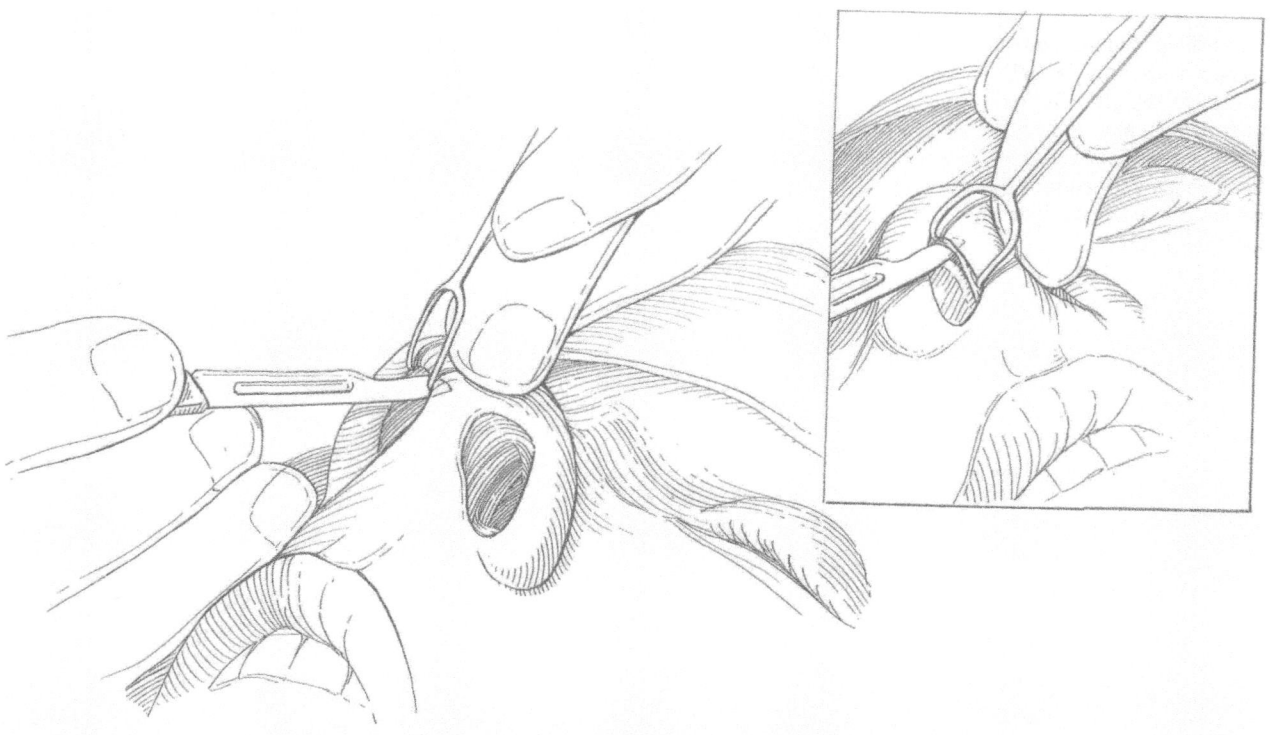

Figure 4-8a, 4-8b
A standard anterior rim incision is extended down the lateral edge of the columella, anterior and inferior to the medial footplate. It is only unilateral so that the lateral side of the tip graft can be placed against the opposite wall of the columella. If alar cartilage reduction is being performed, the classic "bucket-handle" incision is carried out and is in continuity with this incision.

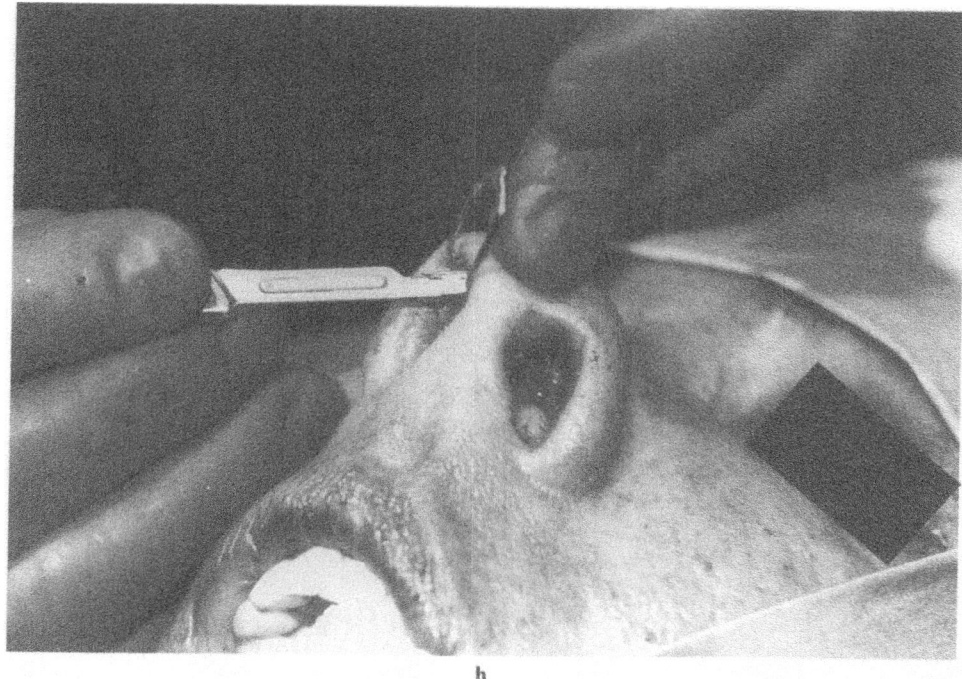

crura (Fig. 4-8a, 4-8b). Only the right side of the columella, anterior to the medial crura, is incised. The right alar cartilage can then be delivered as a bipedicle flap and reduced. At this point, if indicated, excessive tip fat and fibrous tissue can be delivered with the cartilage and trimmed. (See "Thick Nasal Tip Skin and Alar Cartilage Reduction".)

The central inferior soft tissue is then opened with a small scissors and deeply spread (Fig. 4-9a, 4-9b, on page 44). The inferior dissection is made

Figure 4-9a, 4-9b
The entire alar cartilage and tip is undermined, leaving a thick, fatty dermal layer to pad and mask the graft. During dissection, great care is taken to avoid excising mucosa, as a sufficient amount will be necessary for closure. A curved mosquito clamp can be used to bluntly dissect the pocket.

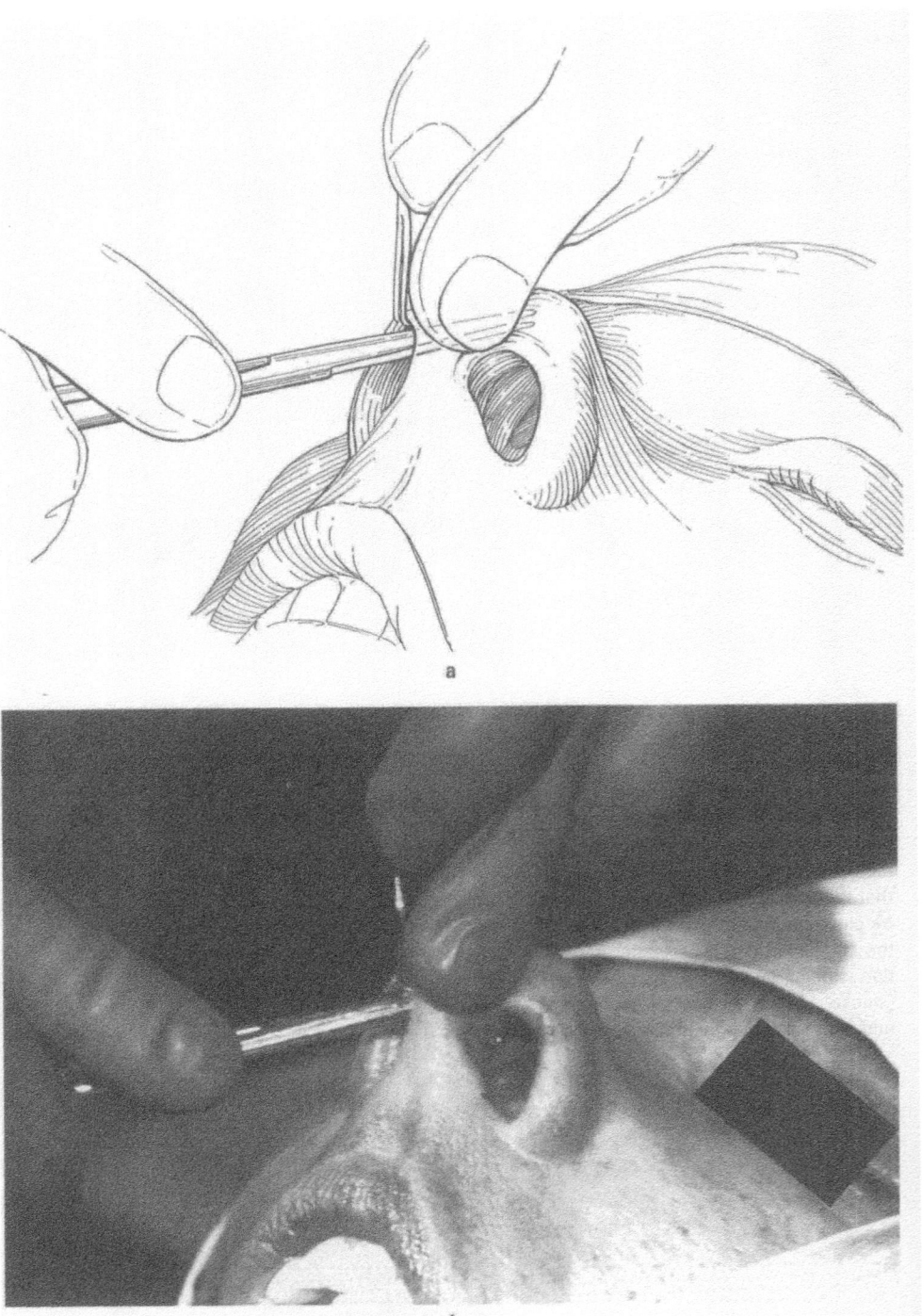

3 to 5 mm above the columellar-labial sulcus and is not extended to the nasal spine. This provides a natural columellar break point. The tip and superior three-fourths of the columella must be undermined sufficiently to allow good positioning and draping of the tip graft. Excessive vestibular mucosa and skin are never excised because they may be needed for lateral graft coverage.

When performing intranasal dorsal dissection (for dorsal grafting), take care to not totally free the nasal bone from the skin, as internasal vault collapse can occur if adequate soft-tissue attachments are not left in place.

Nasal Septum and Turbinates

There are two major causes of airway obstruction in the unoperated nose: (1) septal deviation and (2) turbinate hypertrophy. Congenital septal deviation is quite common in the Caucasian nose but unusual in the black nose. Traumatic septal deviation, however, is common in all races. Vomer spurs are also rare in blacks.

Enlarged turbinates are generally the greater cause of airway obstruction than is septal deviation. Indeed, even in very large nasal vaults the turbinates may be enlarged enough to cause airway obstruction. Diagnostically, one must also rule out sinus obstruction due to ostia blockage as a source of airway problems by a trial of decongestants and aerosolized steroid nasal inhalers in symptomatic patients.

Septum

The septal pocket can be utilized as a reservoir for cartilage excised from either the septum or the ear. Hard tissue can be straightened and placed back into the pocket, along with a thin sheet of ethmoid or cranial bone. Septocartilage is not as malleable as ear cartilage and the presence or absence of the perichondrium may make a difference in terms of its "memory." Nationwide studies are currently underway to determine cofactors associated with cartilage "memory." The possibility of cartilage contortion or bending should be kept in mind when dealing with salvaging sites and cartilage. Another excellent source of cartilage is the alar cartilage/caudal septum and vomer, which can be used for augmentation.

The nasal spine or base of the caudal septum is not found to be substantially enlarged in most ethnic patients, possibly excepting Hispanics, depending on the bony architecture. The maxillary area frequently has to be augmented. And the presence of the nasal spine may be important in providing a degree of maxillary augmentation and modification.

Turbinate Surgery

Surgeons have become more conservative regarding turbinate surgery. It appears that the best time for anatomical examination is after shrinkage of the turbinates with either oxymetazoline hydrochloride (Afrin), Neo-Synephrine, or topical epinephrine spray. Boggy edematous mucosa may be secondary to allergies. Saline irrigations and topical cortisone sprays such as beclomethasone dipropionate (Beconase), two or three times a day, may help to control swelling. A recommended allergy consultation may benefit those patients who are quite symptomatic. Newer antihistaminelike medications without drowsy side effects may be recommended. Many surgeons utilize both topical and oral medications. Dilute steroid injections into the tip of the turbinates may be of benefit for surgery and postoperatively. It appears that turbinate excision and/or excessive cauterization may cause prolonged rhinorrhea. Conservative use of these modalities should be kept in mind. Overresection of turbinates, which decreases normal nasal airflow, may give rise to excessive dryness and/or airway difficulties.

Singers not infrequently "voice" a concern about injury to their voice after septal, turbinate, or rhinoplastic surgeries. It is the author's experience that such detrimental effects have NEVER occurred, while marked improvements have been realized in numerous Grammy Award–winning singers—although the techniques are not recommended as a path to an improved singing voice. But a conservative program can frequently reduce or eliminate abnormal nasal resonance or turbinate obstructions.

Frequently though, the turbinates have to be addressed surgically. When reducing a turbinate, remember that the average width between the turbinate and septum is 2 mm. For the majority of mild-to-moderate turbinate enlargements, simple outfracturing in conjunction with conservative steroid injections may be sufficient.

My personal technique for reducing turbinates is to cross-clamp the tips of the inferior turbinates and to excise the tissue distal to the cross-clamp. Careful injection of dilute steroids into the turbinate remnants can help decrease postoperative turbinate edema. Reduction of the turbinates is often sufficient to satisfactorily improve the airway. After performing turbinate surgery, packing may be indicated. (See Chapter 5: "Postoperative Nasal Packing and Dressings".)

Nasal Dorsum and Bridge

The ethnic dorsum is typically low and concave and the bridge is very wide, as compared to the Caucasian counterparts. Most rhinoplastic patients request a dorsum that is straighter and less concave, with a bridge that is neither too broad nor too thin, but of uniform and moderate width from nasion to alar groove. Most patients want to retain a small degree of concavity.

The most effective way to accomplish these changes is to augment the flat, low dorsum with a long, straight, stable graft (Fig. 4-10a, on page 47) and to narrow the wide bridge through lateral osteotomies (Fig. 4-10b, on page 47). A surgeon can create a nice aesthetic effect with the skilled combination of these two techniques. Simply narrowing a wide bridge often creates the illusion that a higher bridge was constructed. This effect is amplified with the placement of a dorsal graft.

Many patients want to limit the size of the dorsal graft out of fear that their nose will appear too large. When given a choice, most choose a prominent tip over a prominent bridge. Preserving or creating a harmonious relation between the tip and the bridge, with the bridge slightly less prominent, is crucial to the success of the operation.

Dorsal Grafting Preferences

My primary choices for dorsal graft material are autologous layered septal cartilage or ethmoid bone. But neither is amply available in the ethnic nose. Therefore, conchal cartilage and the associated mastoid fascia are often utilized. Other sources of graft material, such as cranium, ninth rib, or iliac

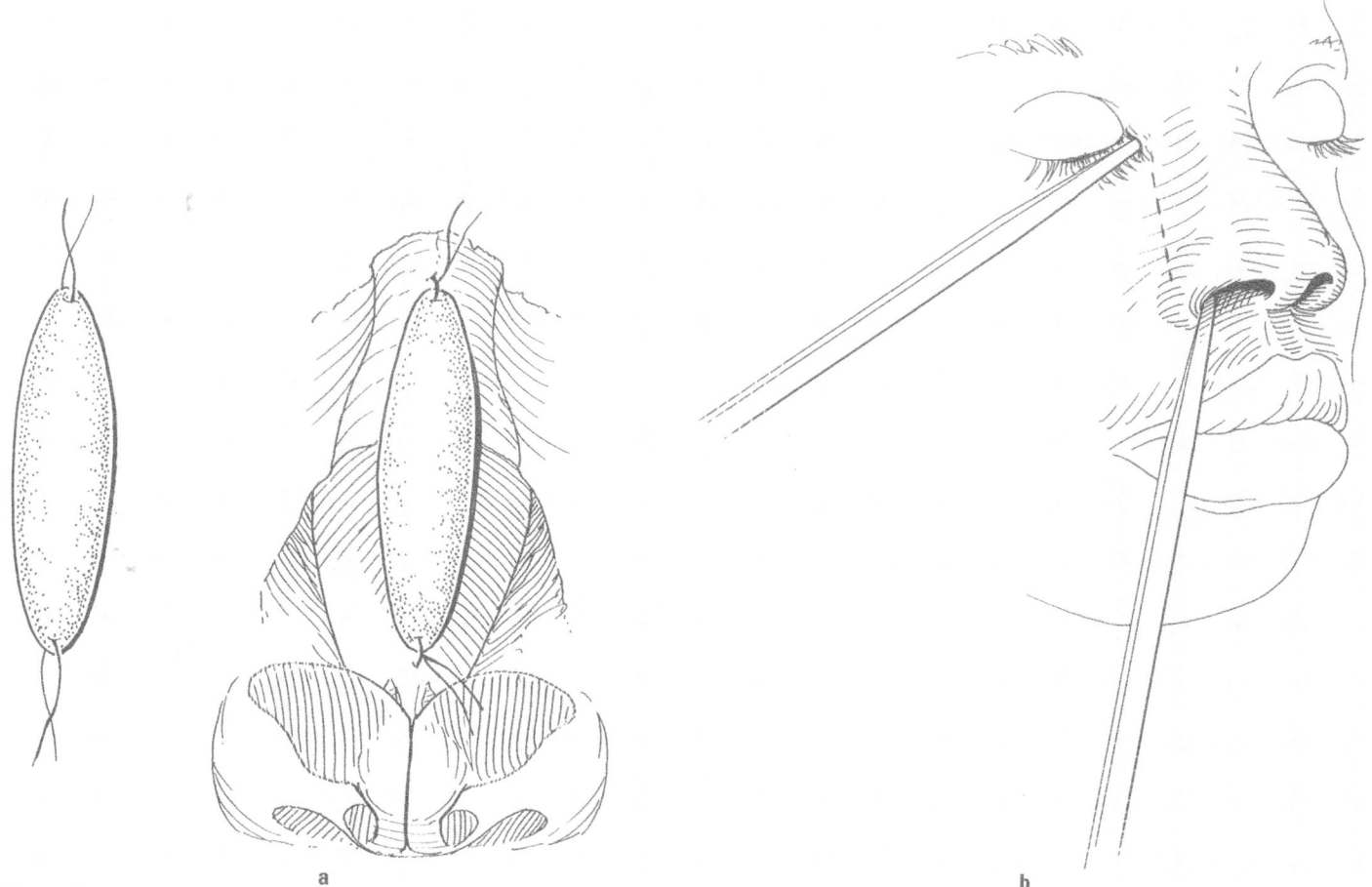

a   b

Figure 4-10a
A fusiform-shaped graft provides less bulk at the supratip area. Beveling the edges, linear scoring, or limited crushing can assist in contouring under thin skin. To ensure viability, the future dorsal graft should also have complete, vascularized, soft-tissue covering. Mastoid or temporalis fascia can also be used to "soften" the edges.

Figure 4-10b
Fine 2-mm osteotomes are used to perform low medial osteotomies; stab incisions are made at the piriform aperture and the medial canthus. Medial canthal incisions heal quite well and provide the extra benefit of a small drainage hole that decreases early ecchymoses. Whenever dorsal cartilage and/or bone grafting are simultaneously performed, the mucosal lining is left intact.

crest, may also be used. It is usually beneficial to use a single graft donor site such as the ear, if at all possible.

Other types of dorsal grafts have been used with some success in ethnic rhinoplasty. Whenever the skin envelope is sufficiently thick and no previous operative procedures have been performed, soft Silastic or Gore-Tex grafts have sometimes yielded satisfactory long-term results. Advantages of Silastic that have been cited include its availability, ease of placement, and smooth straight contour. One particular disadvantage is the tendency of the implant to shift or extrude over a long period of time. Mobility can be decreased by creating a pocket that is just barely larger than the graft. Also, aggressive trimming of mucosa should be avoided to minimize later pocket contracture, which could lead to implant extrusion. Silastic grafts should be reserved for the dorsum and should not be placed in the tip, because of potential excessive supratip fullness, "open" pointing, and high reported rates of extrusion. As a principle, neither should ever be used in either dorsum or tip revision procedures.

Ivory and ceramic were historically used for dorsal grafts, especially in Asia. Most eventually extruded, but a number were retained, probably due to the thicker skin cover of the Asian nose.

Personal Dorsal Grafting Technique

Determine the skin thickness prior to deciding upon a grafting technique. Thick skin can camouflage sharp or irregular graft edges. In thin-skinned individuals, cartilage grafts may have to be laterally contoured and supplemented with mastoid or temporalis soft tissue. If insufficient septal cartilage or ethmoid bone is available, conchal cartilage and/or mastoid fascia

Figure 4-11a, 4-11b
Conchal cartilage is being used to create a medium-sized dorsal graft. 5-0 Dexon sutures are used for both the multilayering of grafts and for stabilization.

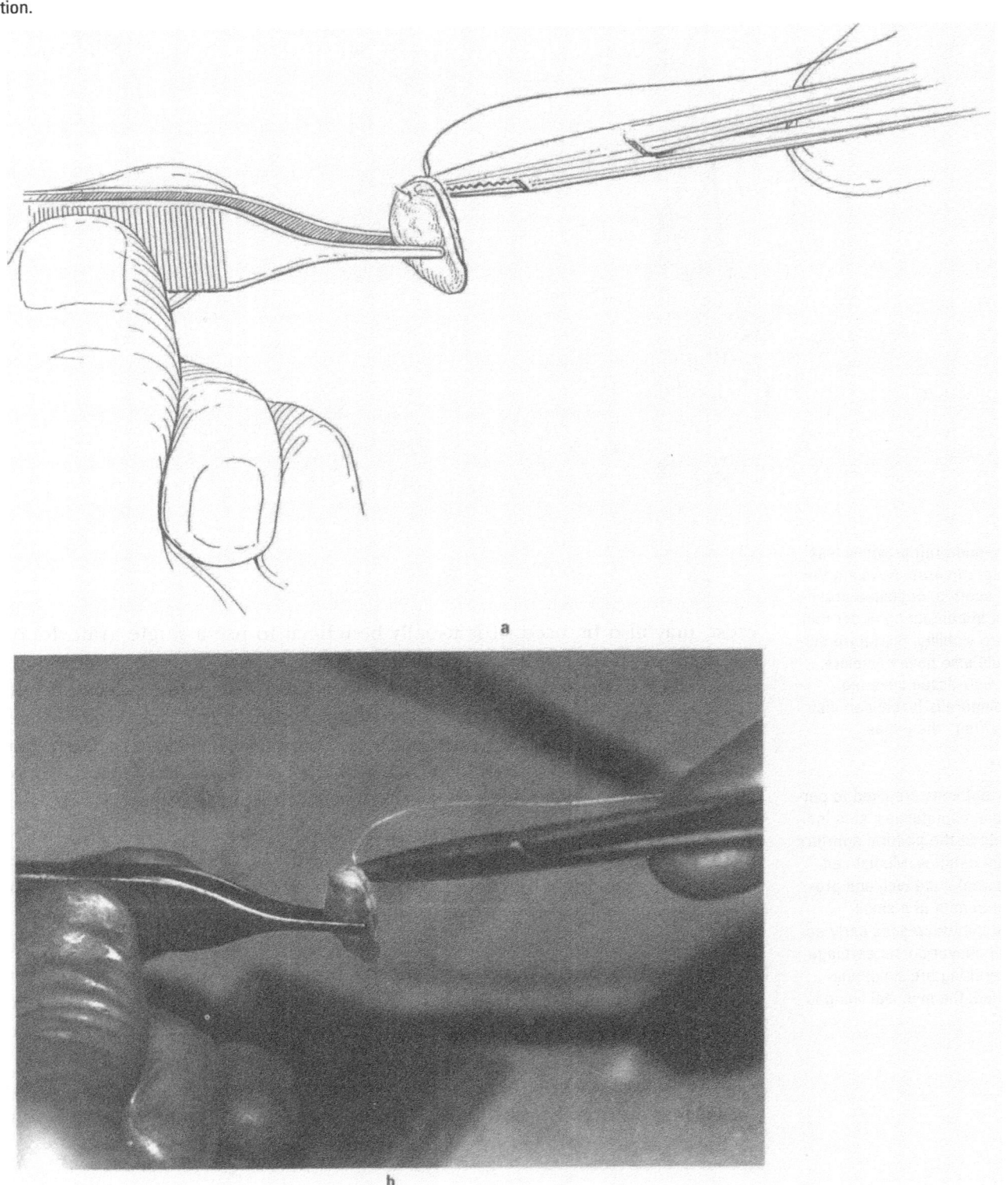

are utilized. Conchal cartilage is usually covered with soft-tissue fascia which can be incorporated with the graft or used as separate soft-tissue covering which assists in camouflaging the sides of the graft. If septal or conchal cartilage is unavailable, cranium, iliac crest, or rib can be used. For limited augmentation, temporalis fascia or carefully prepared dermis provides good graft material, but neither is sufficient for large defects.

Cartilage grafting requirements are estimated before graft material is gathered. The length, width, and height of the desired dorsal graft is measured with calipers and markings are made. These markings are important for graft placement. A larger amount of graft material than needed for the graft itself is harvested to take into account carving and contouring. Once the dorsal pocket has been dissected, construction and placement of the graft(s) are performed.

Cartilage segments are measured, cut, and sutured together with Dexon (Fig. 4-11a, 4-11b, on previous page). The cartilage is then scored with a #15 blade or contoured in the JOST crusher. If fragile, the entire graft can often be wrapped in Dexon or fascia to decrease fragmentation with crushing. The use of the JOST crusher can contribute significantly to proper contouring of the graft (Fig. 4-11c, See chapter 10: "Recommended Instruments"). Linear scoring along the length of the graft can also be of benefit. Severe crushing should be limited because it can contribute to graft resorption. Nasal grafting is performed by attaching both proximal and distal pull-out Dexon sutures to the ends of the nasal graft. These ensure stability and, if necessary, allow repositioning a few days after the bandages have been removed and the alignment has been checked and confirmed. The Dexon needle is straightened and the sharp tip is placed up into the end of a tuberculin syringe (Fig. 4-12a, 4-12b, on page 50). This allows passage through the designated point at the push of the syringe plunger (Fig. 4-13a, 4-13b, on page 51). Prior to placement, the onlay cartilage graft is

Figure 4-11c
The JOST crusher is ideal for the controlled crushing of and contouring of medium-to-large-sized segments of cartilage.

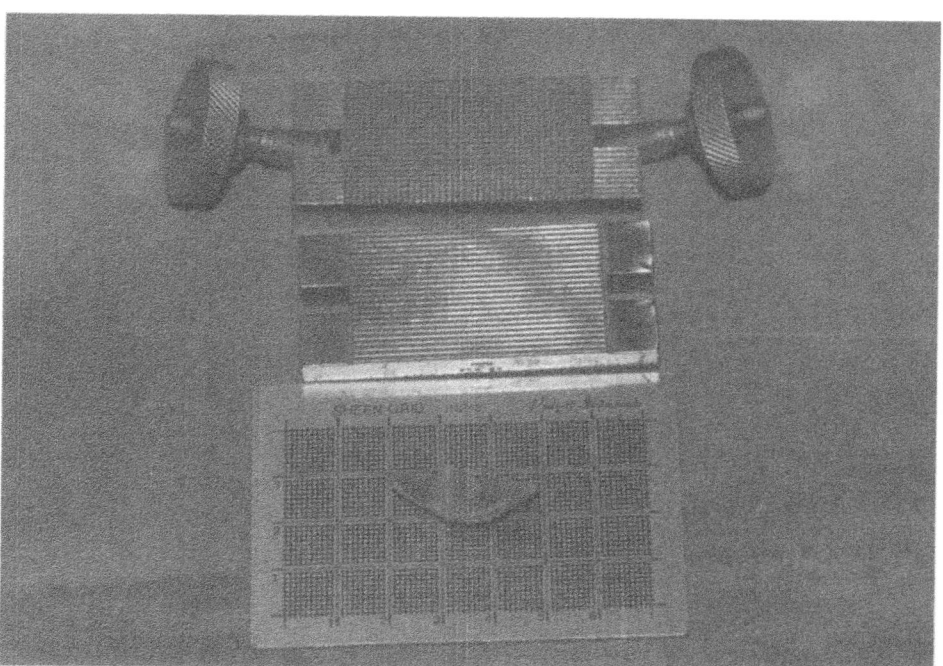

c

Figure 4-12a, 4-12b
Dorsal grafting is performed with the use of a tuberculin syringe. The reverse end of the small suture needle is pushed into the rubber plunger of the tuberculin syringe. The plunger is then pulled back so that the needle point is just within the barrel of the syringe.

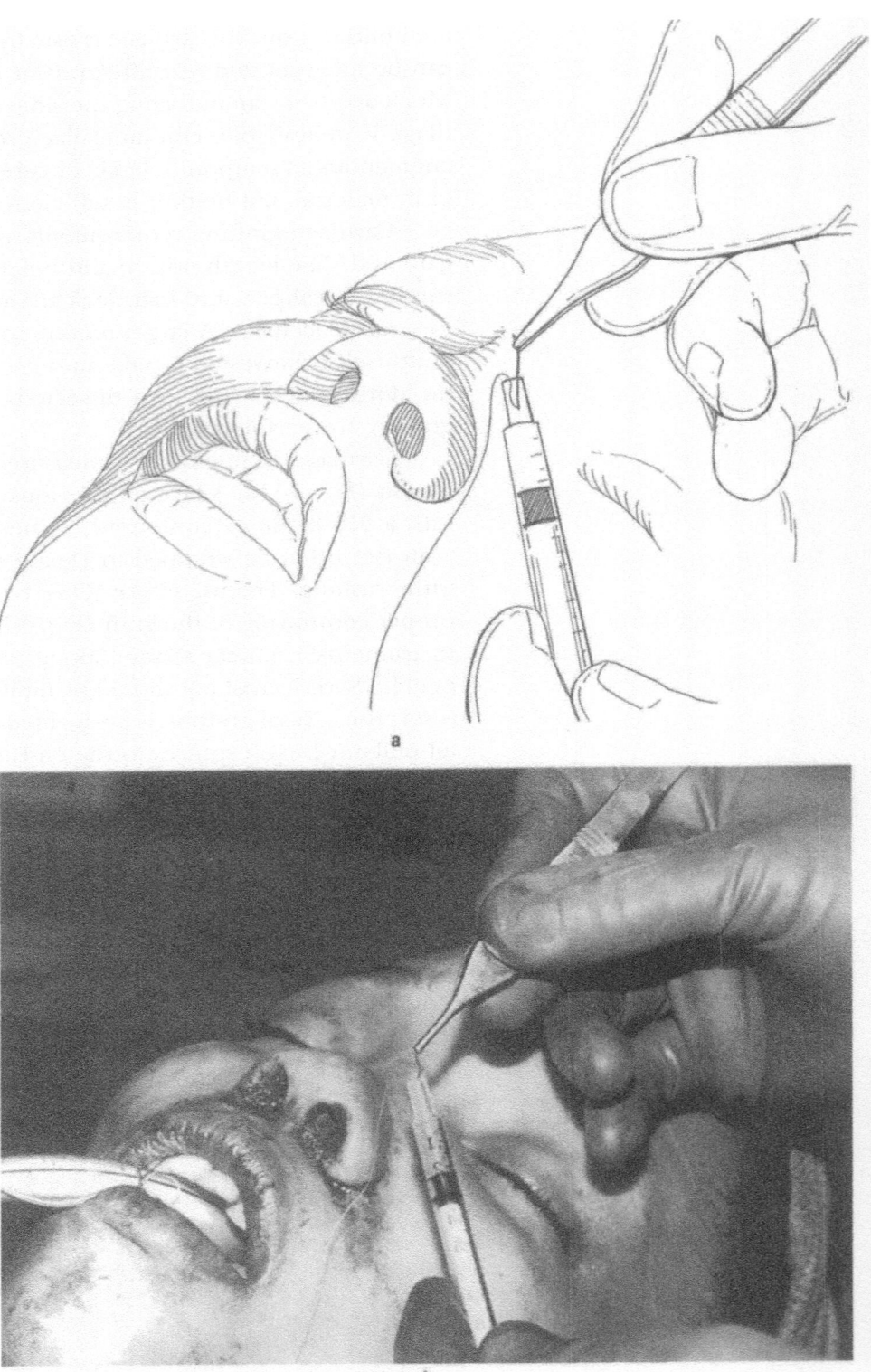

checked for size and stability. When inserted, the graft is placed between the nasal frontal angle and just short of the supratip break (Fig. 4-14a, 4-14b, on page 52). It is not extended any further because excessive fullness in this area could contribute to supratip fullness and deformity. Carrying the graft to the tip of the nose does not provide the definition that can be

Figure 4-13a, 4-13b
The smooth tip and barrel of the narrow tuberculin syringe is placed into
the dorsal pocket so it pushes against
the far end of the pocket. The plunger
is pushed and the needle is delivered
through the end of the pocket, thus
helping to stabilize the end of the graft.

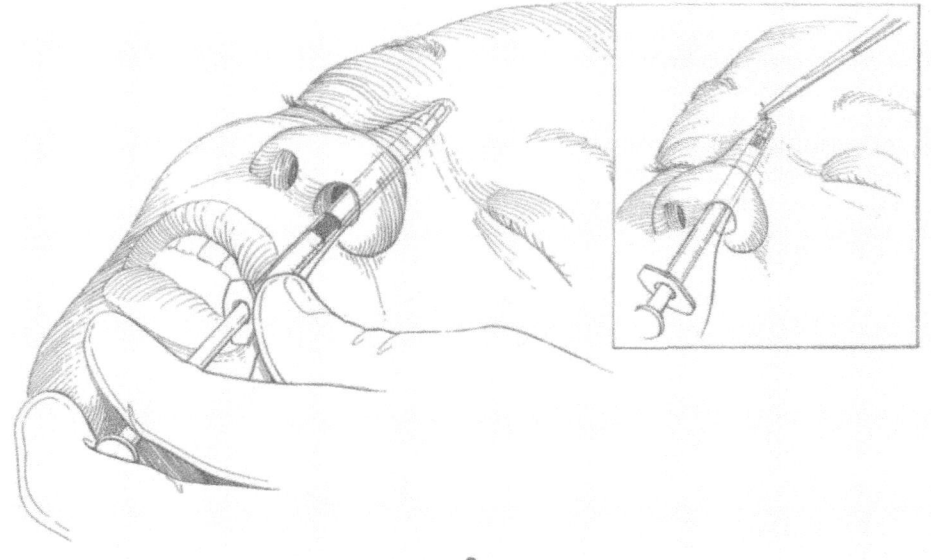

a

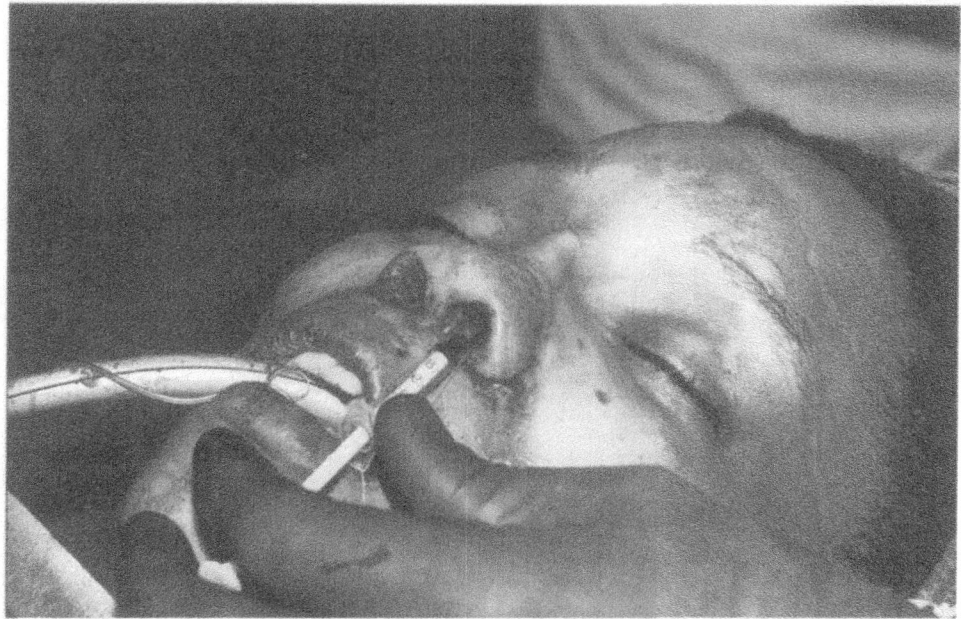

b

achieved with the use of a vertical "pea-pod" graft. A natural depression or
break behind the tip adds to definition. The absorbable skin pull-out sutures are tied at each end for precise localization and greater stability.

Bony Dorsum

Correctly judging the size, shape, and thickness of the nasal bones is key to
a successful examination of the ethnic rhinoplastic patient. Studying actual
skulls or even textbooks on the various races provides insight into the varying bone shapes and thicknesses. Blacks and Asians may have quite small
nasal bones in relationship to their soft-tissue complex, while Hispanic nasal
bones may be quite large in relationship. Intranasal cotton tip appliqués
along the external palpation, with possible use of topical local anesthesia,

Figure 4-14a, 4-14b
The cartilage graft is slowly inserted into the dorsal pocket with bayonet forceps while, at the same time, the suture is being gently pulled to remove slack. The opposite end of the graft is then similarly stabilized, and a loose French knot is tied at both ends of the graft.

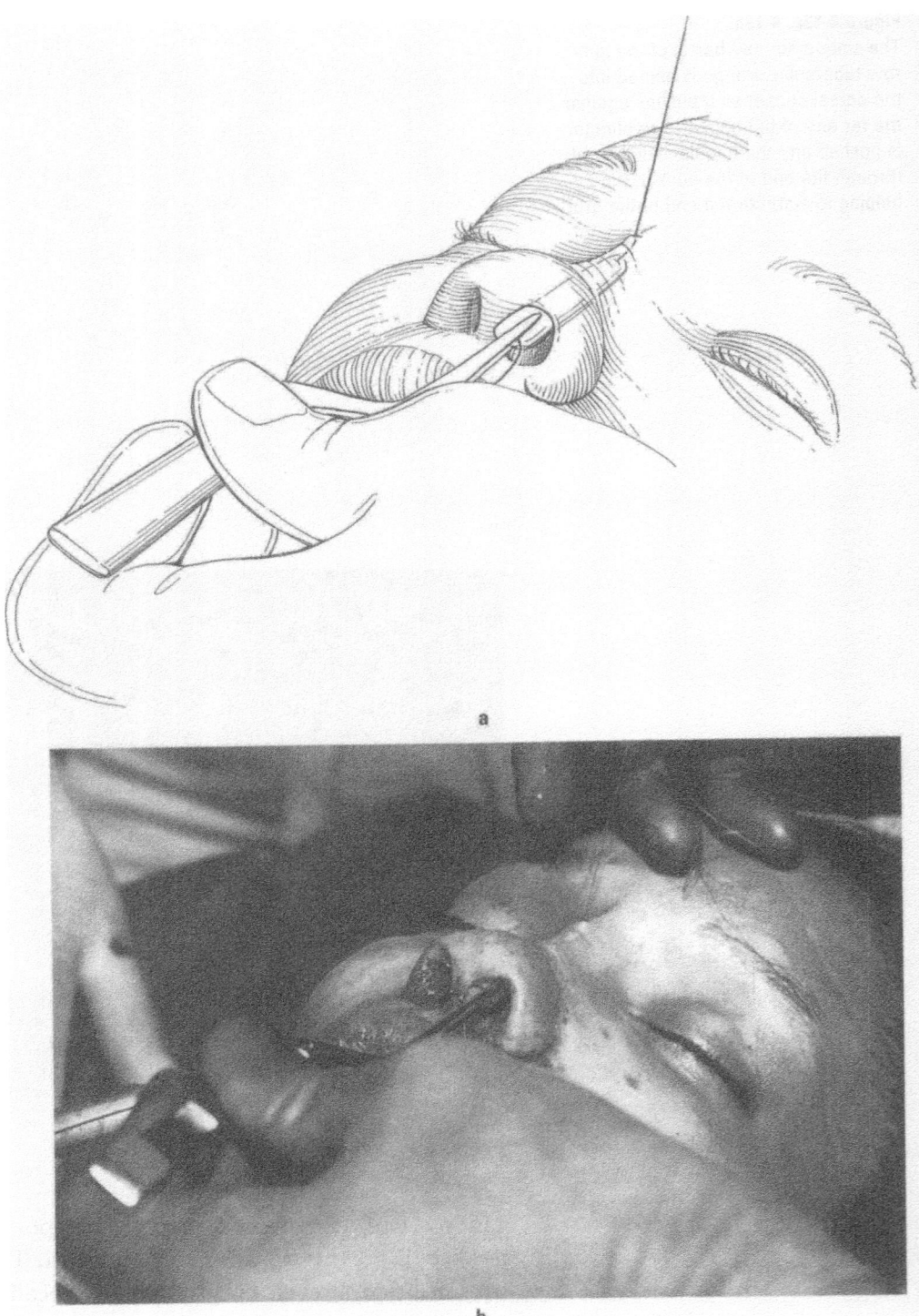

a

b

Figure 4-14c, 4-14d
The patient complained of a prominent nasal dorsum consisting of both prominent nasal bone and dorsal septal cartilage. She also had fullness of slightly asymmetrical alar cartilages. The nasal columellar angle was open. The patient underwent bony rasping and cartilage shaving of the dorsum, alar reduction, and onlay cartilage graft to the tip (the "pea-pod" was not required).

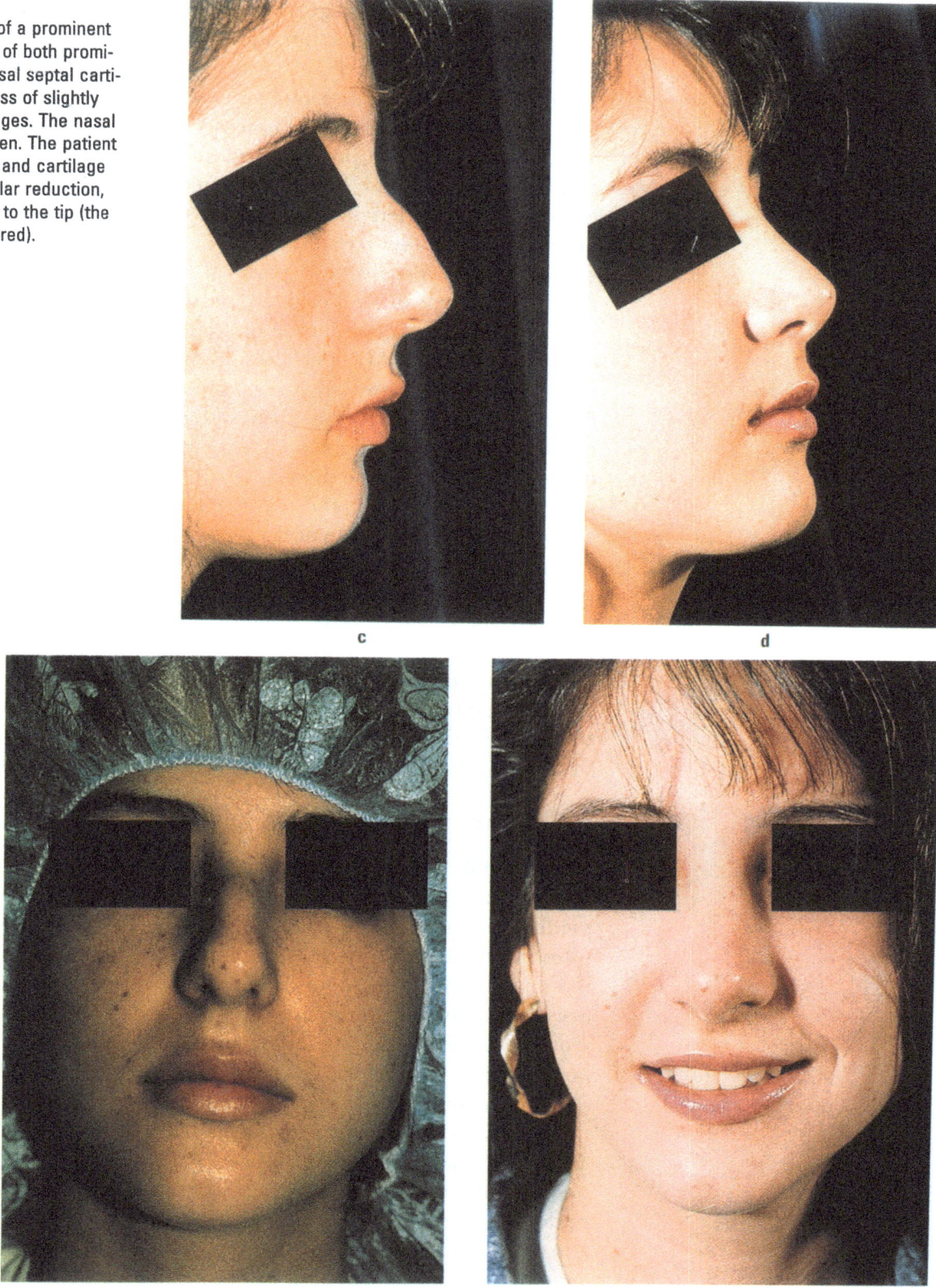

c

d

e

f

Figure 4-14e, 4-14f
On frontal preoperative view the prominent dorsum can be seen. A very sharp double-guarded osteotome can excise both cartilaginous and bony dorsum, and fine rasping and cartilage shaving with a #15 or broken #11 blade can smooth the contour. A minimal medial osteotomy was performed to close the open roof. The distal septum was not excised, to avoid excessive nasal elevation, and the depressor nasi muscle was not divided.

Dorsum

Finer rasps and/or cartilage scrapers can be useful for smooth excision of the bony-cartilaginous dorsum and other unpredictable bony callus formations. In the author's opinion, it is difficult to totally correct bony irregularities. The onlay of a thin sheet of temporalis fascia or thinly crushed cartilage may help to alleviate (at least) palpable irregularities (Fig. 4-14c, 4-14d, 4-14e, 4-14f, on previous page). Nodular scar tissue can occur, particularly when the nose is NOT irrigated and fragments of cartilage, bone, or soft tissue are left in place. Even steroid injections (such as triamcinolone) and applied pressure may not completely alleviate such irregularities. It may be necessary to perform a small open procedure utilizing a small ear curette to remove the extraneous fragments or tissue. It is very important to do a subperiosteal dissection with a Joseph or similar elevator in order to elevate ALL periosteum off the bone. A wet finger is used to determine if there are any irregularities. When irregularities are present, further rasping is performed. When the nose skin is pressed down, if there are any visible depressions or irregularities, small crushed grafts or fascia can be inserted into the area. It is very important with headlight or fiberoptic assistance to look and feel the nasal dorsum. Small irregularities in the bony area can be quite noticeable even when thick dorsal soft-tissue coverings are present. It is of utmost importance that ALL soft tissue be left in place in the nose. In the author's experience, in even the bulkiest of noses, it is extremely rare to reduce the dorsal or lateral soft tissue—with exception of the tip—particularly where abundant fibrofatty tissue is present and thinning will predictably not jeopardize the subdermal plexus. A very prominent frontal bossing may be a source of irritation, and a coronal approach to bony thinning may be considered in the unusual patient—especially burr thinning (Fig. 4-14g, 4-14h, 4-14i, 4-14j, 4-14k, 4-14l, on following pages).

Osteotomies

My personal osteotomy technique is to make a stab incision through the piriform aperture with a 2-mm osteotome. I uplift the periosteum to the medial canthal area and then hold pressure for 2 to 3 minutes. A stepwise osteotomy starting at the piriform aperture is then performed. When there is a small bony-cartilaginous hump, it is removed by rasping with headlight-assisted scalpel excision or rasping with various rasps. A double-guarded osteotome is used to remove large cartilaginous bony humps. Rasping is then performed to smooth the area down.

While some patients do not require osteotomies, the typical ethnic nose, with its low and wide nasal bones, usually necessitates infracturing. This is especially true for blacks and Asians. The balance between the alar base and the bridge width must be ascertained prior to osteotomies being performed (i.e., an exceedingly wide nasal base would not be attractive with a narrow bridge). Low nasal bones, characteristic of the ethnic nasal anatomy, necessitate that low osteotomies (not high) be performed to ob-

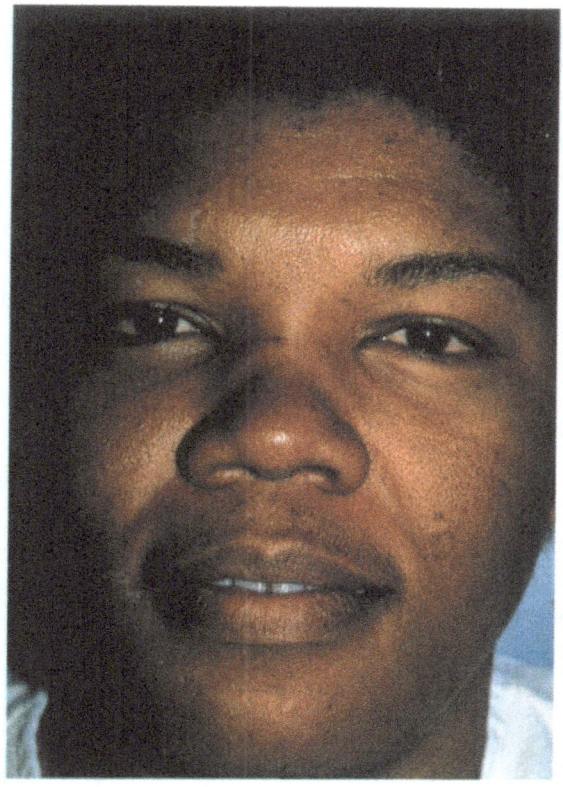

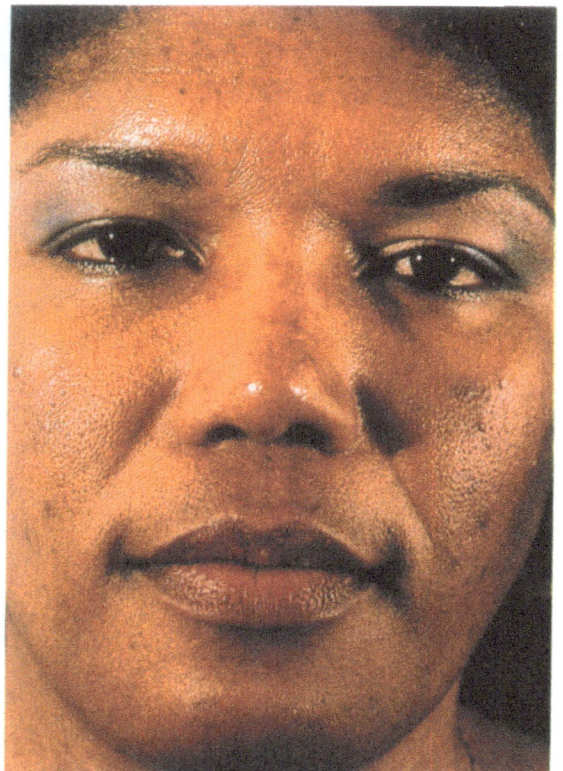

Figure 4-14g, 4-14h, 4-14i, 4-14j
Preoperatively, this patient had a moderately concave dorsum and excessive fullness of the nasal tip. A single piece of conchal cartilage, wrapped with fascia, was used to augment the dorsum, giving more dorsal elevation and balance to the nose. Both piriform aperture and medial canthal osteotomies were also performed.

g

h

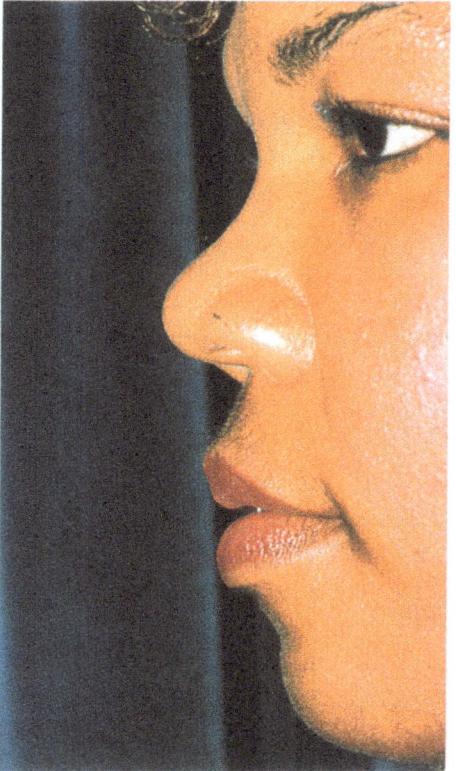

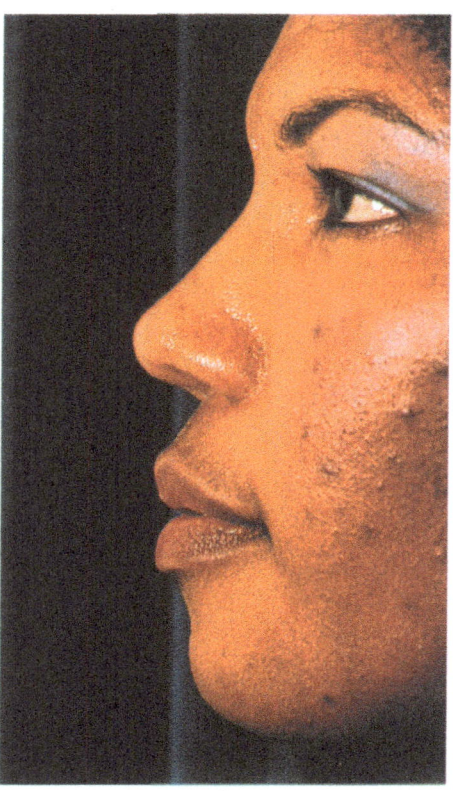

i

j

Figure 4-14k, 4-14l
When only subtle corrections are required, a single-layered septal cartilage dorsal graft can give a slight-to-moderate augmentation. Bone or Silastic grafts may be too prominent.

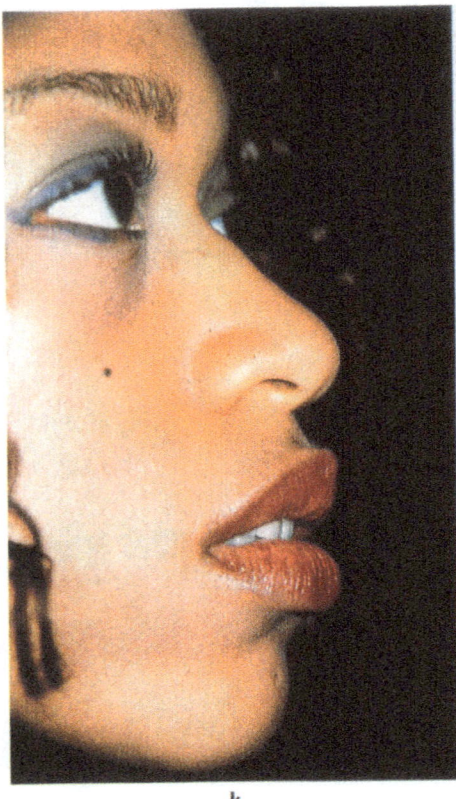
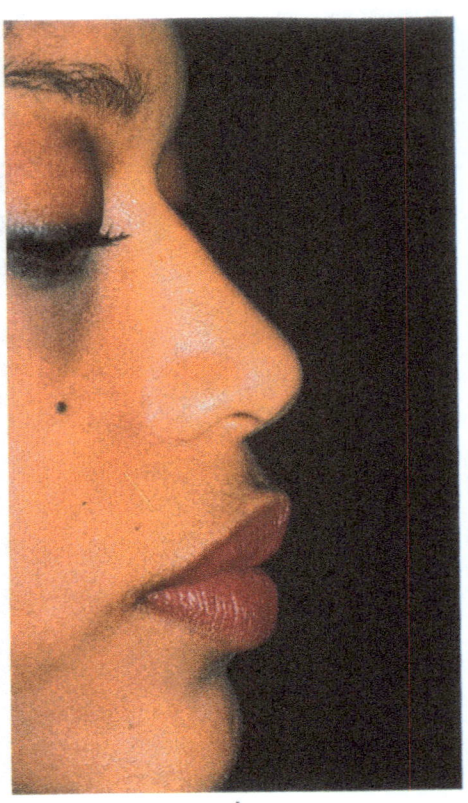

k

l

tain adequate narrowing. Osteotomies that are too high, however, can show step-offs, since the excessively wide and bony base is still maintained. Proper infracturing can likewise result in a thinner nose and the relative appearance of more projection. On the other hand, poorly performed osteotomies, or green stick fractures, often show asymmetry or irregularity of the nasal bridge sidewalls. I have had minimal difficulty with autologous dorsal grafting (bone, cartilage, fascia) in association with properly performed osteotomies.

My technique for performing osteotomies is as follows: A 2-mm osteotome can be placed through the intranasal approach and a stab wound placed into the piriform aperture intranasally (Fig. 4-15a, 4-15b, on page 57). The periosteum at the low lateral aspect of the nasal bones is elevated to the medial canthal area. Pressure is applied for 3 minutes. The thinness and delicacy of the 2-mm osteotome is advantageous in specifically placed osteotomies. These are followed, if indicated, by bilateral percutaneous osteotomies at the level of the medial canthus (Fig. 4-16a, 4-16b, on page 58). Again, a 2-mm osteotome is used. The osteotome is introduced through the very thin medial canthal skin for very precise osteotomies. This is particularly beneficial if the piriform approach appears difficult. Ethnic nasal bones may be quite small, but oftentimes they are very thick. For this reason, two different approaches help to ensure successful infracturing. These techniques have resulted in the greatest degree of accuracy in my hands. Frequently, if the dorsum is intact, there may be some difficulty in obtaining complete osteotomies and great care must be taken not to fragment the

Figure 4-15a, 4-15b

If osteotomies are indicated, a 2-mm osteotome is punched through the piriform aperture. The periosteum is then elevated with a Freer elevator, and stepwise low nasal bone osteotomies are performed bilaterally.

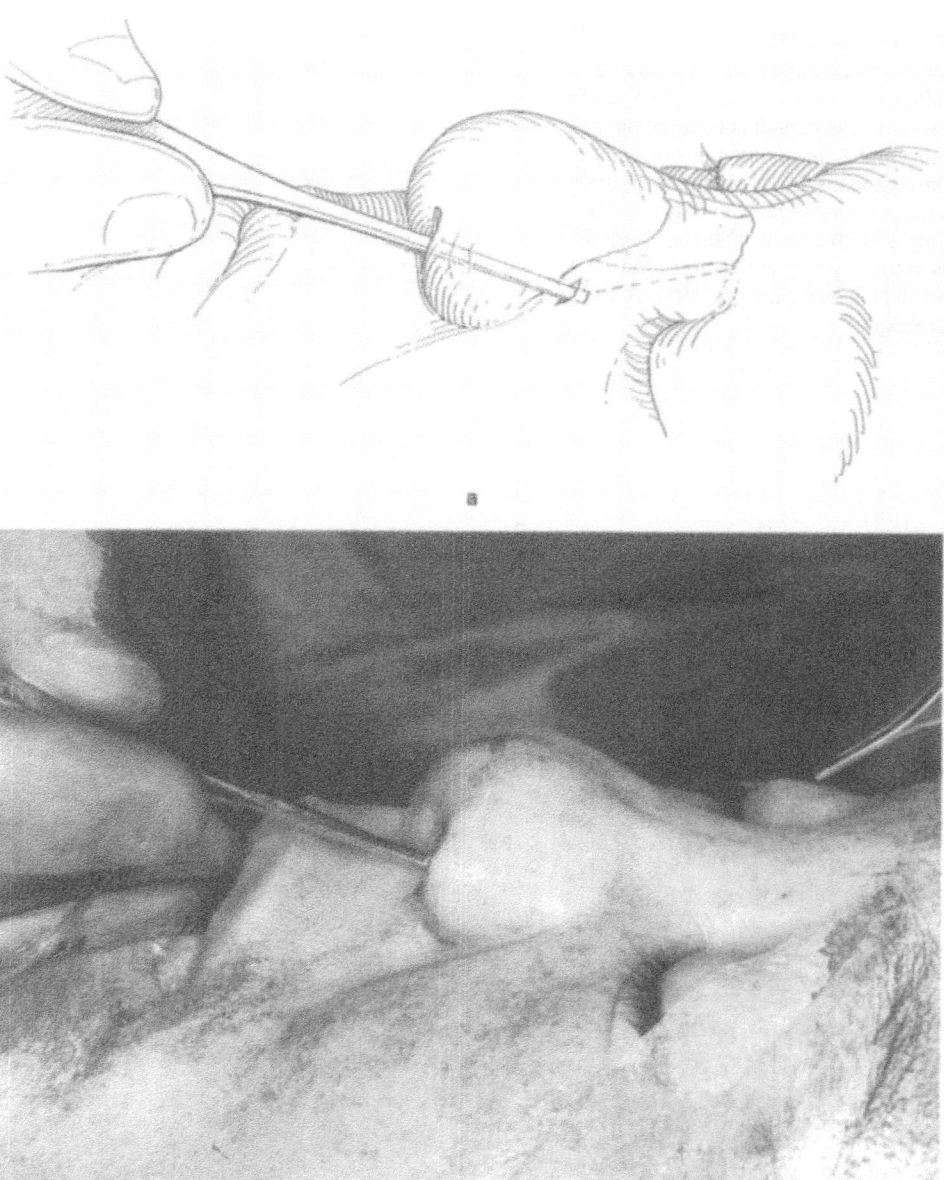

a

b

bones. A standard 2-mm osteotome can easily pinpoint-fracture the bony side walls at the correct level, leaving the nasal mucosa intact, while a single-guarded osteotome, when not placed correctly, can tear the medial bony periosteal and mucosal lining. The resultant loss of mucosal continuity can lead to excessive bleeding, bruising, and delayed healing. Routinely, osteotomies are followed by applying digital pressure to the nasal bones to reduce them medially (Fig. 4-17a, 4-17b, on page 59). Bimanual palpation can also be used to determine any areas of irregularity or subtotal reduction. Five minutes, or the patient's bleeding time equivalent, of digital pressure substantially helps decrease bruising and swelling after osteotomies. In addition, injecting the turbinates with an epinephrine-containing local anesthetic and dilute steroids prior to performing osteotomies helps decrease bruising and swelling postoperatively.

Figure 4-16a, 4-16b
Where nasal bone reduction may be difficult, an additional osteotomy site is chosen. This patient is undergoing medial canthal infracturing by means of a percutaneous 2-mm osteotome. A stab wound at the medial canthus is made with a #15 blade. Noticeable scarring is extremely rare in this area. The small puncture sites are left open for drainage.

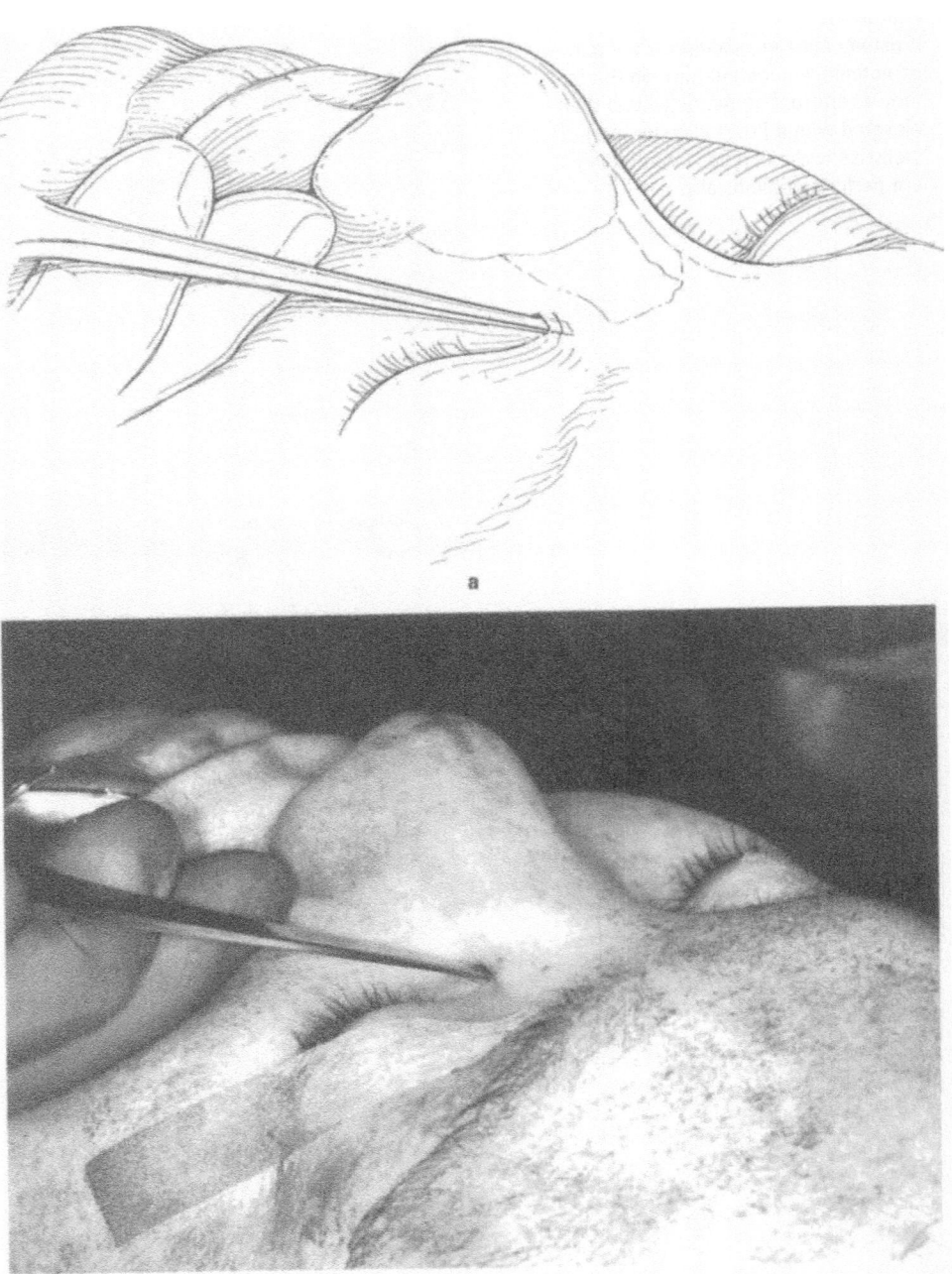

This 24-year-old Hispanic female desired a more defined attractive nose (Fig. 4-17c, 4-17d, 4-17e, 4-17f, on page 60). Examination revealed a depressed nasion, full wide nasal bridge, prominent osteocartilaginous hump, wide alae, nondefined nasal tip, and hanging columella. She had airway obstruction with a deviated left nasal septum and bulky turbinates. The patient's nasal tip became ptotic when she smiled, caused by the depressor nasaii muscle.

The preoperative surgical plan was as follows:

1. A limited septal excision and anterior turbinate reduction to improve the nasal airway was planned.

Figure 4-17a, 4-17b
After osteotomies are performed, digital thumb reduction of the nasal bones can assist in symmetrical medial reduction. Dorsal grafting and limited osteotomies can often be performed at the same time.

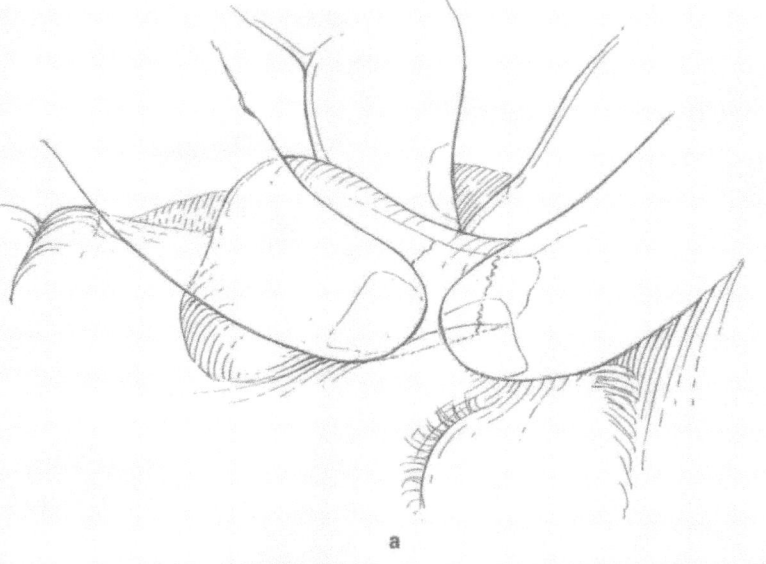

a

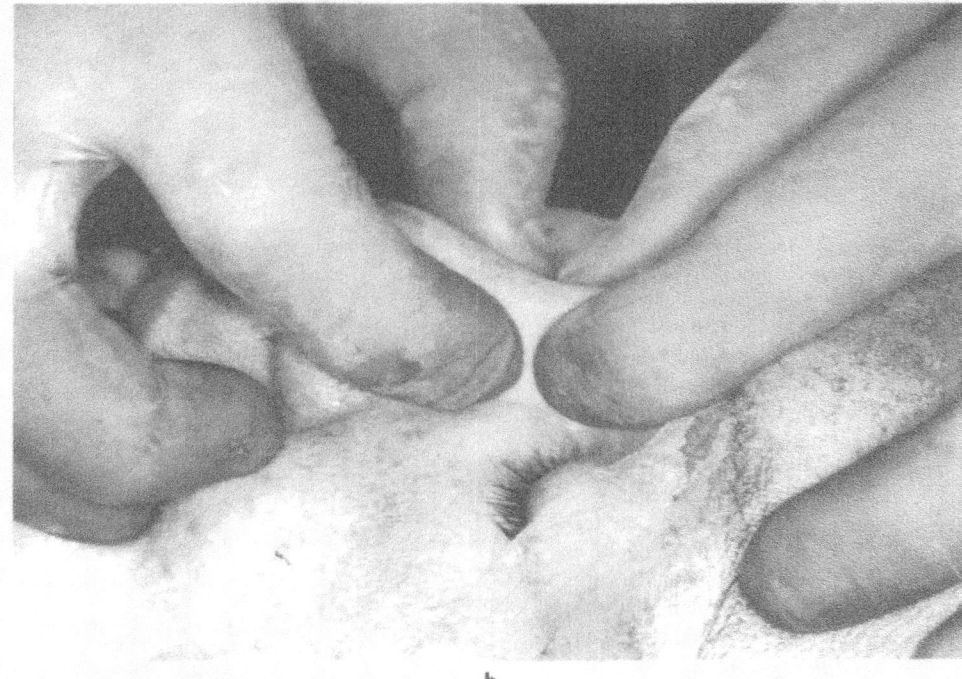

b

2. Since the patient desired more nasal definition and a well-supported tip, a sizable "pea-pod" tip graft would be implanted.

3. Auricular cartilage of the left ear would be used (the patient used her right ear talking on the phone for several hours of the day).

4. The dorsal bony-cartilaginous hump would be excised with a double-guarded osteotome and rasped smooth.

5. Piriform aperture osteotomies would be performed. As the alar cartilages were thought to be quite flimsy, no alar reductions would be performed, but the depressor nasaii muscle release would be performed.

6. Crushed cartilage would be used to fill in the nasion depression.

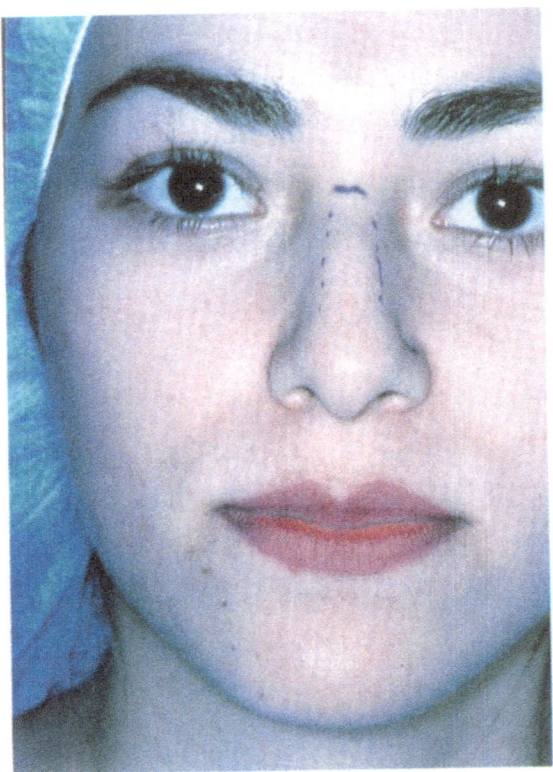

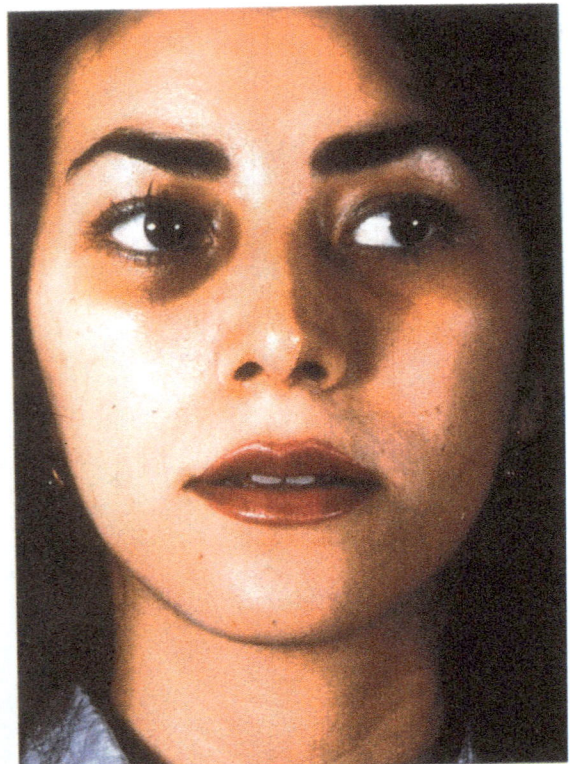

c

d

Figure 4-17c, 4-17d, 4-17e, 4-17f

This patient was concerned about the preoperatively depressed nasion and prominent nasal bridge and width of the alae and tip. She desired a straight dorsum. A double-guarded osteotome excised the bony-cartilaginous hump, and fine rasping and fine cartilage scraping were then performed. The skin was quite thin and a very thin layer of temporalis fascia was used to cover the area to avoid any palpable irregularities. Medial osteotomies were performed. Alae were reduced and alar cartilage thinned. No tip graft was necessary. Preoperative and measurement markings may be of benefit when determining the amount of bony dorsum to excise. A crushed cartilage nasion graft was inserted. The bony dorsum was slightly reduced and the alae were reduced. The osteotomies were performed to close the roof after excision of the dorsal hump. Onlay maxillary grafts of cartilage were used over the anterior maxilla. It may often be of benefit to use the patient's autogenous bony-cartilaginous tissue to augment the anterior maxillary wall or nasal spine when necessary.

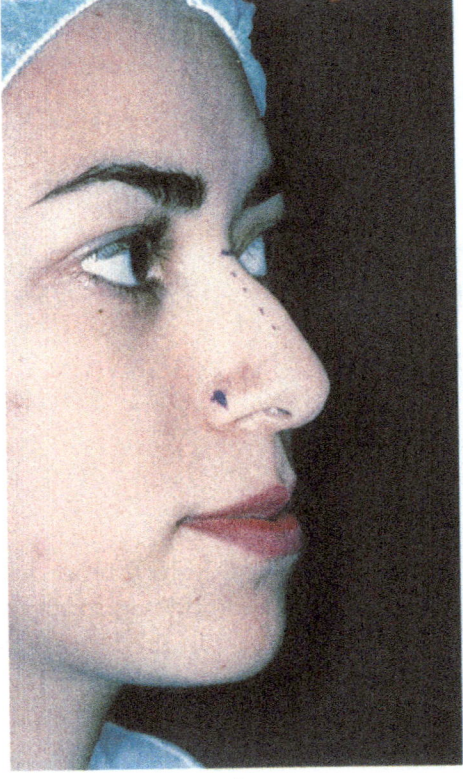

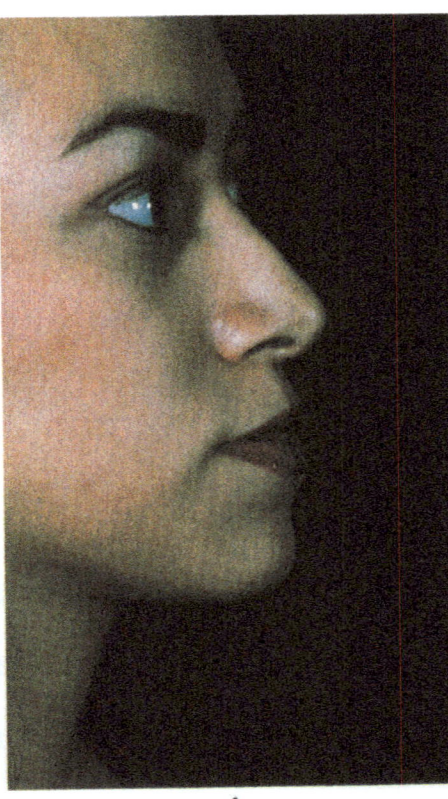

e

f

Operative Procedure

1. A general anesthetic was administered. Eight milligrams of intravenous Decadron and 25 mg of intravenous diphenhydramine hydrochloride (Benadryl) with 1 g of cephalosporin was administered.
2. Rim incisions were made and a dorsal skeletonization performed. The hump was removed with a double-guarded osteotome.
3. Through the alar incision line, a piriform stab incision was made with a 2-mm osteotome.
4. The periosteum was elevated with a Freer.
5. The junction between the nasal bones and maxilla was determined and stepwise osteotomies were performed from piriform junction to medial canthal area. (When there is difficulty at the frontal nasal bone junction, a medial canthal stab with a 2-mm osteotome can be performed and stepwise horizontal osteotomies performed. This is rarely necessary.)
6. Digital pressure was utilized to fracture the nasal bones medially.
7. Although dorsal osteotomies and/or dorsal rasping are performed prior to the osteotomies, it may be necessary with wet-finger palpation to determine any irregularities after the osteotomies. Further rasping is then performed.
8. Digital pressure is utilized for at least 5 minutes to decrease bruising and swelling.
9. I have not found intraoral or intranasal single-guarded osteotomes to be of benefit. The stepwise 2-mm osteotome excision has been much more controlled and exact through the piriform aperture.
10. Firm intranasal packing before osteotomies reduces turbinate swelling which can otherwise occur due to bleeding into turbinate soft tissue.
11. Tretinoin (Retin-A) and 4% hydroquinone cream (Eldoquin Forte) were used around the alar incision sites to decrease pigmentation and improve healing. Due to slight hyperpigmentation, the patient continued tretinoin (Retin-A) for some months.

Postoperative Comments

The patient had a hump removed and conservative narrowing of the nose. The projection and definition are improved. The osteotomies resulted in more balance to the frontal nasal appearance. Not performing infracturing would have resulted in a very flat dorsal or open-roof deformity. I specifically discussed the desire for or against a narrower nose with the patient.

Nasion Grafting

Nasion grafting in noses where the graft requirements are especially sizable and the skin is thin can be a challenge when cartilage is being used. Even when the cartilage is crushed and the graft is perfectly positioned, visualization and palpation of the graft are potential problems. I have found that temporalis fascia or mastoid fascia often provide good augmentation with proper contour, but without palpable or visible edges.

Alar and Nasal Base Reduction

Correcting large, thick, and/or asymmetric alar bases with attendant nostril flaring can represent a formidable challenge to the rhinoplastic surgeon. It can be difficult to create a desirable aesthetic shape with normal alar and alar base contours. Overreduction, which can be exacerbated by later retraction, must be avoided. Scarring must be kept to a minimum. To complicate matters further, a hypoplastic nasal spine and maxilla may require augmentation, while a thickened columella and/or alar wall may demand narrowing.

As previously mentioned, nostril shape usually falls into one of three categories: (1) central-round, (2) medial horizontal-oblique, or (3) lateral horizontal-oblique. The ideal nostril contour tends to be pear-shaped with a medial vertical-oblique orientation, occupying approximately two-thirds of the distance from the subnasale to the tip-defining points. The remaining one-third consists of the infratip lobule. Tip grafting in conjunction with alar reduction helps to reorient the nostrils into this more vertical position.

Figure 4-18a, 4-18b
Alar base reduction is performed with a wide curvilinear incision usually located approximately 1 mm above the alar crease in order to provide a small rim for proper alar suturing. A natural curve that sweeps the sill floor will provide a more natural appearance than squaring-off the incision and creating a notch.

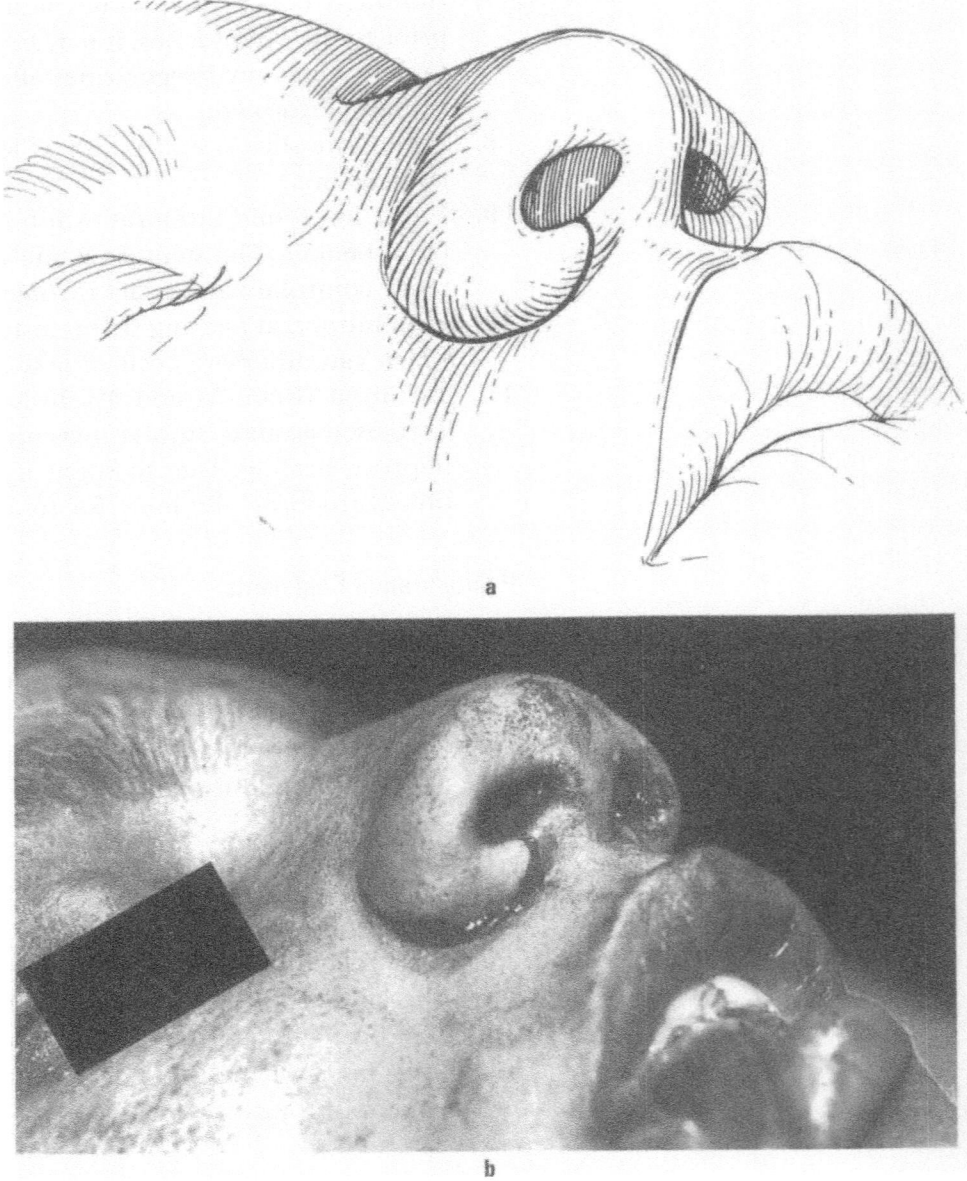

a

b

Before interrupting the alae, the alar cartilages are reduced, and the fibrofatty tissue is removed. That allows accurate and symmetrical adjustments of the alae and nasal base.

Cartilage-splitting or retrograde eversion techniques do not secure good release of the nasal tip in ethnic patients. Both cartilage-splitting and retrograde eversion techniques leave tissue attachments medially in the alar roof, which may result in retractions when a highly projecting tip graft is placed. Complete bipedicle alar cartilage exposure is necessary to release these attachments to the alar cartilage and allow for more definition and projection for the "pea-pod" graft. In addition, trimming the alar cartilages is best done under direct vision to ensure that they are not overresected, which could lead to subsequent retraction and buckling.

My preferred technique for alar reduction begins with a full-thickness incision made approximately less than a millimeter above the alar crease, parallel to the cheek skin (Fig. 4-18a, 4-18b, on previous page). In thick-

Figure 4-19a, 4-19b
Symmetrical markings of the width of the alar base, using calipers, are performed prior to actual excision. It is recommended that less than the full amount is excised and a trial closure of a deep, buried suture performed to ascertain the degree of desired correction. Overreduction is extremely difficult to correct, where underreduction is usually easily correctable.

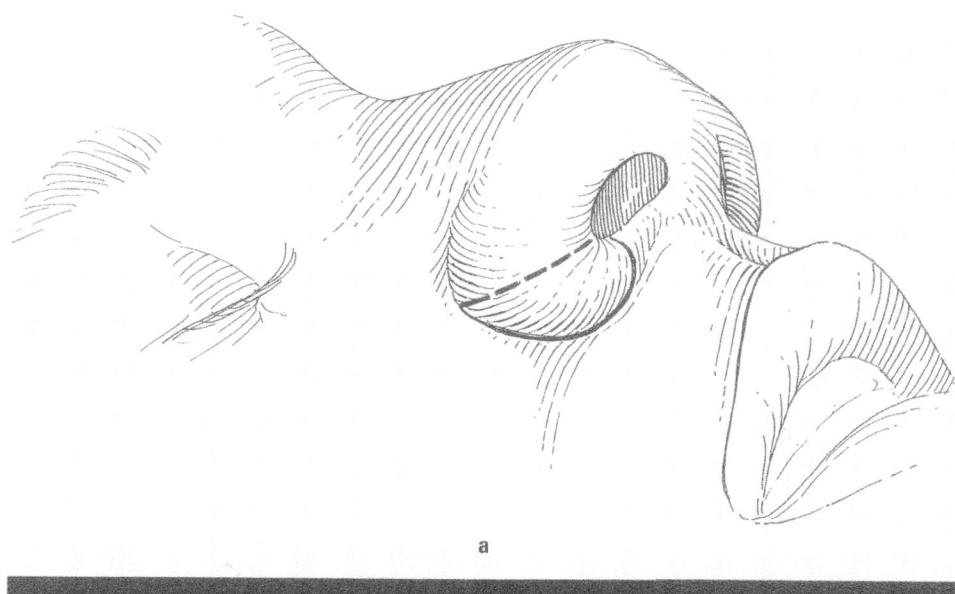

a

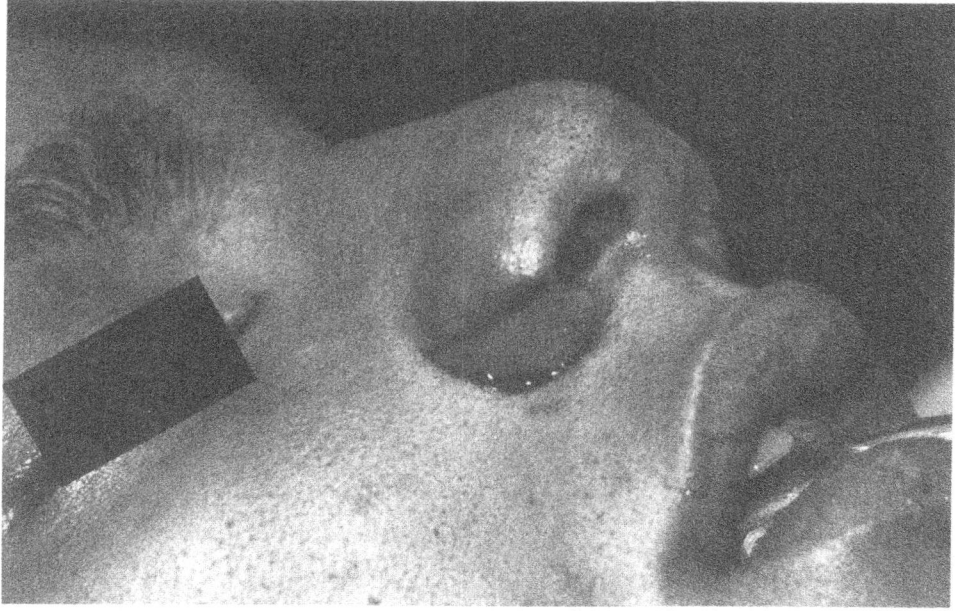

b

Figure 4-20a, 4-20b

A full-thickness angled excision of alar tissue is performed in the alar wall. The angulation of the blade at the alar base will determine the degree of bulk. Leaving a concave dissection will decrease the bulk, whereas a concave dissection leaving more internal soft tissue will add to the bulk. Not infrequently, an internal excision of further soft tissue can be performed to decrease the width. Care must be taken to do this symmetrically and to leave as much thickness underneath the dermis as possible in order to decrease dimpling and irregularity.

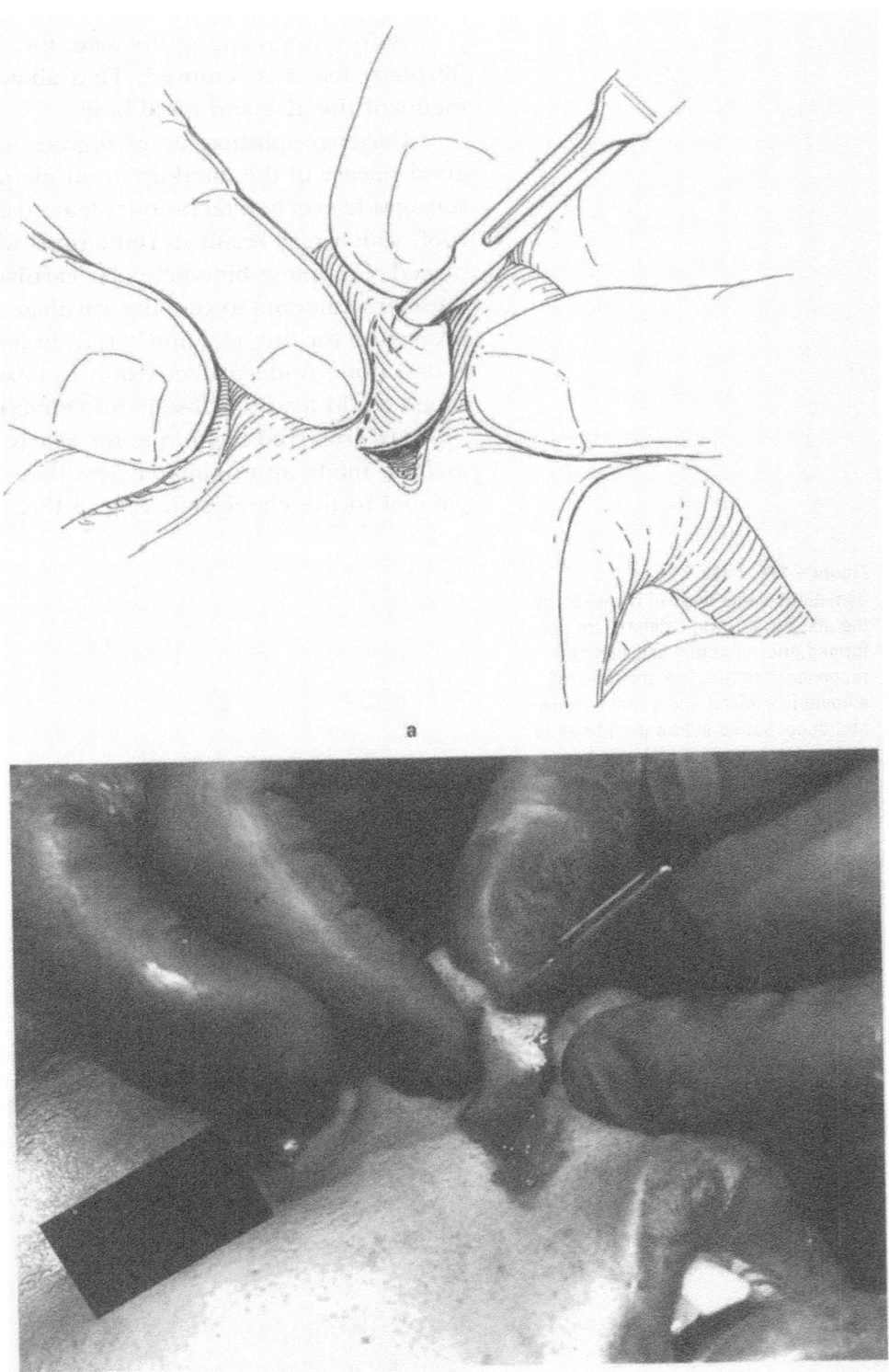

a

b

skinned patients with large pores, an incision less than a millimeter above the alar crease allows for easier closure. After the amount to be resected has been determined, a curvilinear excision-line is marked for accuracy in the alar side wall (Fig. 4-19a, 4-19b, on page 63). With the excess amount determined, a second full-thickness "angled" incision is made and the intervening segment is excised (Fig. 4-20a, 4-20b). The incision is angled to

Figure 4-21a, 4-21b
The central core is exposed for any additional soft-tissue removal. It is not necessary to resect the skin superior to the base. Hemostasis is performed.

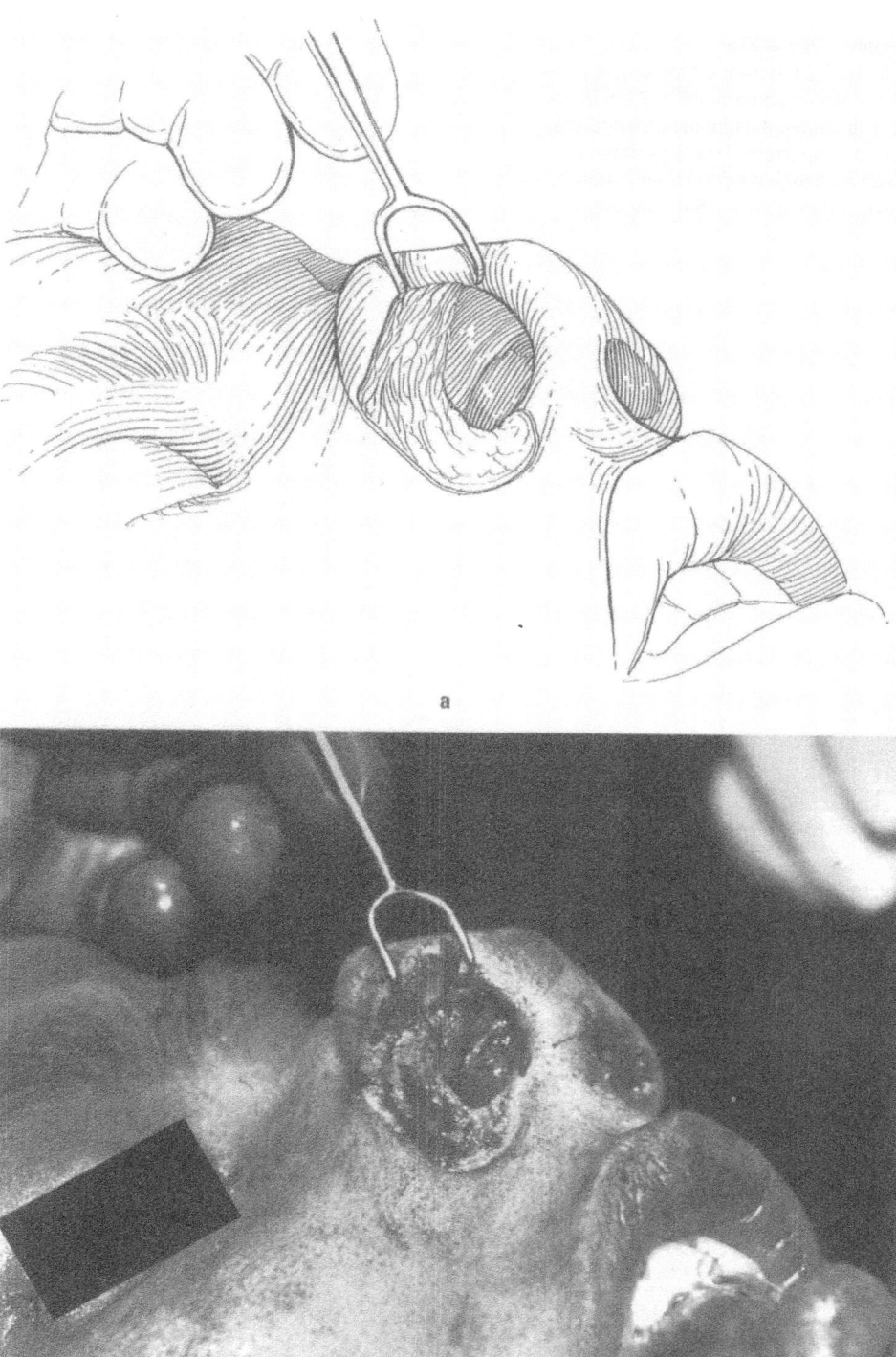

a

b

leave more soft tissue laterally at the alar base, resulting in a more normal contour. Less tissue is removed medially (mucosa) than laterally (skin). Remember that the initial excision should be somewhat smaller than desired, and great care should be taken to not overresect the alae. If the area is overresected, it is often uncorrectable. After a full-thickness alar excision has been completed, the central core of excessive alar soft tissue can be excised (Fig. 4-21a, 4-21b). It is not necessary to resect the skin superior to the base.

Figure 4-22a, 4-22b
The residual defect on the cheek-maxillary skin is undermined 1–2 cm in order to allow advancement toward the piriform aperture. This is performed with an adequate dermal lip that allows suturing with a 5-0 PDS suture.

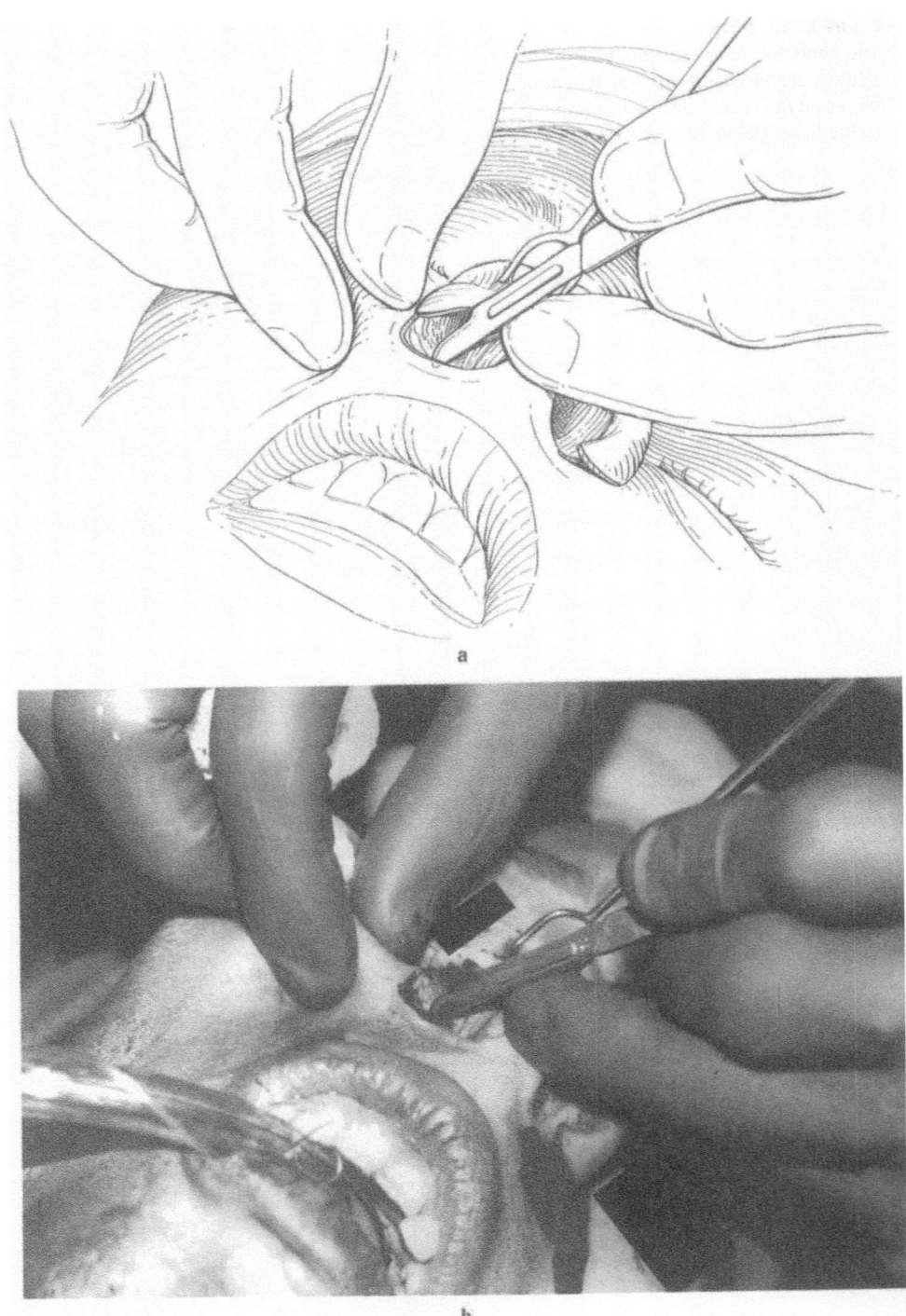

a

b

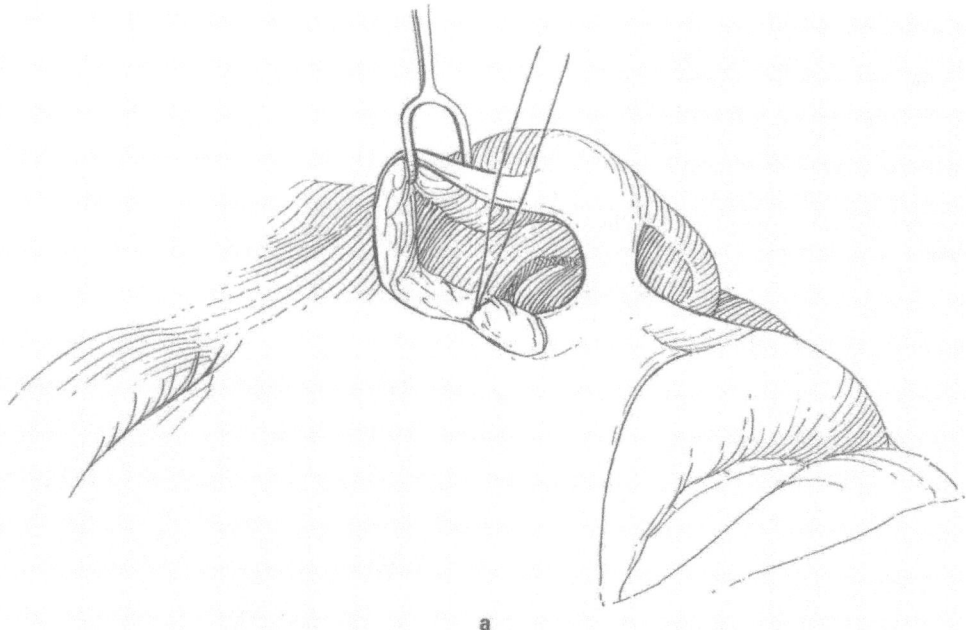

a

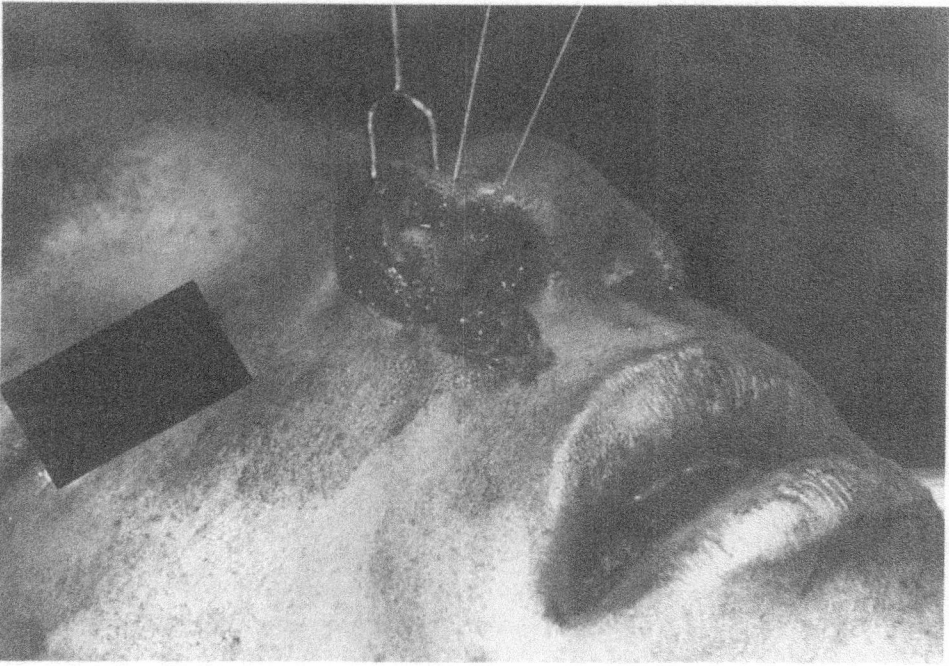

b

A #15 blade is used to undermine the skin lateral to the alar base a minimum of 1 to 2 cm onto the cheek (Fig. 4-22a, 4-22b, on previous page). The cheek and lateral alar base are advanced medially toward the vestibule and sutured to the soft tissue and/or periosteum of the vestibular segment with 5-0 PDS suture, solidly anchoring the alar base into position (Fig. 4-23a, 4-23b). This both narrows and medially advances a wide base. PDS suture is preferred because it lasts approximately 6 weeks, which is enough time to allow good tissue stabilization to occur. The use of 5-0 nylon suture is also acceptable, but nylon can extrude, leading to tract formation or becoming palpable with overlying fibrosis. Dexon and catgut sutures are not

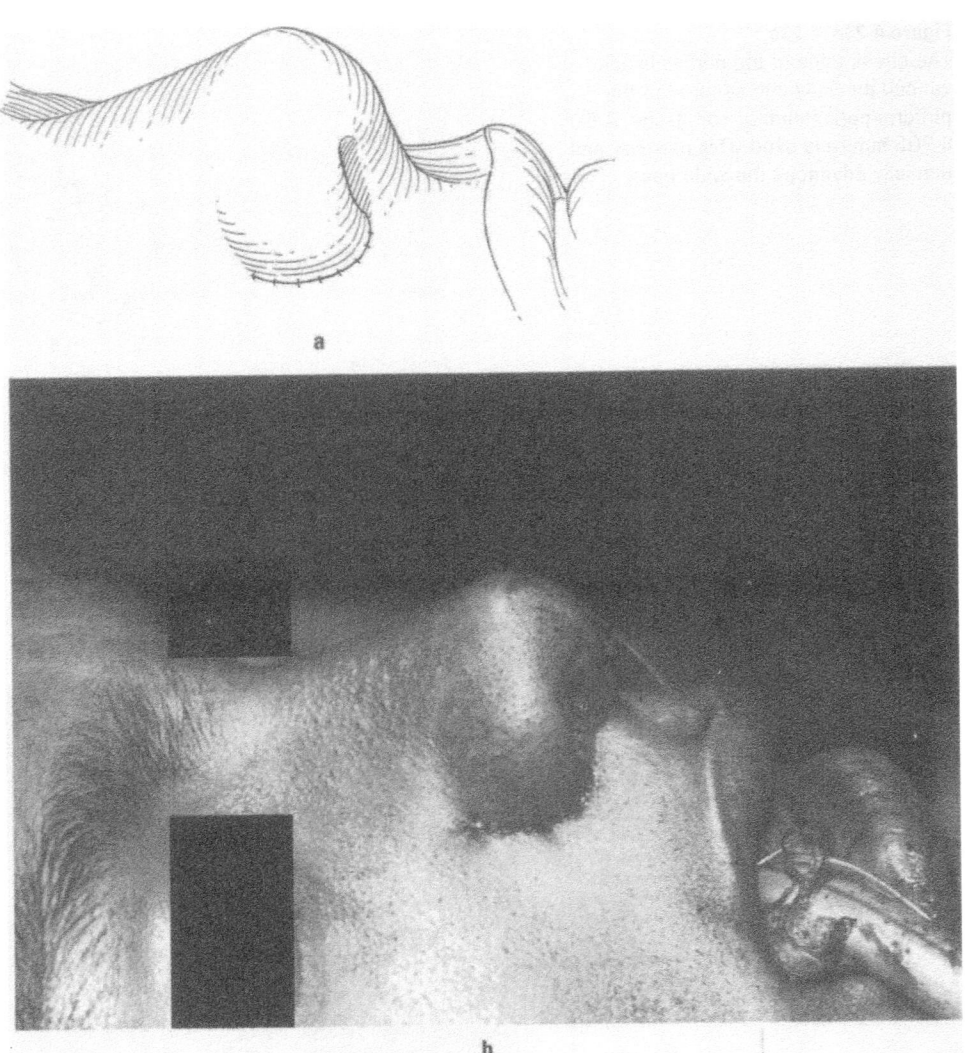

recommended because of their propensity for local reaction and extrusion. Dexon and catgut sutures also do not maintain enough tensile strength to offset the lateral pull of facial musculature and its widening effect on the alar crease incision. Medial advancement of the alar base helps not only to decrease the tension on the repair but also to eliminate the telltale flat, wide, triangular-shaped alae that are seen all too often. If the cheek skin is not advanced medially, the alar base will result in a lateralized and flattened appearance. (See chapter 7: "Risks, Complications and Revisions".) A standard closure is performed. Medial advancement of the tip of the alar soft tissue is accomplished by suturing the alae to the periosteum near the piriform aperture, using one or two deep sutures. The skin is then carefully closed with either interrupted or a continuous 6-0 nylon suture (Fig. 4-24a, 4-24b). I have found that vertical alar floor excisions or transalar cinching sutures result in either an abnormal alar configuration or in eventual spreading with loss of correction. A thickened columella can be narrowed through an incision in the membranous columella. The cartilaginous medial crural footplates are reduced and the area is conservatively defatted. The incision is carefully closed with mattress sutures.

While alar crease incisions have been frowned on by some because of the potential for widened scarring that may result from the lateral pull of the facial musculature, deep PDS stitches prevent that problem. Alar crease incisions are absolutely essential to narrow the base and to alleviate tension at the skin closure site. In some patients, the alar excision sites may be prone to hypertrophic keloid formation, although I have rarely encountered it. There appears to be a "safe triangle" from lateral canthus to nasal base to lateral canthus that is relatively immune to keloid formation. We have had no cases of true keloids. However, hyperpigmentation has been problematic. There is some evidence that pretreating the surgical sites for 2 to 4 weeks with daily tretinoin (Retin-A) 5% cream at night and hydroquinone 4% in the morning decreases postoperative inflammation and pigmentation.

Alar sutures are removed in 5 to 7 days, depending on the amount of tension. Patients with thick skin and enlarged pores tend to develop epithelialized tracts, and therefore the sutures should be removed earlier. In those patients, a subcuticular closure is ideal. Once the sutures are removed, Steri-Strip support can be used for a few days. Unacceptable scars or asymmetries should not be revised for 6 to 12 months.

Alar Resection

Preoperative planning of alar resections is paramount. The curvature of the incision and the degree, size, and volume of resection are all preplanned. This is especially true when asymmetries are present and the injection of local anesthetic may distort the tissues. Calipers, permanent marking pen, and three-dimensional multiangled visualization markings are critical to the planned surgical procedure/s. In the author's opinion, following step-by-step procedures is important—including even temporary partial closures and visualization before further resection is advisable. Excessive resections are extremely hard (if not impossible) to correct.

Significant reductions of very wide alae, which bring in the alar base medially, can result in notching of the roof of the alar nasal orifice. Such notching may be prevented by relaxing incisions in the cartilage and the addition of overlay cartilage grafts. When notching is seen postoperatively, a small revision procedure can be carried out after a few months.

Maxillary and Nasal Base Augmentation

Craniofacial and orthogenetic evaluation techniques have highlighted the importance of maxillary retrusion when assessing the rhinoplasty patient. Due to the frequently greater maxillary retrusion in ethnic patients (especially of African and Asian descent), maxillary retrusion needs special consideration to achieve an improved result. It is the author's opinion that augmentation is frequently of benefit and should be discussed with the patient. Alloplastic materials, although initially appearing quite successful, have proven to be very susceptible to extrusion, infection, and palpability problems over time. The author prefers the simplest materials, such as sep-

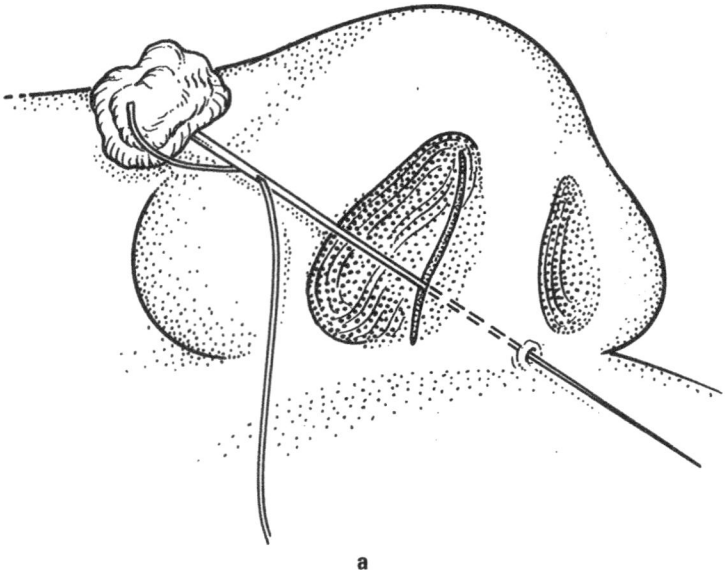

a

tal tissue, auricular cartilage, rolled mersilene, and possibly temporalis fascia.

During facelift procedures, fascia from the postauricular area and even fat injections may be of benefit, but a pocket must be developed which is free of excessive bleeding. Starting the dissection prior to the rhinoplastic procedure, a very light packing may allow time for assured hemostasis. Placement of the graft should be exact, frequently secured with sutures.

Minor degrees of retrusion without associated dental or masticatory abnormalities may require only onlay augmentation with crushed cartilage, cranial bone, or synthetic mesh. More severe retrusions, particularly those with dental abnormalities, may require formal maxillary advancement procedures. There are many forme fruste facial abnormalities that may require formal evaluation and cephalometric measurements.

Nasal base augmentation, alone or in combination with maxillary augmentation, may be necessary. The nasal base and/or maxilla are augmented with onlay auricular cartilage grafts or rolled mersilene mesh when indicated (Fig. 4-25a). It has been my experience in thick noses, however, that nasal base augmentation does not significantly improve nasal tip projection, even with large grafts (Fig. 4-25b, 4-25c, 4-25d, 4-25e, 4-25f, 4-25g, 4-25h, 4-25i, 4-25j, 4-25k).

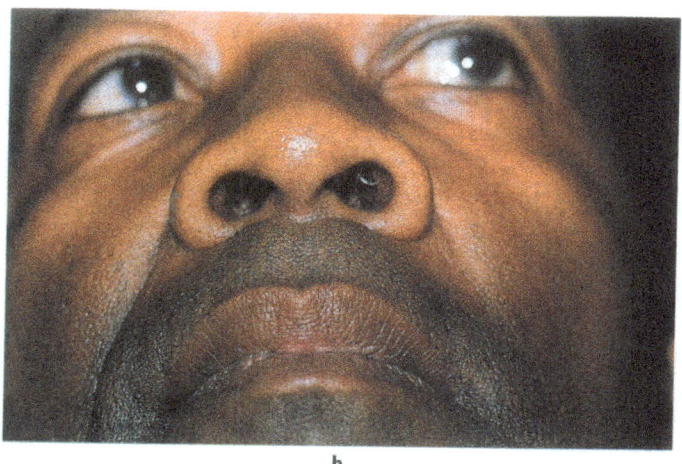

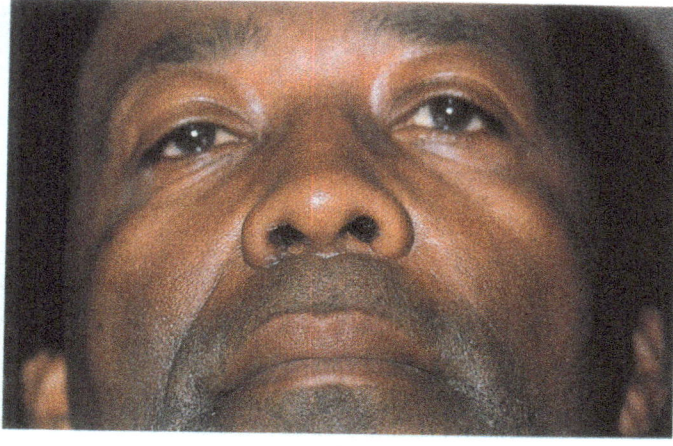

Figure 4-25b, 4-25c
Lateralized excessive alar fullness was reduced with a 1-cm excision at the alar base. The alar base was undermined and advanced medially. Again, without the advancement the lateral wall would be flattened and laterally retracted. It is also essential to maintain a natural, curved contour to the alae.

Figure 4-25d, 4-25e
This patient had minor excision of the alar base and medial advancement of the cheek skin. The alar flaring was corrected and the shape of the nostrils modified. The use of an ultrasupportive tip graft was also of paramount importance in obtaining the postoperative result.

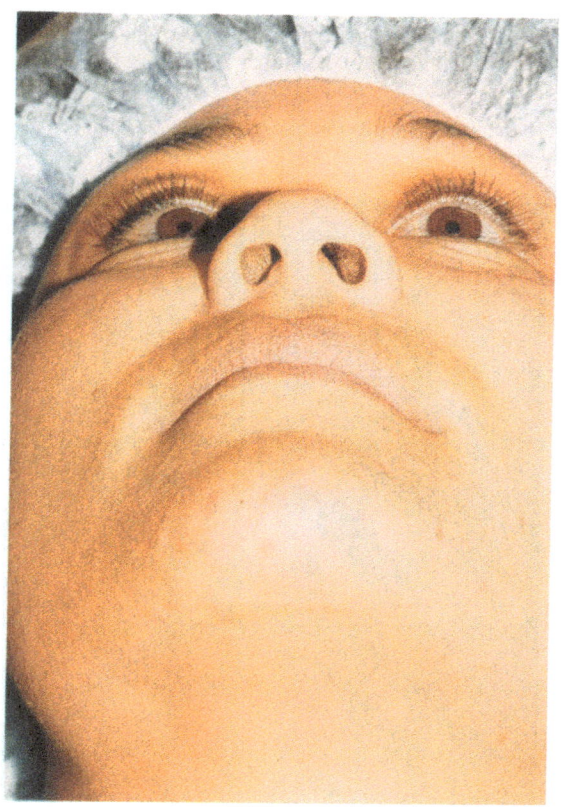

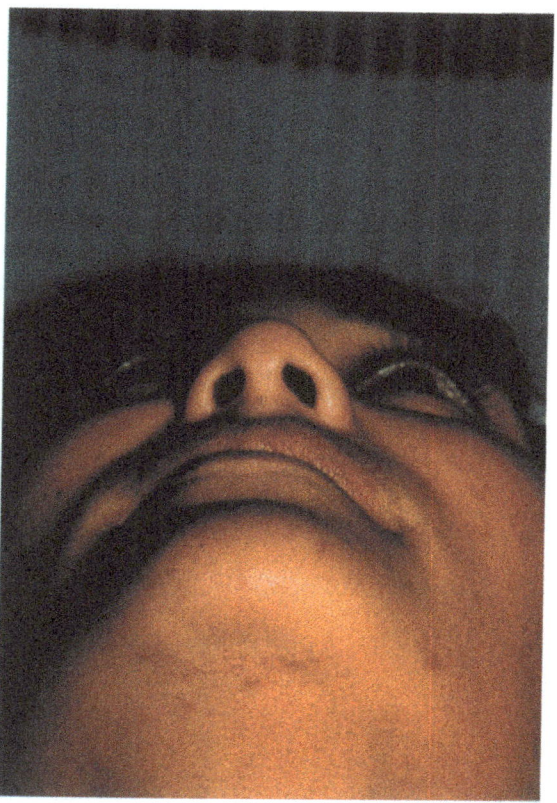

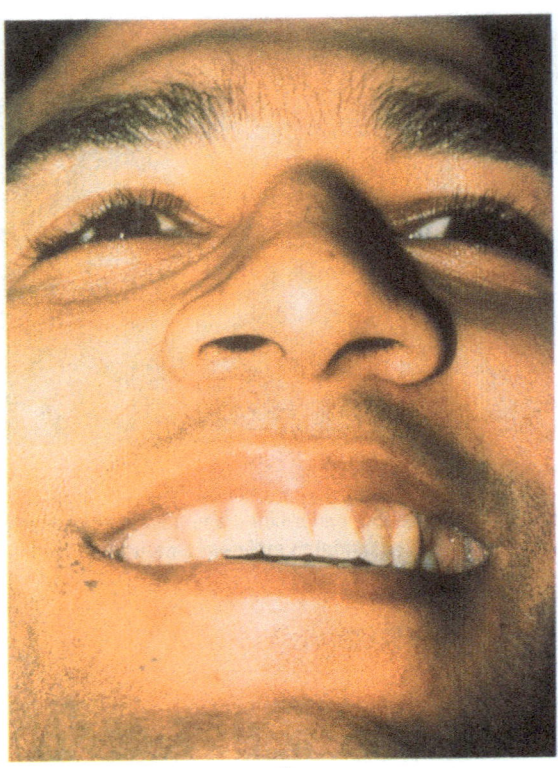

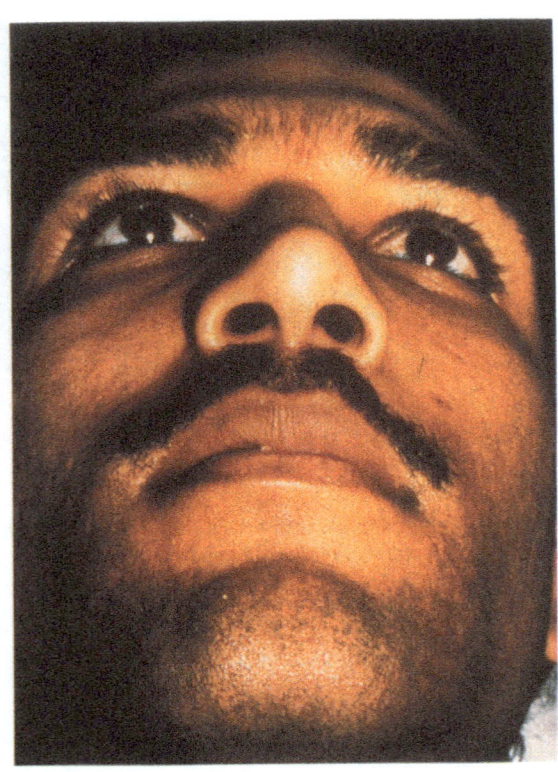

f g

Figure 4-25f, 4-25g (above)
Major excision of the alar base with medial advancement of the cheek skin resulted in a more natural convex curvature to the lateral alar wall. He also underwent central thinning of the alar walls. This was performed by excising a central wedge of soft tissue. Marginal excisions can be made to the skin and soft tissue—but are unnecessary in the author's opinion—to obtain adequate thinning of the alae.

Figure 4-25h, 4-25i (below)
Alar base resection, medial advancement, and a 3 cm × .75 cm "pea-pod" tip graft were employed to give the illusion of a much thinner tip. Notice how the nostrils have changed from a horizontal to a more medial-vertical orientation.

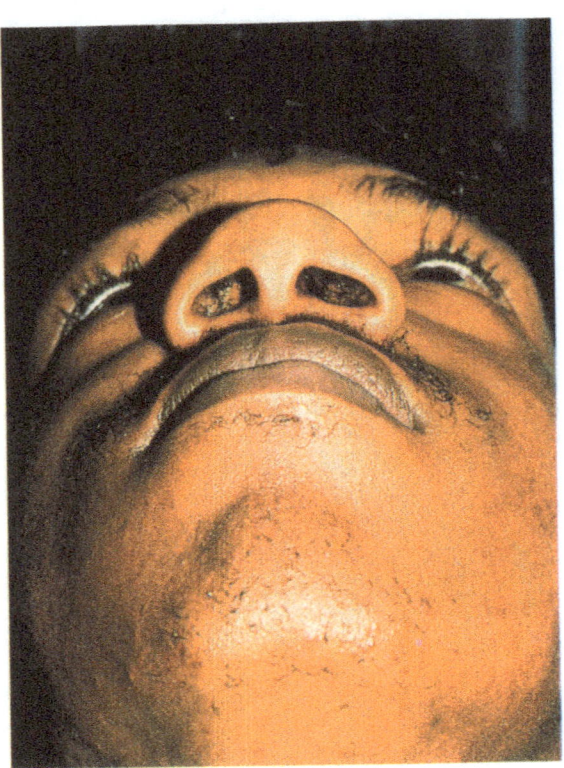

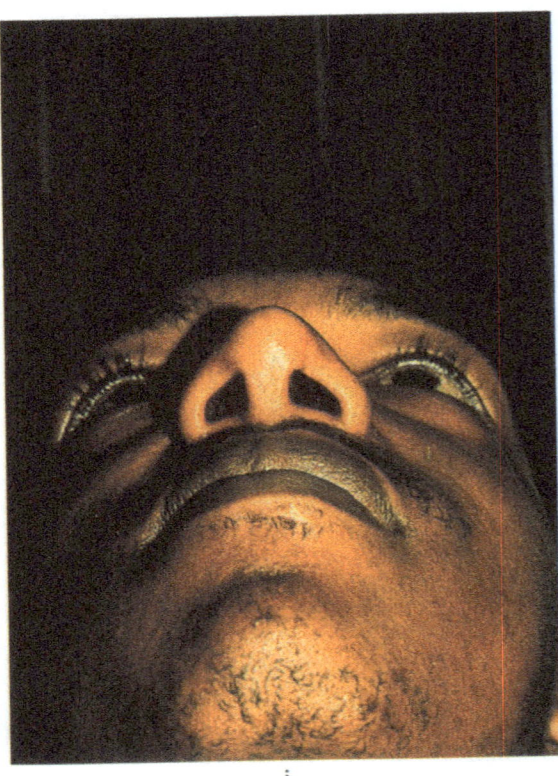

h i

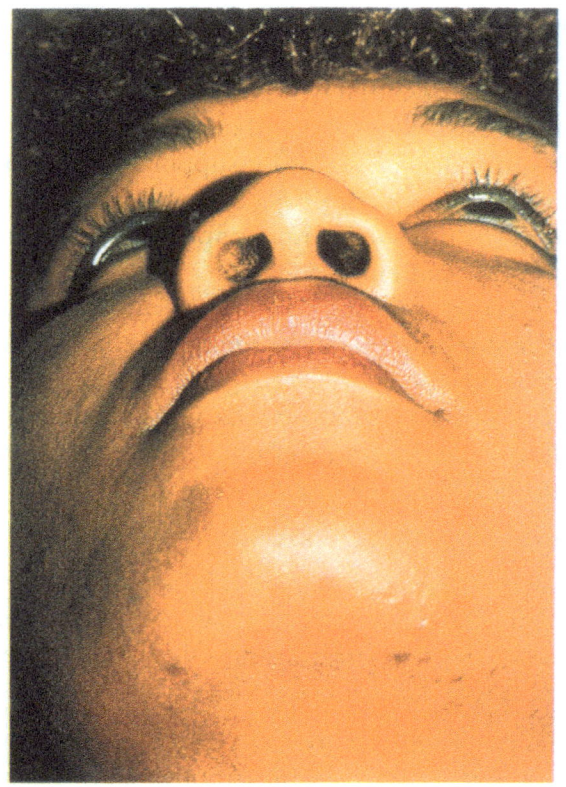 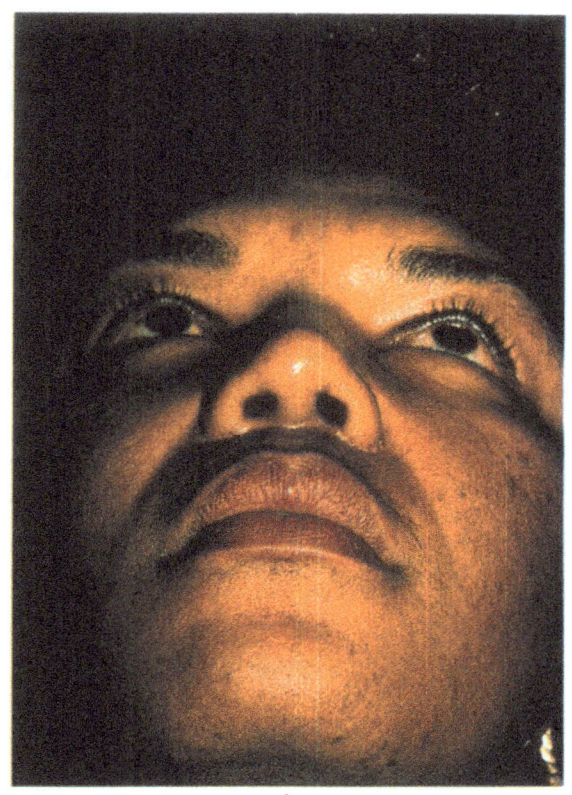

Figure 4-25j, 4-25k
The goal of a narrower nasal base was met with standard alar base excision and medial advancement of the cheek skin. However, it must be noted that a 3 cm × .75 cm "pea-pod" graft was placed to give a more triangular appearance.

Nasal Tip and "Pea-Pod" Graft

Non-Caucasian noses (Asian, black, and Hispanic) have historically presented a formidable challenge to the rhinoplastic surgeon. Whereas the Caucasian nose is usually corrected by standard reduction techniques and occasionally by the incorporation of a Sheen-type shield or Peck onlay graft, the different anatomical structure of the non-Caucasian nose necessitates new approaches.

Before the augmentation techniques of Sheen, Peck, and others, it was the techniques of reduction rhinoplasty as popularized by Ashley, Diamond, and Reese, etc., that served as stimulant for my "pea-pod" technique.

In addition to a short columella, thick skin, and wide bridge and alae, the flat, bulky, somewhat ptotic nasal tip is a most troublesome area to cor-

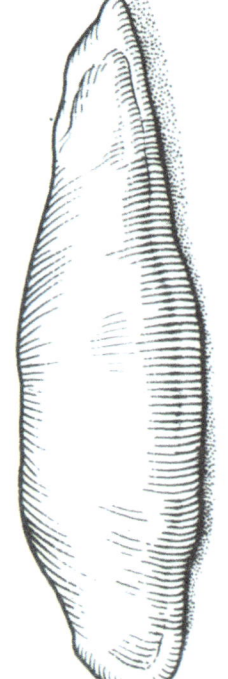

Figure 4-25l
The "pea-pod" graft closely resembles a vegetable pea-pod. It may be of minor historic note that the first record of the vegetable pea-pod coincides with the first total nasal reconstruction. Both occurred in India during the fifth century B.C.

rect. Standard reduction techniques alone show only minimal improvement, and all too often lead to overreduction as well. While some defatting of the tip is possible and quite helpful, it is essential that overreduction be avoided. After much trial and error in this area, I have found what is required is an innovative, special type of graft—one that is firm, ultrasupportive, autologous, and capable of providing a high degree of projection and definition. I feel that increasing tip projection is the single most important factor in achieving the results desired by ethnic patients.

I have developed a special graft to meet the demands of these particularly difficult tips. Because it is molded into a shape similar to that of the vegetable pea-pod, I have named it the "pea-pod" graft (Fig. 4-25l, on page 73). The final constructed shape is also akin to two hands approximated in prayer. The "pea-pod" has sufficient projection, definition, strength, and durability and is composed of the following elements:

Double (and if indicated, triple) layers of conchal cartilage.

Two opposing pieces of conchal cartilage that are press-sutured together, face-to-face, concave-to-concave into the shape of a pea-pod. If even greater projection is desired, then the concave side can be sutured to the convex side by bending it anteriorly and tilting the concave side forward.

The "pea-pod" shape allows for a high degree of projection and the multiple layers provide extreme firmness and support. Approximating and forcing together the opposing surfaces ensures long-term strength and security, while the natural curvature of the conchal cartilage yields a very natural-looking contour.

Conchal cartilage possesses at least eight advantages over septal cartilage for use in thick-tipped noses: (1) thickness, (2) strength, (3) abundance, (4) natural curvature, (5) ability to incorporate mastoid soft tissue, (6) resistance to suture tearing, (7) a somewhat roughened texture, allowing it to hold its position and support the nasal tip, and (8) ease of harvesting.

The "pea-pod" tip graft is the author's preference for difficult ethnic noses. But having a full command of the various nose tip grafts and other opinions is always vitally important for the rhinoplastic surgeon. Combining cartilage with soft-tissue "caps" and appropriate stabilization is essential.

Although open procedures in the ethnic patient may heal well, it is the author's opinion that a more extensive consideration of potential hypertrophic scarring is essential. Keloids or hypertrophic scars are not routinely a significant problem. Hypertrophic scars may be better alleviated with cosmetic tattooing rather than surgical revision. There are many modalities to decrease hypertrophic or keloid scars: from simple pressure and topical silicone-containing creams or gels; Silastic sheeting; injections of triamcinolone acetonide suspension 10 mg/ml (Kenalog), further diluted; combinations of Kenalog, verapamil hydrochloride, and 5FU; all the way to excision and radiation therapy. Radiation's high unpredictability requires that it be used only with highly refractive cases. Utilizing bone or ethmoid grafting, except at the base of a cartilage graft, may not be best for tip support. Firmness and palpability under thin or softened tip skin may be disconcerting for the patient, and the "pea-pod" graft with its concave-to-concave surface provides substantial stiffness and support while giving palpability.

Figure 4-26a, 4-26b
A standard "bucket-handle" delivery
technique is used to expose the alar
cartilage. Fibrofatty tissue is removed
prior to cartilage excision.

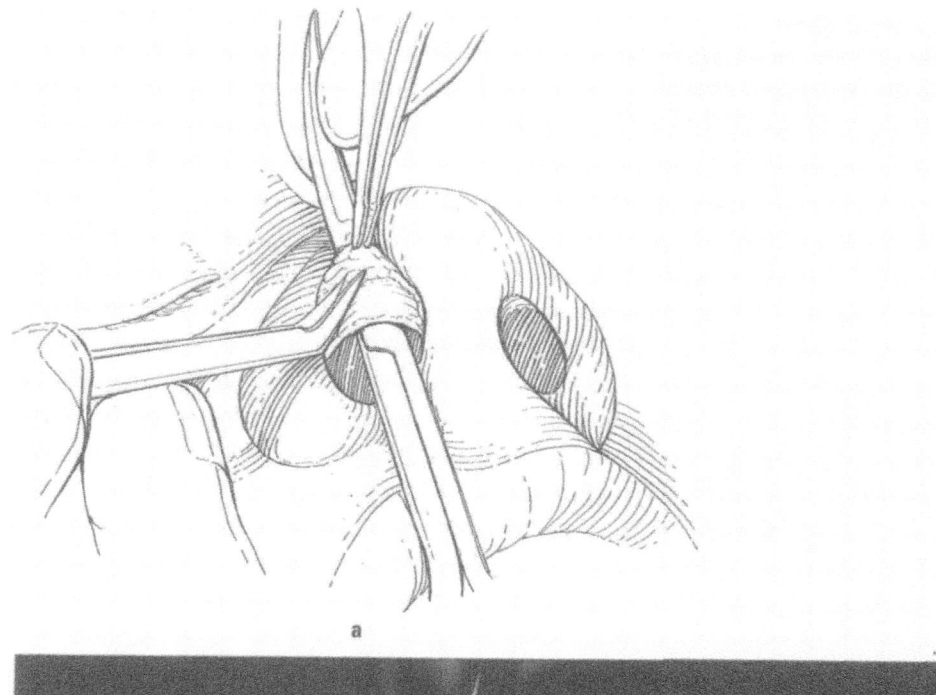

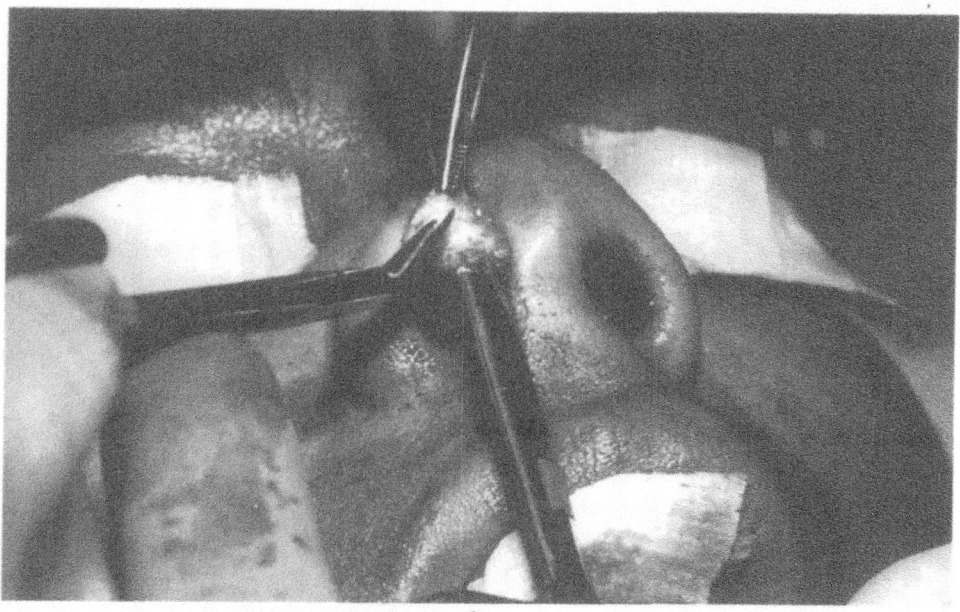

Thick Nasal Tip Skin and Alar Cartilage Reduction

The thick ethnic nose usually contains a limited amount of alar cartilage, but a moderate-to-large amount of fibrofatty tissue. Limited anatomical defatting is therefore beneficial. A bipedicle eversion technique is used on the tip and alar cartilages.

A rim incision is made, along with an intercartilaginous incision, and the alar cartilages are exposed through a "bucket handle" approach. The preferred technique is a dissection utilizing Ragnel scissors over the dome of the alar cartilage attempting to incorporate as much fibrofatty tissue as possible. Upon delivery, geometric sculpturing of the tip is first performed by selectively trimming the fibrofatty tissue off of the cartilages (Fig. 4-26a, 4-26b). A triangular incision (five-eighths of the cephalic portion of the alar

Figure 4-27a, 4-27b
A triangular incision is made on the cartilage. Typically, the upper five-eighths of the lower lateral cartilages are excised.

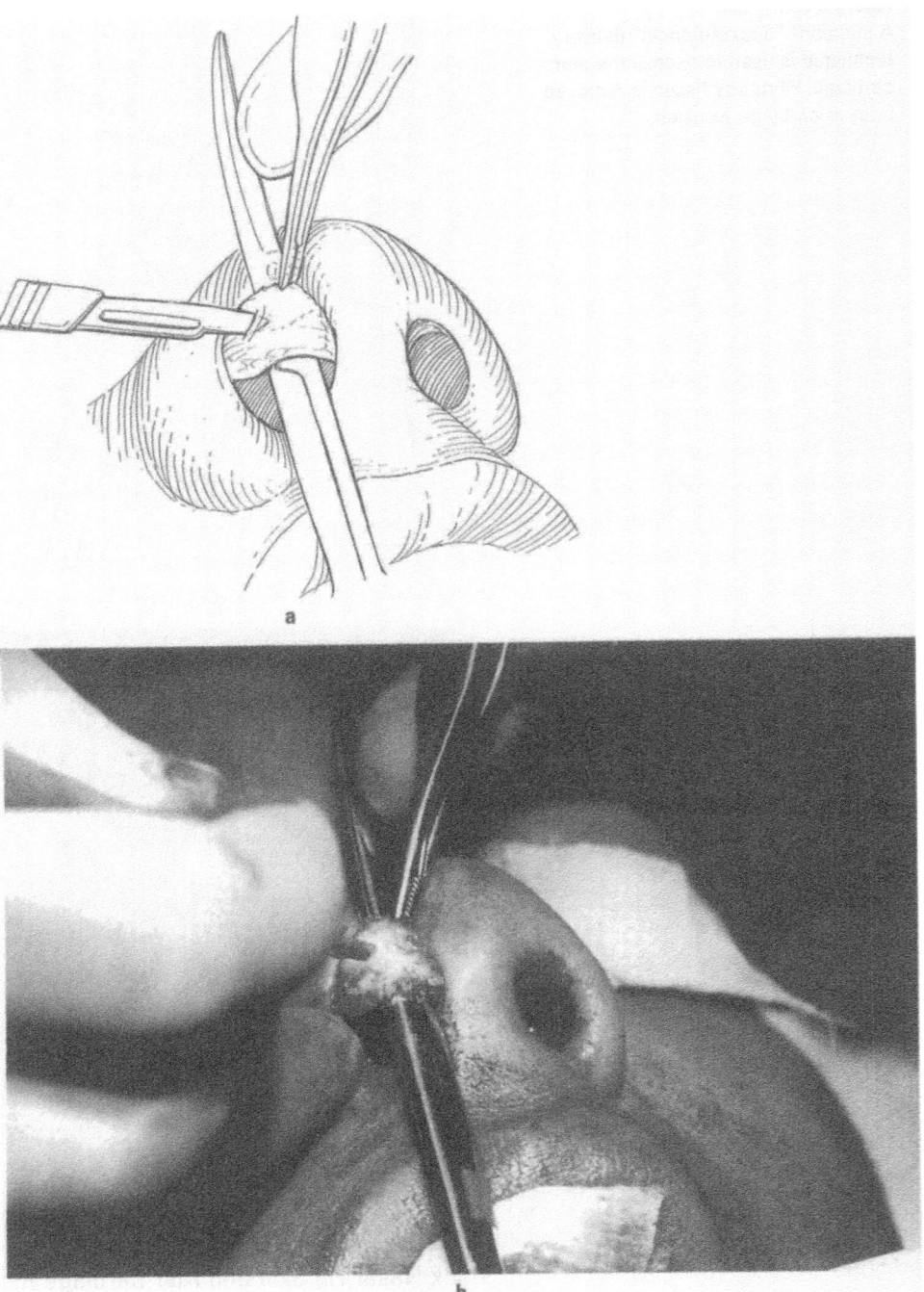

cartilage) is then made (Fig. 4-27a, 4-27b). The cartilage segment is then excised, leaving ample support (Fig. 4-28a, 4-28b, on page 77). The lateral apical cartilaginous areas are retained to reduce the risk of retraction. The triangular segment of the medial fat directly under the central tip is also retained for padding. Even though the entire tip area is dissected in a sub-dermal fashion, attempts at separately overdefatting the tip can result in re-tractions, vascular compromise, and irregularities.

The difficulty in using standard techniques to augment a nose is apparent when one checks and sees the thick ethnic tip. A parallel is a bed with a very thick comforter or blanket over it. When lying in bed, if one "tents" an end of the comforter by raising one's toes, the material appears

Figure 4-28a, 4-28b
Triangular excision of the cephalic portion of the alar cartilage leaves a small triangular segment of medial fat directly under the central tip for padding.

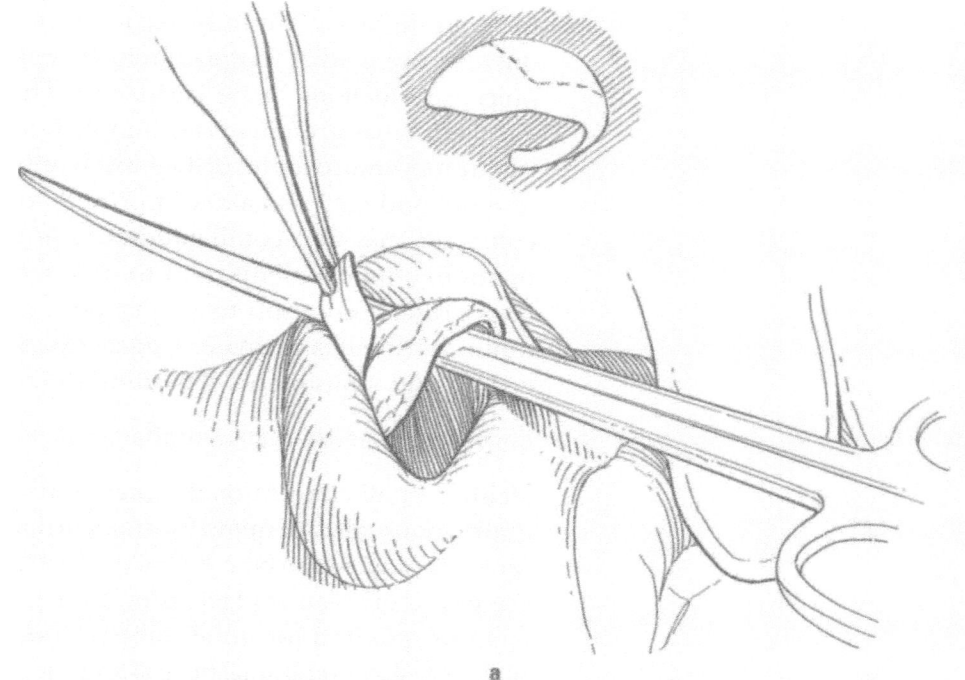

a

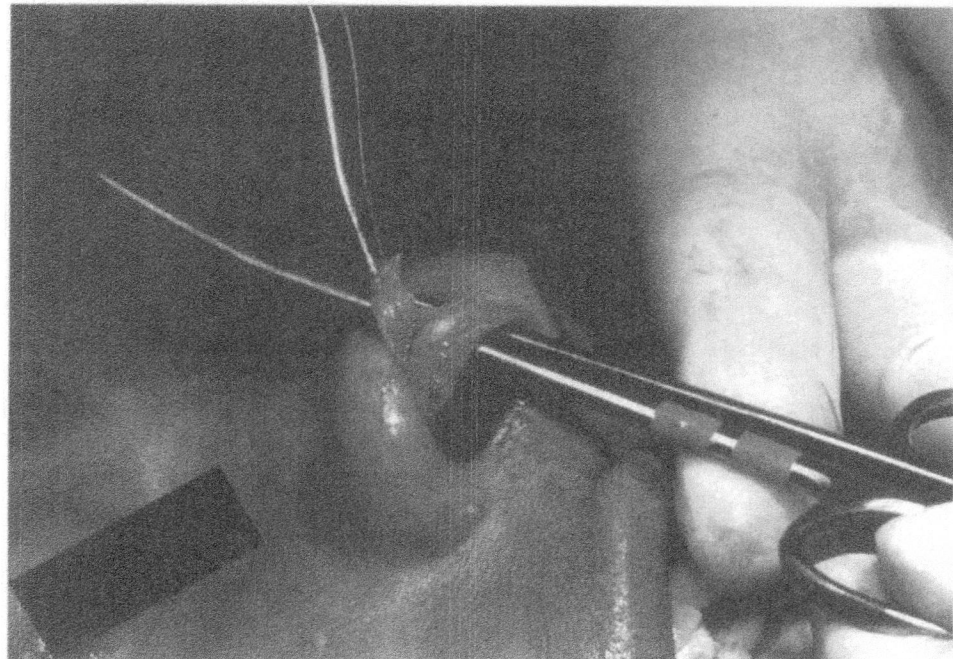

b

to be much thinner than when it is lying flat with no underlying structural definition. The "pea-pod" graft acts much like a tent pole, with acceptable tension, providing definition and increased projection. The "tent-pole" starting point is the base of the columella with some tension present, which may explain the very low rate of resorption and high degree of graft retention.

Malposition of alar cartilage is not seen as often in the black nose as in the Caucasian. Malposition does appear more frequently in the Hispanic nose. It is beneficial to eliminate the malposition of the alar cartilage by repositioning. Great care must be taken to appropriately diagnose the need for delicate dissection in order to avoid cartilaginous distortion. Not infrequently, the medial footplate may be either asymmetric or protuberant, requiring reduction. These cartilage portions should be saved as they make excellent onlay graft material. Simple horizontal mattress sutures of 4-0 plain catgut may improve the orifice when approximated together with moderate tension, and may also allow improved anatomical symmetry. The "hanging" columella may be a combination of soft tissue and cartilage. In the author's opinion, ethnic patients tend to have more soft tissue, which may require a larger resection of soft tissue just posterior to the columella edge than one would normally anticipate. Staged excisions during the first operative procedure and adjustments according to the results may be necessary.

Conventional or Alternative Grafts

Neither small conventional septal grafts nor alternative L-shaped alloplastic grafts are usually adequate for transforming bulky, ptotic nasal tips. Although septal or single-layered conchal grafts are ideal for Caucasian noses (and for the non-Caucasian bridge), they do not provide the projection, strength, or contour required for non-Caucasian noses. Likewise, alternative techniques such as L-shaped alloplastic grafting have a tendency to extrude and thus do not yield safe, long-term projection. Nor does the L-shape itself give a natural appearance to the tip; it provides excessive fullness to the supratip area and often does not give separate definition to the anatomical tip.

Separate nasal dorsal and tip grafts are necessary to provide the retrotip or supratip with a tip "break," which is crucial for creating a profile with an attractive contour. Moreover, this effect can often be achieved only by a large, highly supportive tip graft. Solely reducing the alar cartilages or adding an onlay dorsal graft is usually insufficient.

Aesthetic Results of the "Pea-Pod" Graft

Few other grafting techniques can compete with the high level of tip projection and definition provided by the "pea-pod" graft, in my opinion. Several aesthetic problems are solved by the proper placement of a "pea-pod" graft. Rather than making the nose appear too large—as some patients initially fear—this graft, particularly in conjunction with the effects of alar reduction, actually creates the illusion of a thinner, better projecting tip. Two key aesthetic transformations are achieved by the combination of both techniques: the interdorsal distance is narrowed and the transverse alar orifice is shifted to a more vertical position.

Moreover, the old puzzle of how to provide a "pointed" tip or tip with definite projection in noses with a broad interdomal distance is finally resolved by the use of the "pea-pod" graft. Previous attempts at creating two domes with a normal bidomal light reflex often only added width to the tip, while the unidomal central point and reflex created by the "pea-pod" graft results in a thin, well-defined tip.

The "pea-pod" graft is constructed in such a way that when positioned, it is able to tent the thick tip skin and provide a high degree of definition. It must be noted that these results are usually optimal only in thick-skinned tips. When used in noses with thin-skinned tips, such as those characteristic of fair-skinned Caucasians, the "pea-pod" graft may provide a tip that is

Figure 4-29
In the thin-skinned Caucasian nose, highly projecting, pointed tip grafts give an unnatural appearance. Conversely, these are ideal in difficult, bulky, thick, or depressed nasal tips. A standard tip graft, such as an onlay graft, would have provided a more natural appearance.

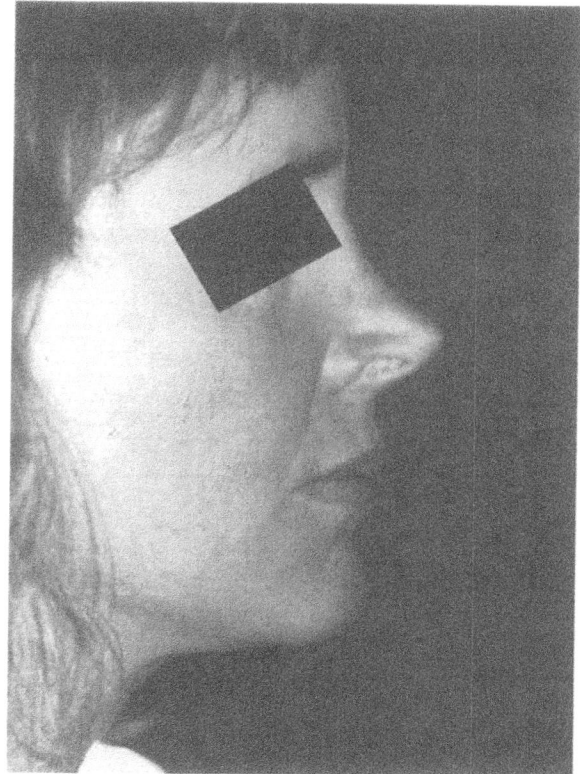

too pointed (Fig. 4-29). But the "pea-pod" graft has tremendously increased the satisfaction of my ethnic rhinoplasty patients.

When nasal tip "tenting" occurs as a result of inserting the "pea-pod" graft, the supratip area usually has some "dead space." Past attempts to close this space using small suction drains have been relatively unrewarding owing to the extended time required for contraction.

When a watertight closure is performed in the nasal tip area, a substantial accumulation of blood serum and resultant organized fibrosis usually occur. Leaving supratip mucosa edges open often results in mucosal wall upgrowth, resulting in further fibrosis. While placing a large dorsal graft to tent the tip does result in good nasal contouring and shape, it will not completely prevent or eliminate dead space.

When loosely closing mucosal edges, the author's practice has been to ensure that any significant dead space is filled with crushed cartilage grafts. This procedure is followed by long-term nighttime taping for at least 2 to 4 weeks in order to ensure contraction of the area. If fibrosis is predicted, the author gives a maximum of three injections of triamcinolone acetonide suspension 10 mg/ml (Kenalog) further diluted into the tip and supratip areas. Injections are usually 0.125 to 0.25 cc of 5 mg/cc triamcinolone into the area, each followed by another minimum 2-week period of taping.

Estimating the Graft Size

Before obtaining the cartilage graft, the size of the tip graft and the amount of desired projection must be determined. To estimate the length, a mosquito clamp is placed at the apex of the tip and elevated to the desired position. The distance is measured with calipers, down to 0.3 and 0.5 mm above

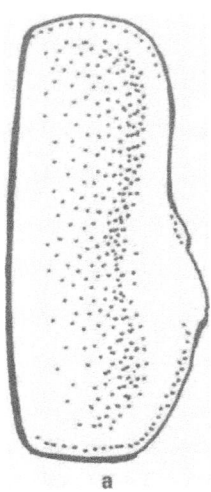

Figure 4-30a, 4-30b, 4-30c, 4-30d
A large segment of conchal cartilage is excised to form two opposing grafts. Ivory and Silastic nasal tip augmentation (as well as dorsal) have a higher-than-acceptable rate of extrusion and infection. Again, autologous tissue is our preference for the nasal tip.

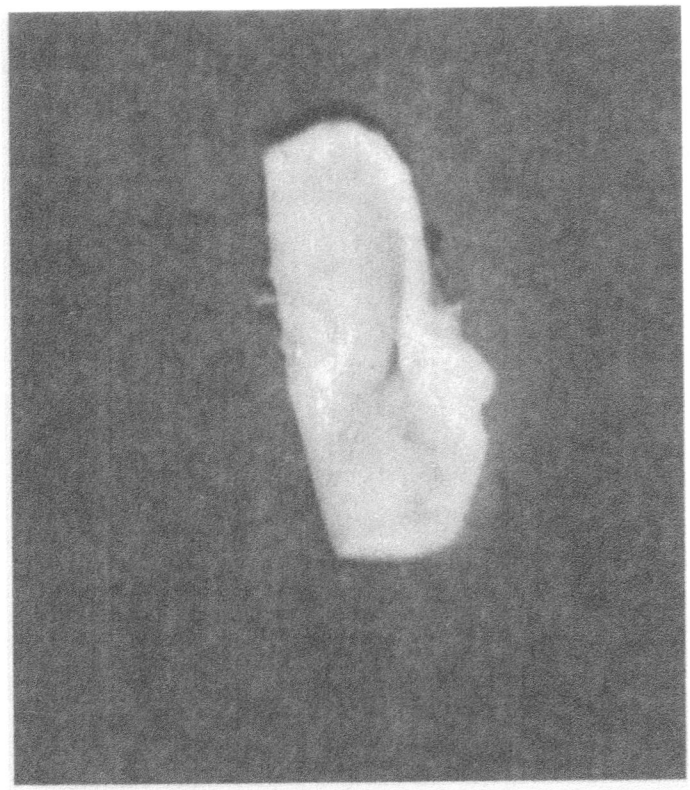

b

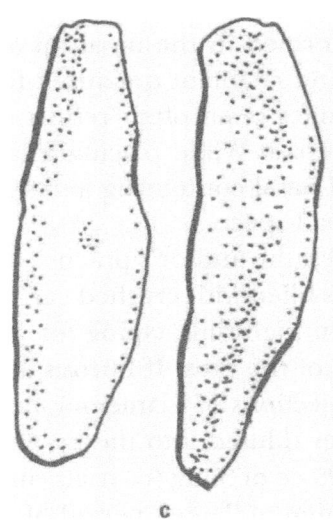

c

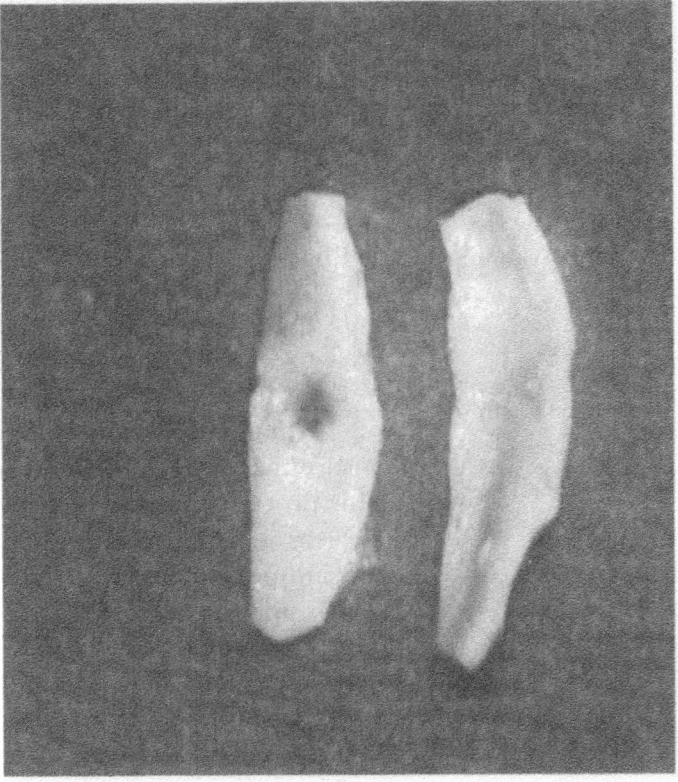

d

the columellar-labial crease. It is important that the measurement ends there and does not extend to the nasal spine. The desired width is then determined. The estimated tip projection should be confirmed by again placing the tip of a curved clamp under the tip skin and elevating it to its desired height. The desired tip projection apex is then marked. It is recommended that the initial nasal tip marking be placed 2 to 3 mm anteriorly. When finally placed, the apex of the graft may have a tendency to shift posteriorly, giving convexity to the supratip, and the tip skin will automatically shift superiorly and posteriorly. Frontal and lateral views are checked to ensure optimal marking.

Constructing the "Pea-Pod" Graft

After a large segment of cartilage from the concha has been removed, graft construction can begin. The segment of curved conchal cartilage is first cut into two equal pieces (Fig. 4-30a to 4-30d, on previous page). Two solid pieces of opposing cartilage of proper size must be used, and sometimes a third piece may be necessary for extra support. The edges of the cartilage

Figure 4-31a, 4-31b
The two pieces of cartilage are sutured together with the concave sides facing each other, using a 5-0 Dexon at each end. The 5-0 Dexon sutures at each end of the graft will later serve as the percutaneous stabilization sutures.

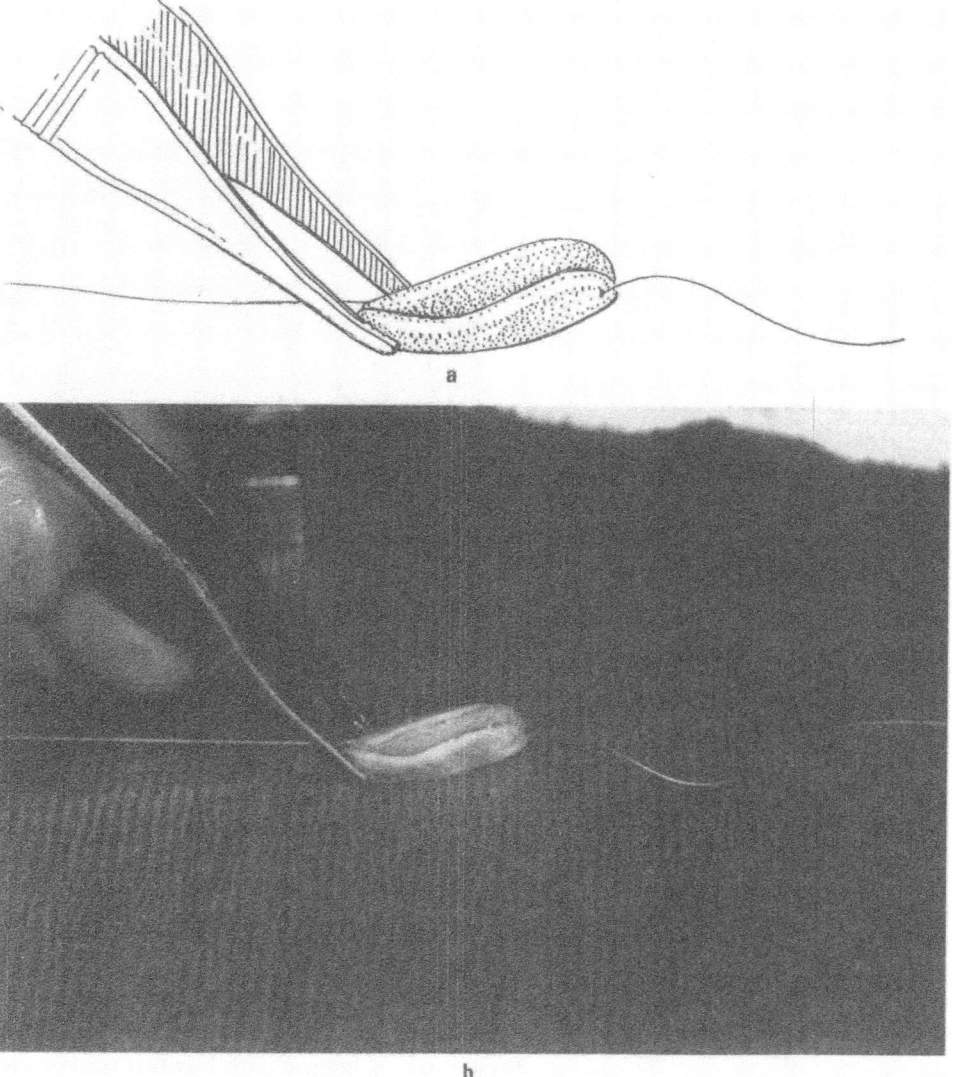

Figure 4-32a, 4-32b
If further stabilization is required, an additional 5-0 Dexon can be wrapped circumferentially around both grafts. The width of the graft is approximately 6 to 7 mm and can be narrowed later if necessary, but the stabilization suture wrapping should then be reinforced.

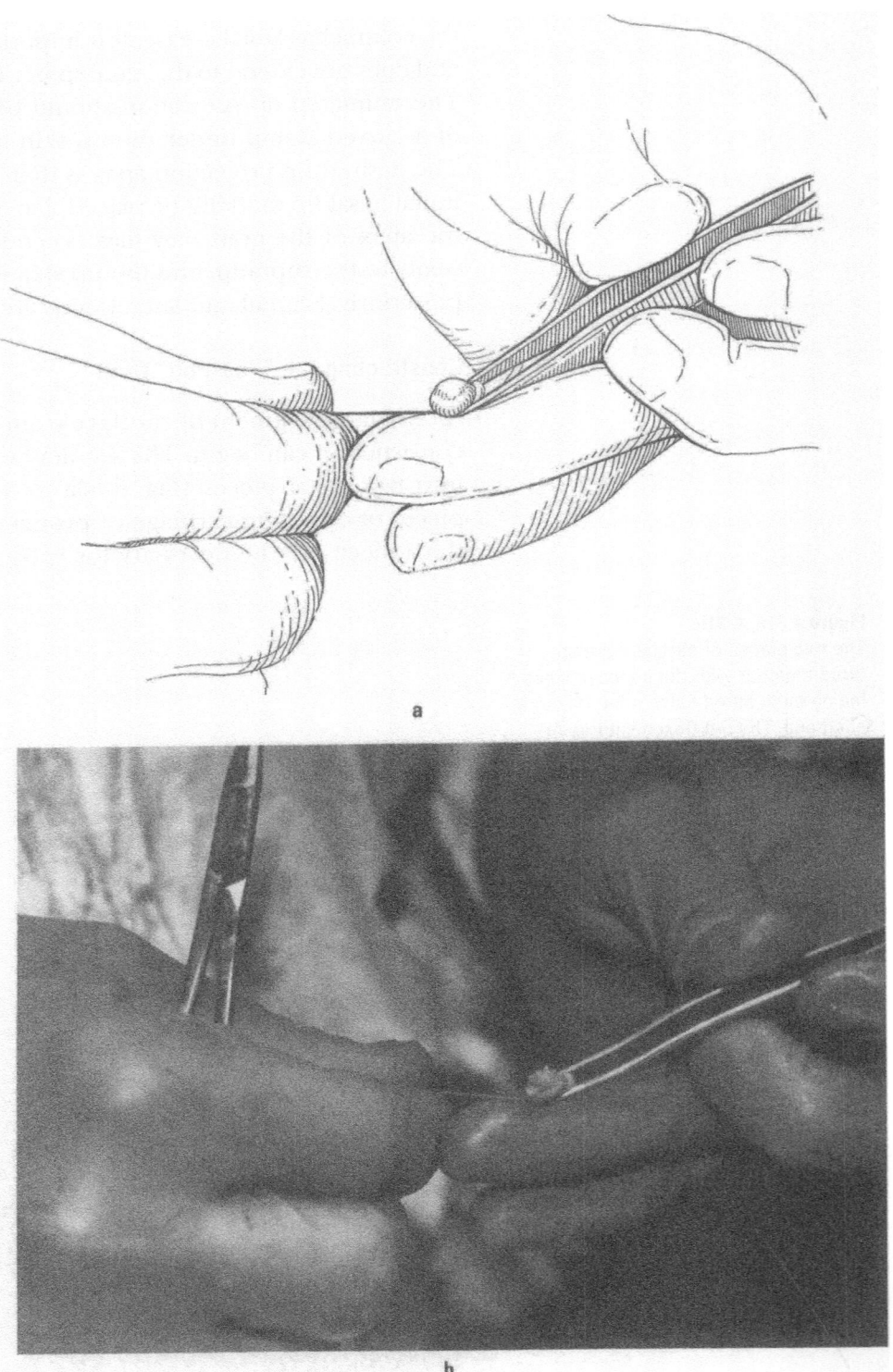

segments are trimmed evenly, and the two opposing pieces of conchal cartilage are press-sutured together, face-to-face, concave-side-to-concave-side, with 5-0 Dexon (Fig. 4-31a, 4-31b, on page 81). Approximating the two sides together in this fashion gives a large, yet firm, ultrasupportive graft. A septal cartilage graft of this size is often a problem to construct. It requires even more layers, which often make it too straight, sharp, easily fragmented,

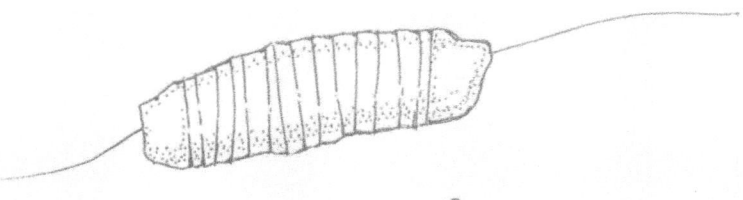

a

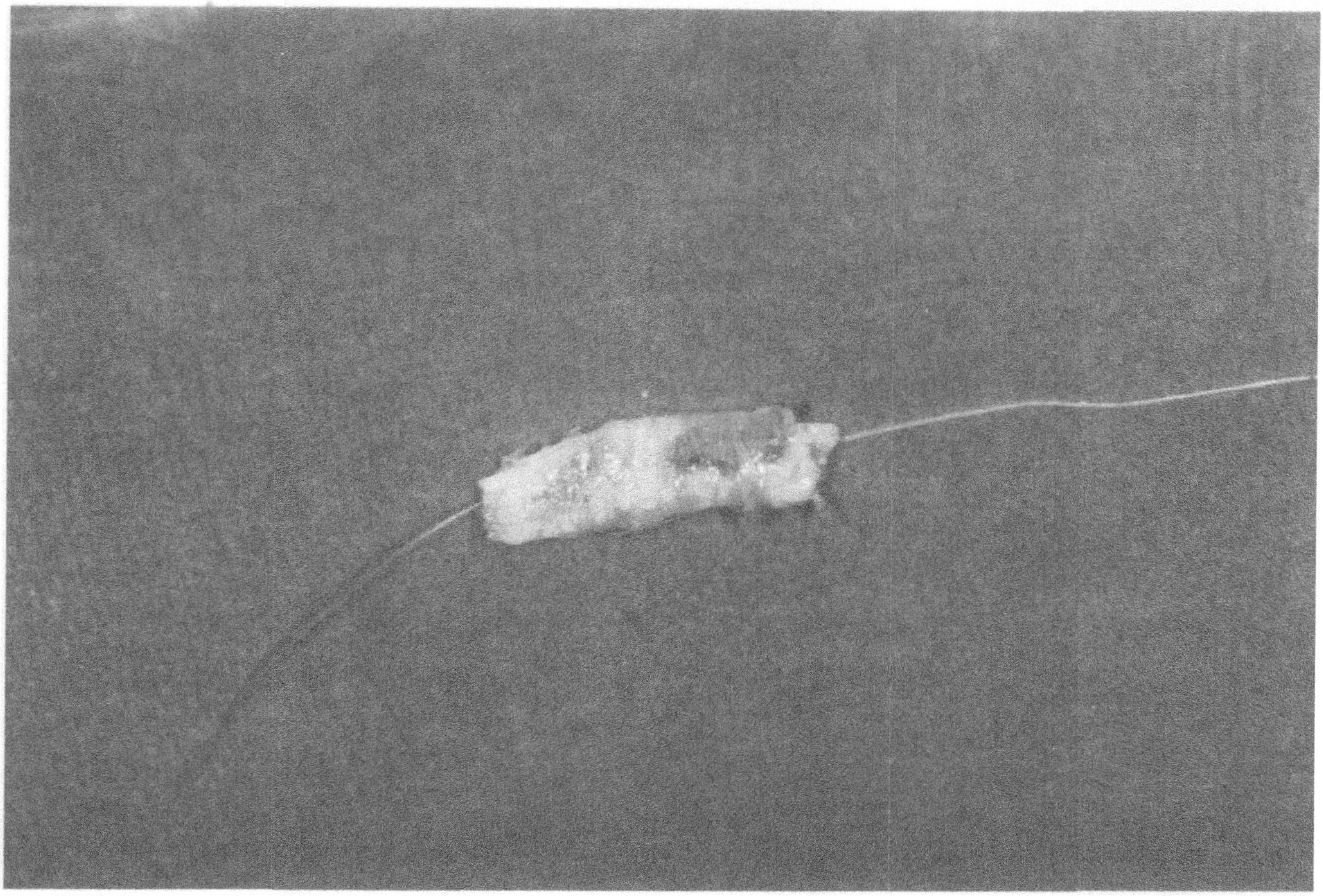

b

Figure 4-33a, 4-33b
The standard "pea-pod" graft consists of two curved pieces of conchal cartilage sutured together with the concave surfaces facing each other. This shape is ideal for thick, bulky nasal tips; it is strong and very supportive. If the graft creates an excessively pointed tip, mastoid fascia can be added to the end of the graft.

and lacking in normal anatomical curvature. External 5-0 Dexon stabilization sutures are placed. (These pull-out sutures are very important for the final positioning of the graft. Prior to cutting the pull-out sutures at skin level, small readjustments, if necessary, can be made a few days after surgery by applying temporary tension to the sutures.) If greater security is indicated, additional 5-0 nylon sutures may be placed or Dexon can be wound around the grafts (Fig. 4-32a, 4-32b, on page 82). More frequently than not, the graft appears larger than one would have estimated (Fig. 4-33a, 4-33b). Again, it looks like two palms placed together in prayer.

The "pea-pod" graft can be easily adapted to fit particular needs while being constructed. If, for instance, more nasal projection is desired, then the concave side can be sutured to the convex side by bending it anteriorly and tilting the concave side forward (Fig. 4-34a, 34b, on page 84). Ninety percent of "pea-pod" grafts are sutured concave-side-to-concave-side.

Figure 4-34a, 4-34b
The degree of anterior projection can be adjusted by either concave-to-concave or concave-to-convex suturing. Ninety percent of the grafts are sutured concave-to-concave. The concave-to-convex arrangement provides greater tip projection than the concave-to-concave arrangement and may be needed in tips that are unusually bulky and poorly projecting.

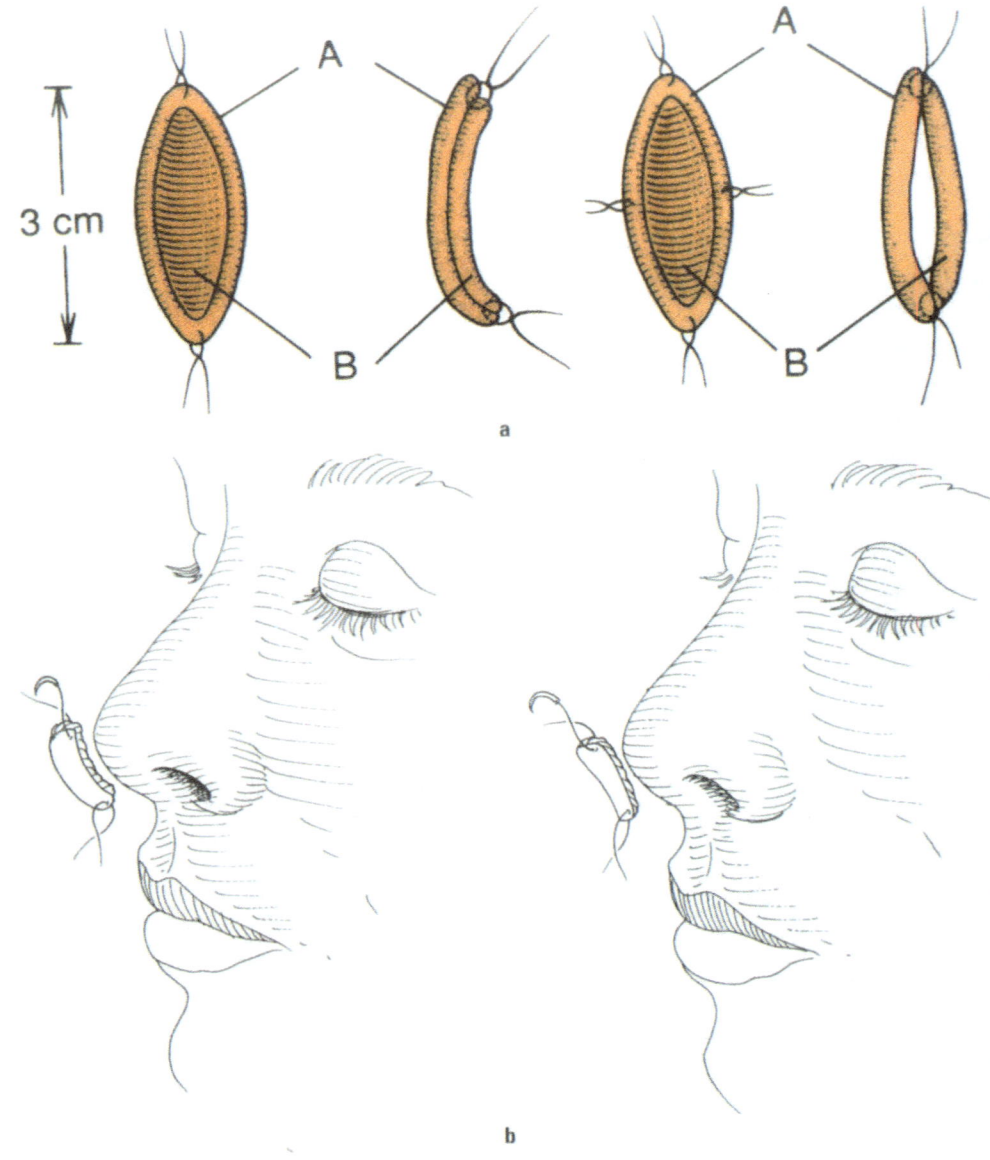

Positioning the Graft

Preoperatively, this patient had a low dorsum and wide bridge. She had a nondefined nasal tip, with low tip point. There was slight hanging of the columella. The tip cartilages appeared moderately supportive, and the columellar-labial angle was not open (Fig. 4-34c, 4-34d, 4-34e, 4-34f, on page 85).

When the "pea-pod" graft has been constructed and a rim-columellar incision is made (the tip is first exposed as described in "Exposure and Incisions"), the graft can then be placed. Again, the "pea-pod" graft should initially be carved approximately 3 cm in length to allow for adequate projection (Fig. 4-35a, 4-35b, on page 86). Prior to inserting the "pea-pod" graft, either or both of the skin pull-out sutures are placed for graft positioning. Depending upon ease of placement, the superior aspect of the graft will sometimes be placed into the pocket for stabilization first, followed by the

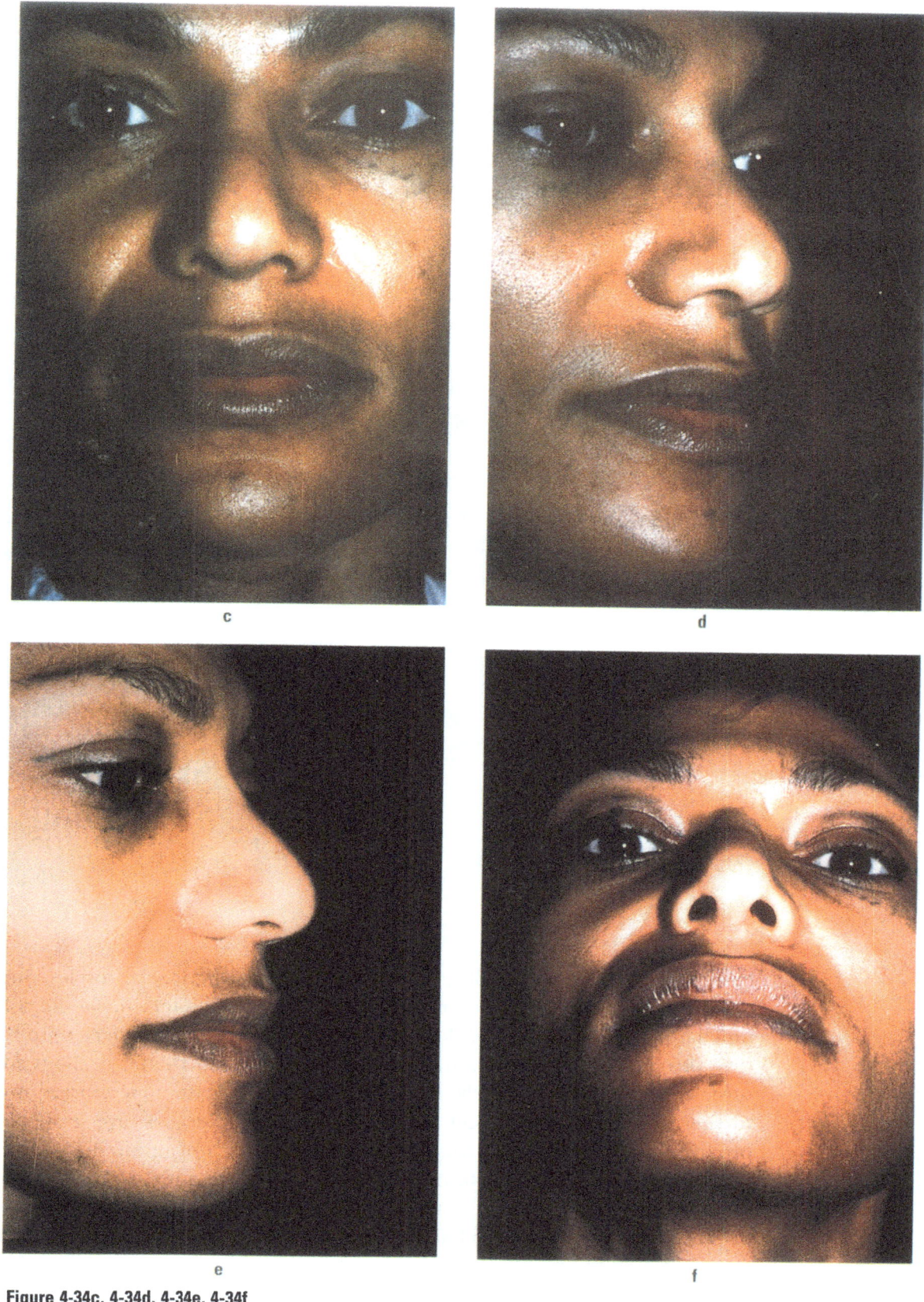

Figure 4-34c, 4-34d, 4-34e, 4-34f
This black female had a flat, unsupported nasal tip.

Figure 4-35a, 4-35b
The final graft is cut approximately 25% larger than needed and sutured together (with additional pull-out stabilization sutures at each end) to allow for trial placements and size adjustments to be made and checked for size and projection prior to placement.

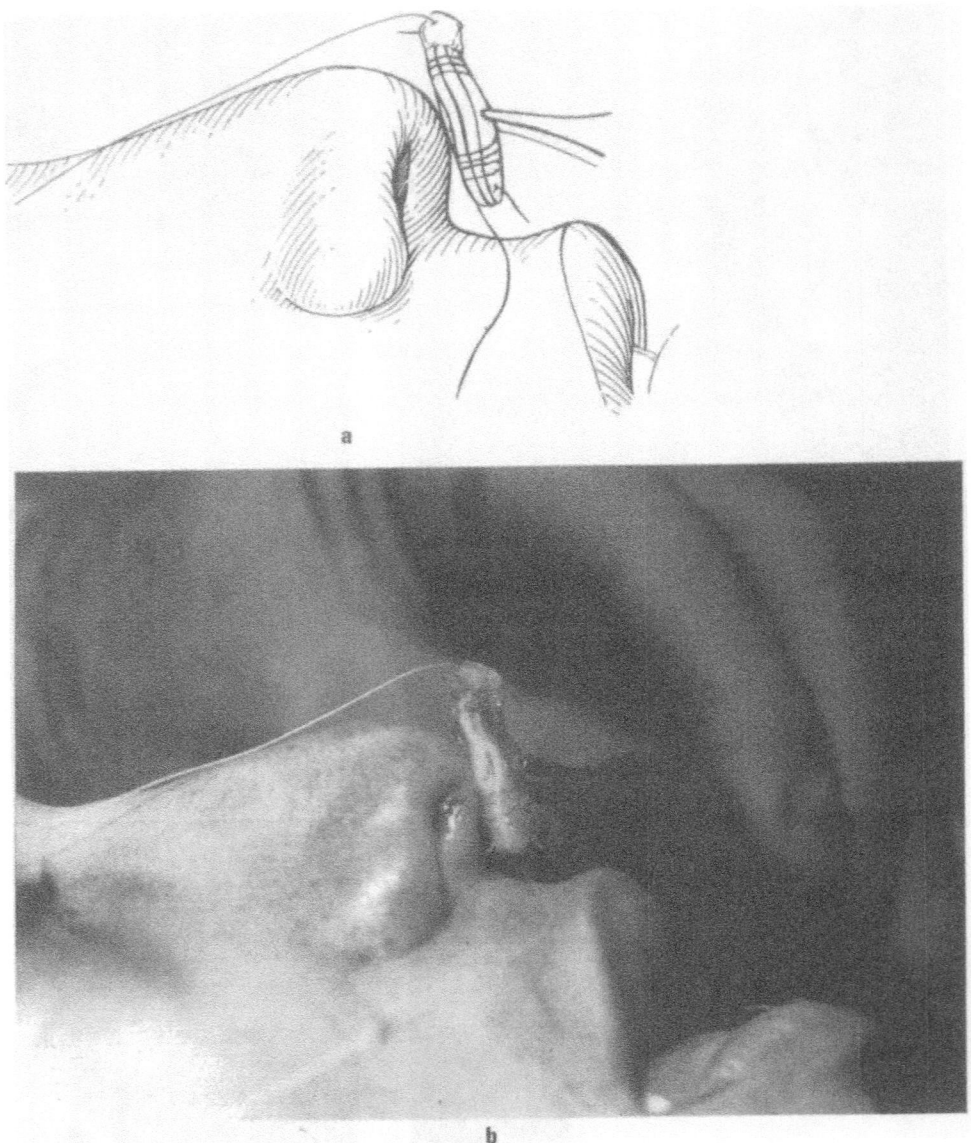

base, or vice versa (Fig. 4-36a, 4-36b). To provide a more natural-looking tip, the base of the proposed graft is placed a few millimeters above the columellar-labial junction—*not* down at the nasal spine. The superior tip of the "pea-pod" graft is positioned with the use of a 5-0 Dexon pull-out suture. This is pulled anteriorly and superiorly under reasonable tension until the graft is in the correct location. The concave-to-concave graft approximation gives a very firm, highly supportive, strong graft that allows good tip projection. Definite pressure against the tip apex is often necessary for proper projection; however, not so much that vascularity is compromised. The appropriate balance between the two must be reached. A few additional interrupted absorbable sutures can be placed along the edge between the columellar soft tissue and the graft for further stabilization. The final graft is oriented so the edges are lateral and the concave-to-concave face of the graft is anterior to posterior (Fig. 4-37a, 4-37b, on page 88).

Figure 4-36a, 4-36b
In this case, introducing the superior aspect of the graft first and utilizing double-hooks to superiorly retract the nasal tip will allow introduction of the inferior portion of the graft.

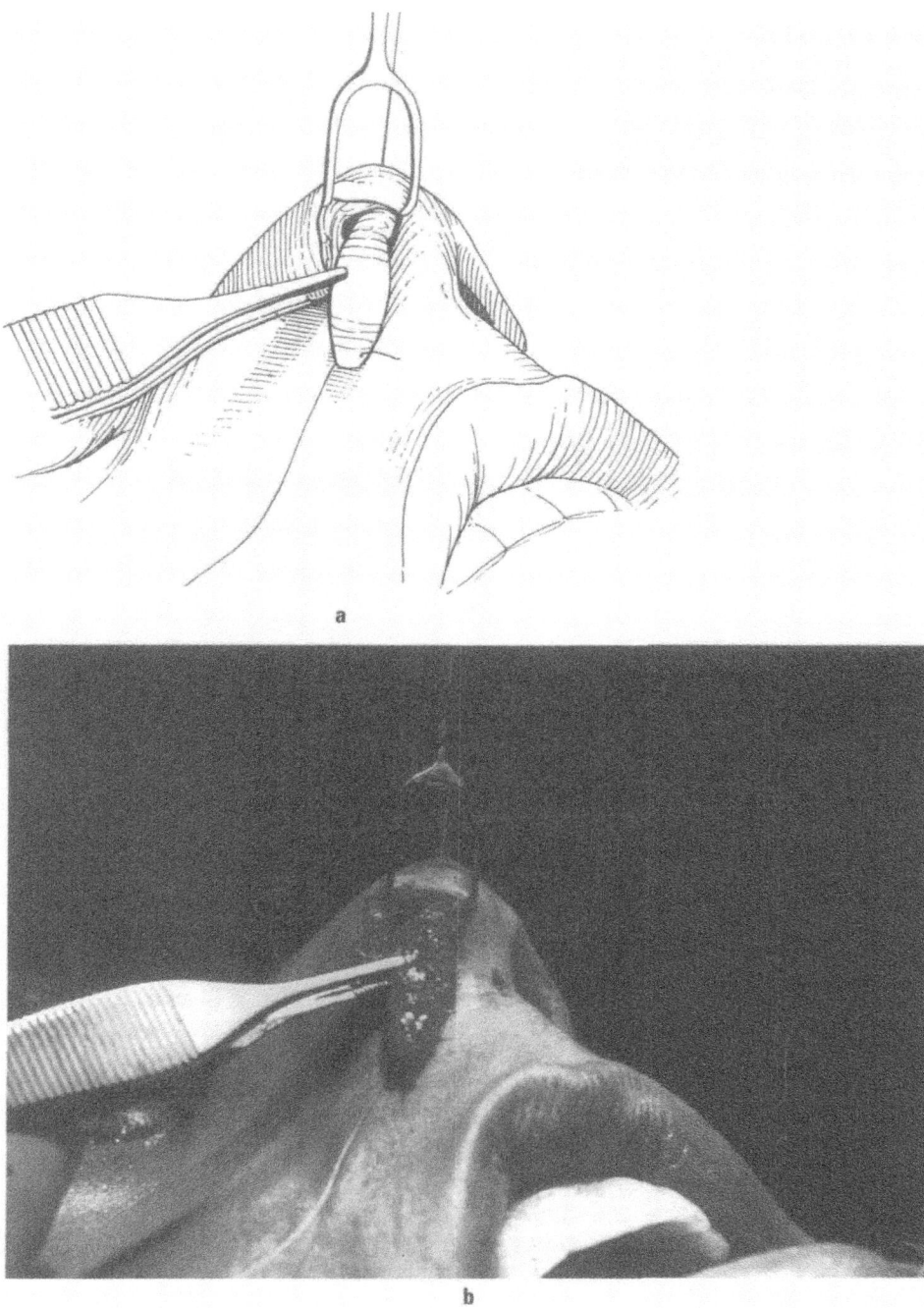

a

b

Figure 4-37a, 4-37b
The graft is placed with slight-to-moderate tip tension. In addition to the pull-out sutures, several absorbable stabilization sutures can be placed through the deep columella soft tissue to further stabilize the graft.

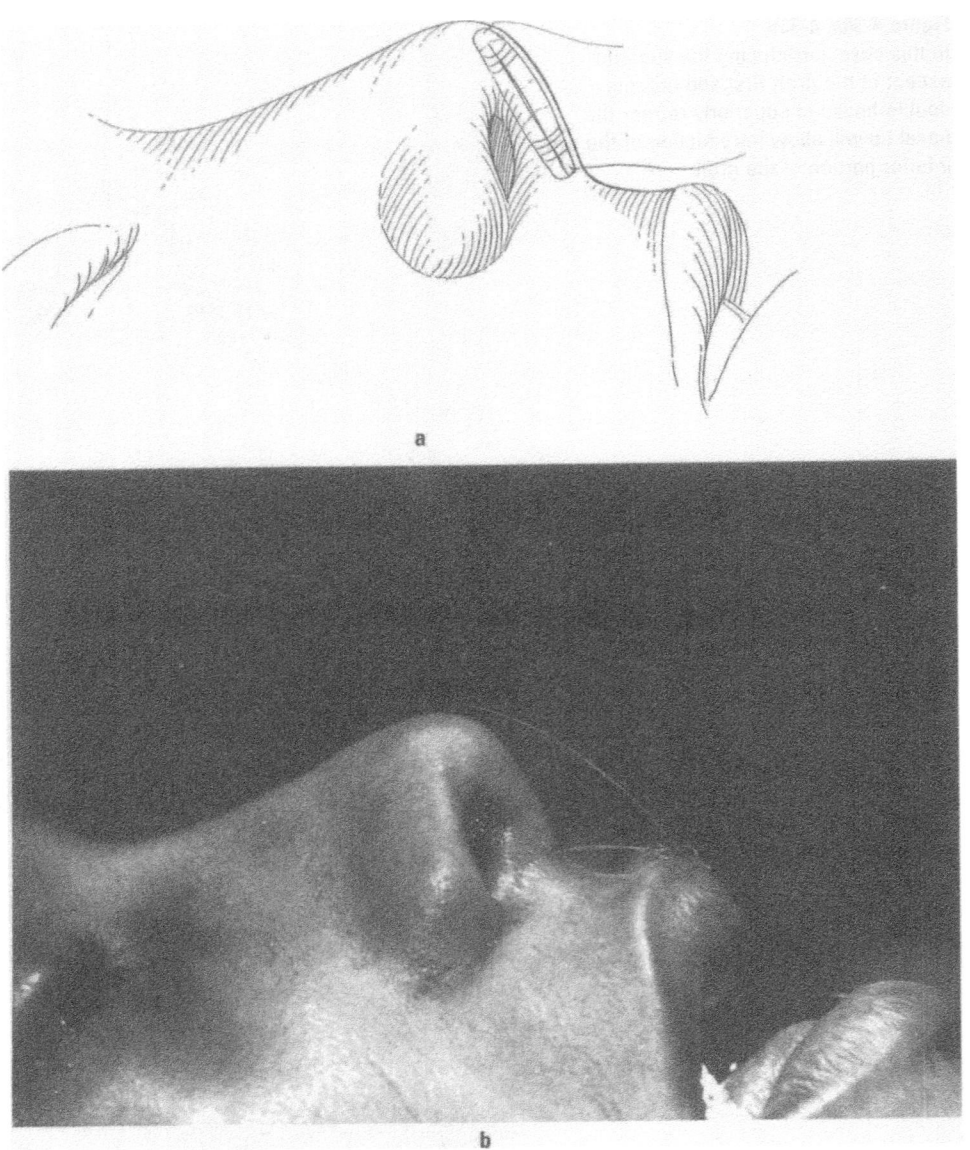

It is essential that the graft is midline (Fig 4-38a, 4-38b). After irrigation, complete soft-tissue closure is mandatory. The inferior medial crural footplates are approximated with the use of 4-0 chromic catgut. The intervening tip graft cartilage is incorporated in the suturing for positioning and stabilization.

This patient had a flat, undefined tip. A "pea-pod" tip graft and crushed septal cartilage to the dorsum were placed. Crushed septal cartilage was also placed over the maxilla at the nasal spine (Fig. 4-38c, 4-38d, 4-38e, 4-38f, on page 90).

This was the patient's second rhinoplasty. Medical records were not available and details of the initial procedure were not known. The previous procedure overresected the dorsum and alar cartilages, resulting in a loss of support. The patient had a low dorsum, supratip fullness, and hanging

Figure 4-38a, 4-38b
The base of the graft is placed 3 to 5
mm above the columella-labial crease
to create a normal "break."

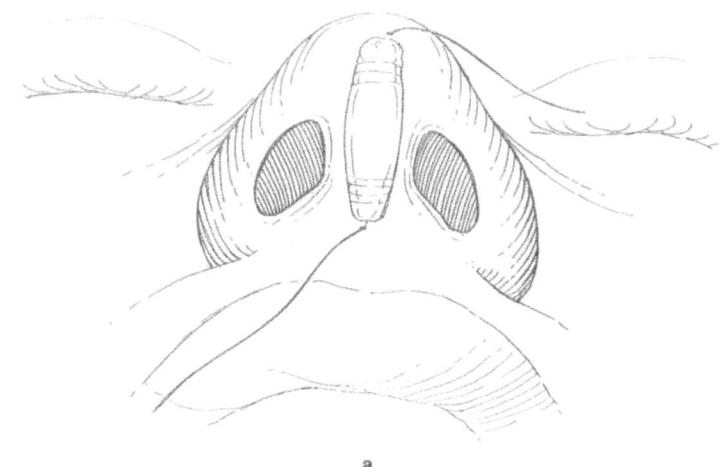

a

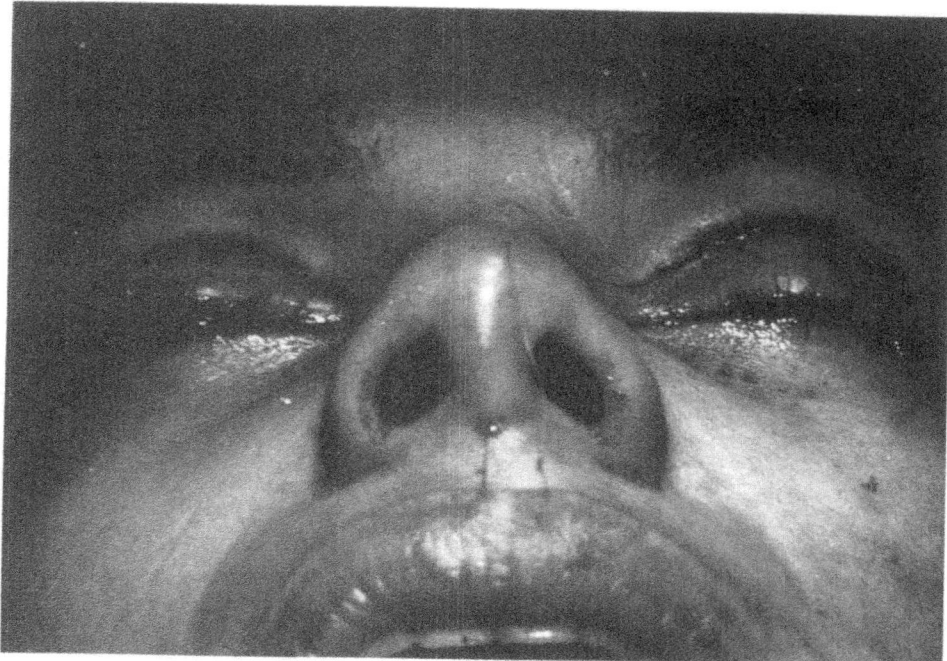

b

columella, as well as a shortened upper lip with a 90-degree columellar angle and a flattened, nondefined tip point (Fig. 4-39a, 4-39b, on page 91).

The "pea-pod" nasal tip graft was created using two 3 cm × .75 cm convex conchal cartilage segments wrapped in Dexon with pull-out sutures placed through the apex and base. A right rim-columellar incision was made just behind the medial footplate, but anterior to the alar cartilages. Any incision scar anterior-inferior to the cartilages is hidden, very similar to the "open" technique, but without any columellar incision. The tip graft was then placed into the pocket with the tip pull-out suture placed at the desired apex. The graft base was then placed approximately .25 cm above the nasolabial junction (when not possible, the soft tissue base is placed at or near the columellar-nasal junction to create a break point) (Fig 4-39c, 4-39d, on page 92).

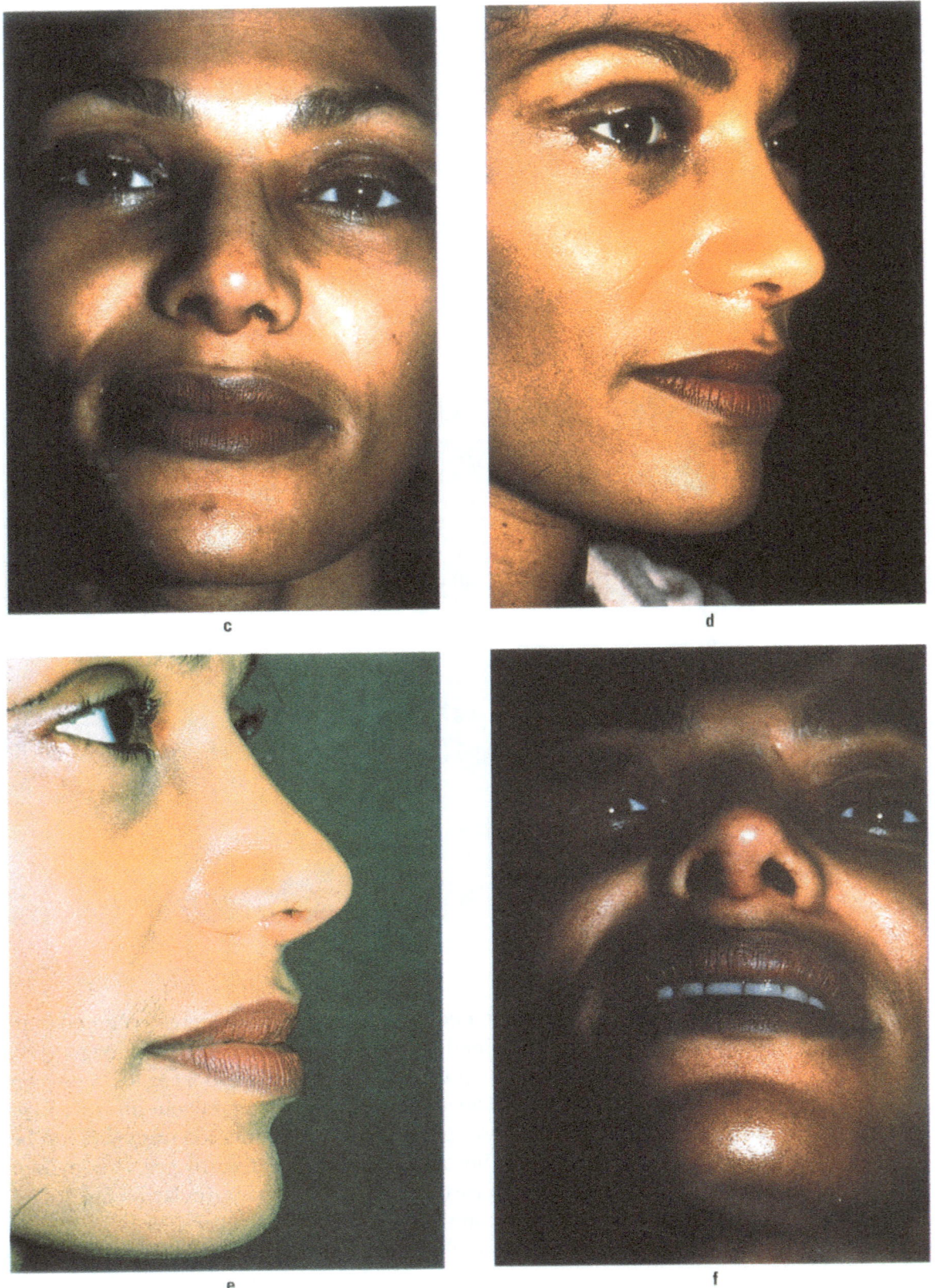

Figure 4-38c, 4-38d, 4-38e, 4-38f
The nose has greater projection due to
the placement of the "pea-pod" graft.

Early intraoperative results show a slight increase in the patient's dorsum, as desired. The "pea-pod" tip graft is in place, rotating and projecting the tip superiorly and at the proper tip point. The tip break point is seen, created by the tip graft. Stabilization of the graft was performed by mattress sutures of 4-0 plain catgut, and secured with 5-0 Dexon and 5-0 plain catgut. The aesthetic results of the "pea-pod" tip graft show increased tip projection and a semblance of a thinner, more angular, and defined tip (Fig. 4-39e, on page 93).

Postoperatively, the patient has a thinner, but more projecting bridge. The tip is better defined, with the tip point at the placement of the apexed pull-out suture. The alar wedge resections were conservative. The columellar-labial angle is open. The "pea-pod" tip graft has added stabilization, definition, and angulation to the tip. The "tenting" effect creates a semblance of a thinner tip without thinning the skin or dermis (Fig. 4-39f, 4-39g, on page 93).

Graft stabilization sutures are normally pulled up and trimmed 5 days after surgery. If any graft movement or distortion has occurred, adjustments can be made by applying tension to the suture and then waiting another 2 to 3 days before trimming. These stabilization sutures can also be incorporated with additional deeper sutures that go from the graft to the surrounding soft tissue and alar cartilage. This will help to avoid lateral or posterior drift of the tip graft.

Figure 4-39a, 4-39b
Preoperative views of flat, unsupported nasal tip prior to placement of the "pea-pod" graft. This patient had a thick, poorly projecting tip.

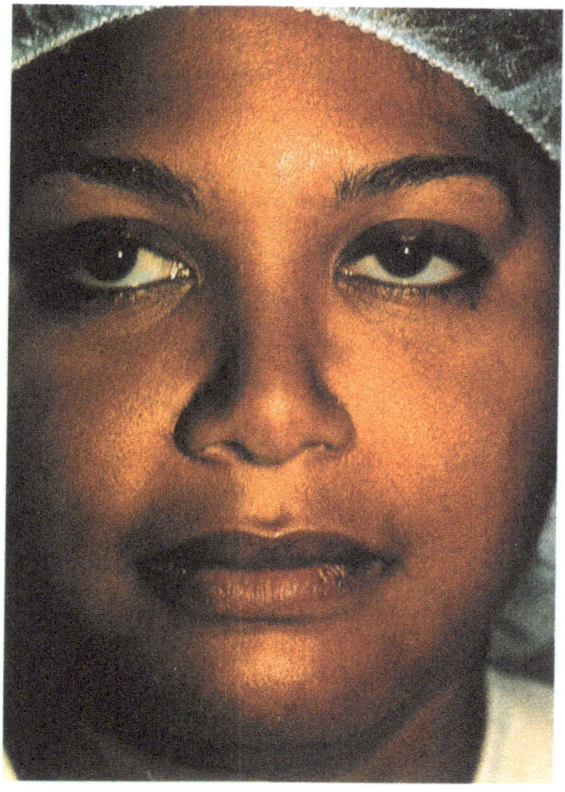

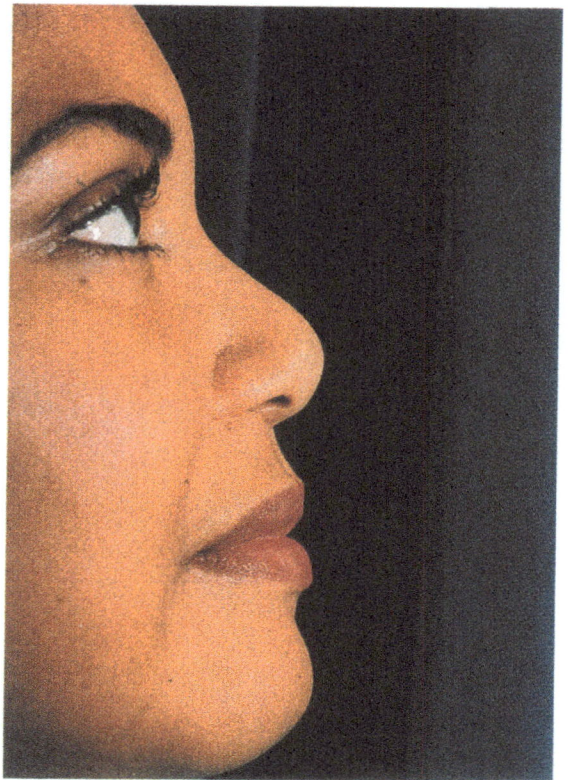

a

b

Figure 4-39c, 4-39d
Placement of 3 cm × .75 "pea-pod"
graft through a right rim incision.

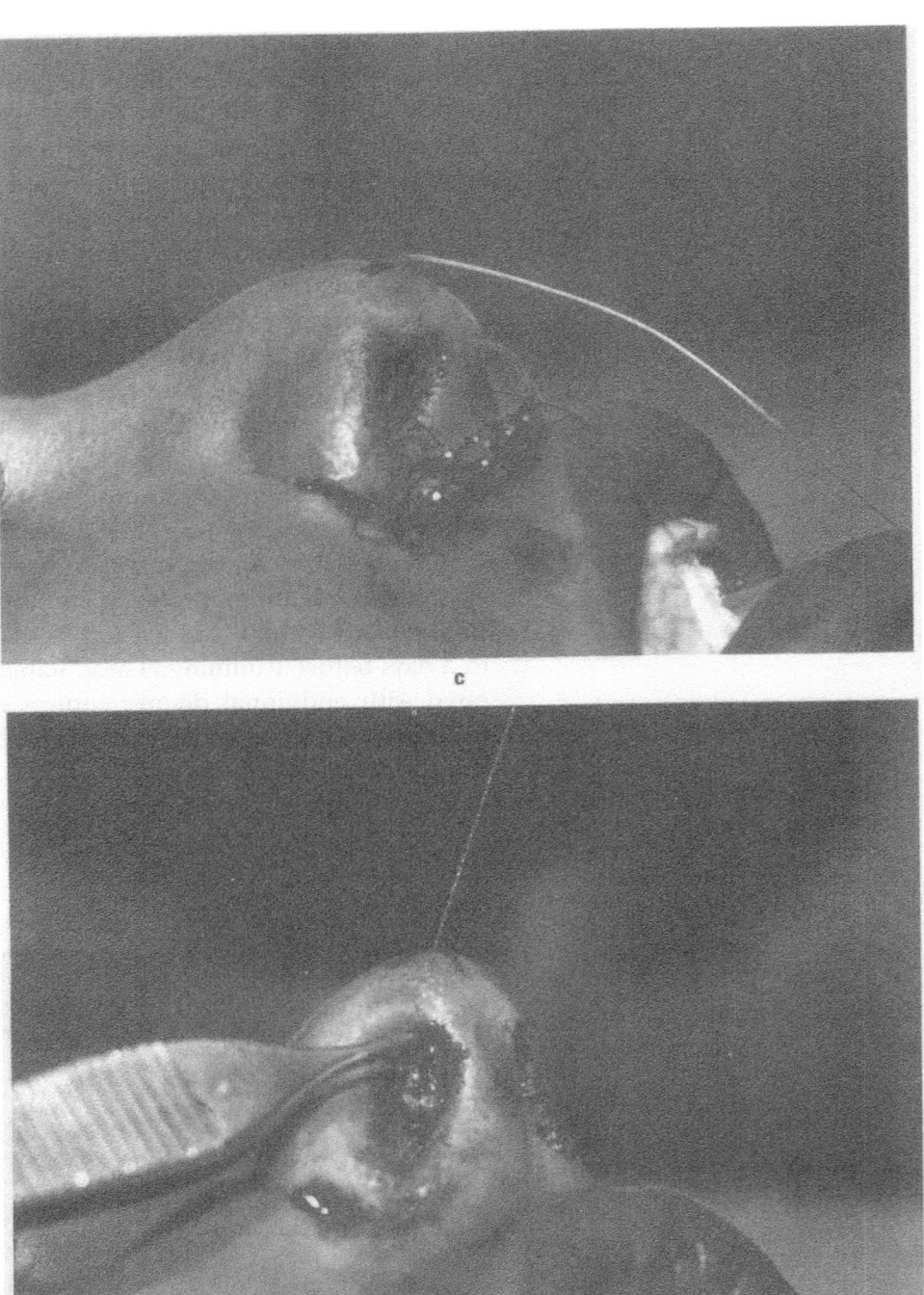

c

d

Chapter Four   **Personal Ethnic Rhinoplasty Technique**

Figure 4-39e
Placement of 3 cm × .75 "pea-pod"
graft through a right rim incision.

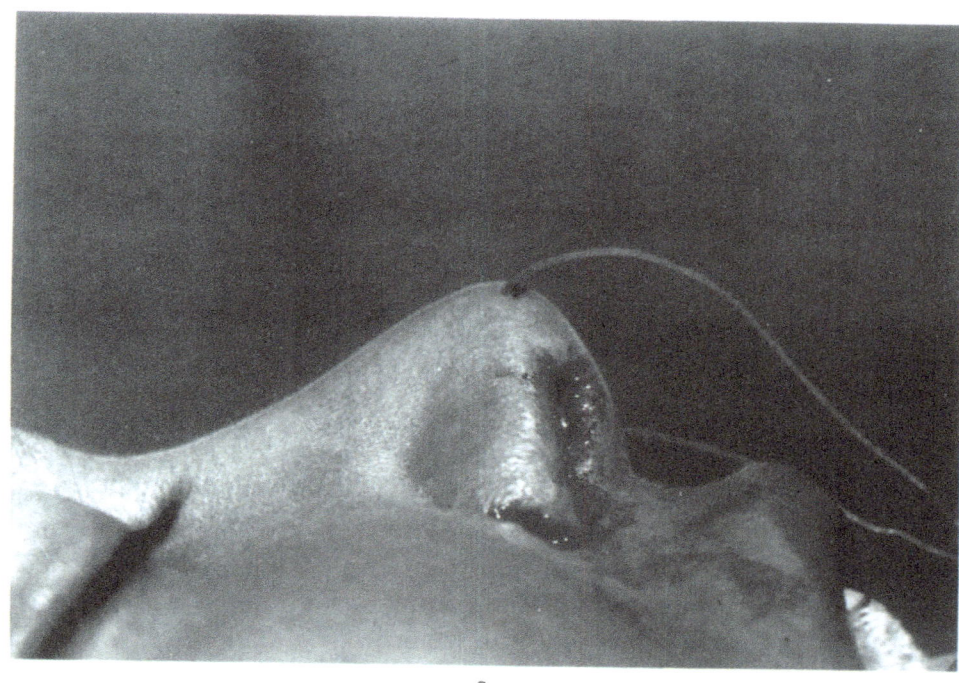

e

Figure 4-39f, 4-39g
An early postoperative result shows
that the "pea-pod" graft gives good
projection and definition, despite the
presence of edema. Aesthetic results
of the "pea-pod" graft: increase in tip
projection and the semblance of a thinner, more angular nose.

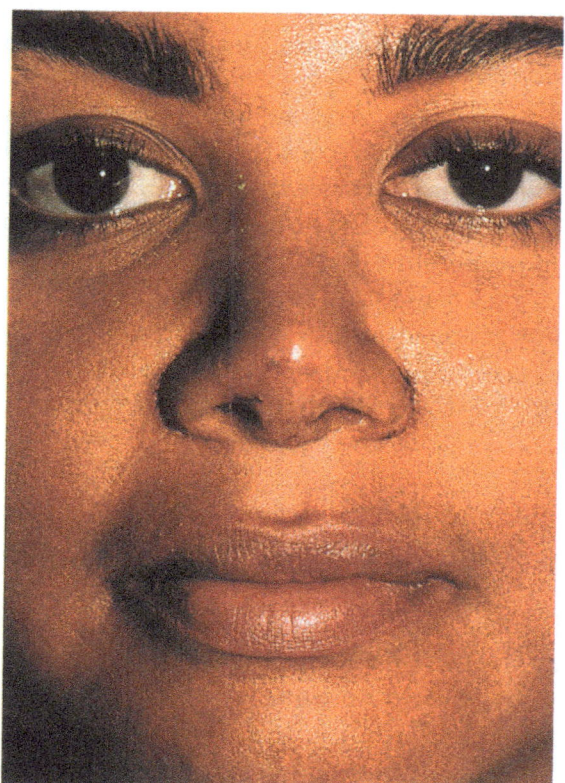

f

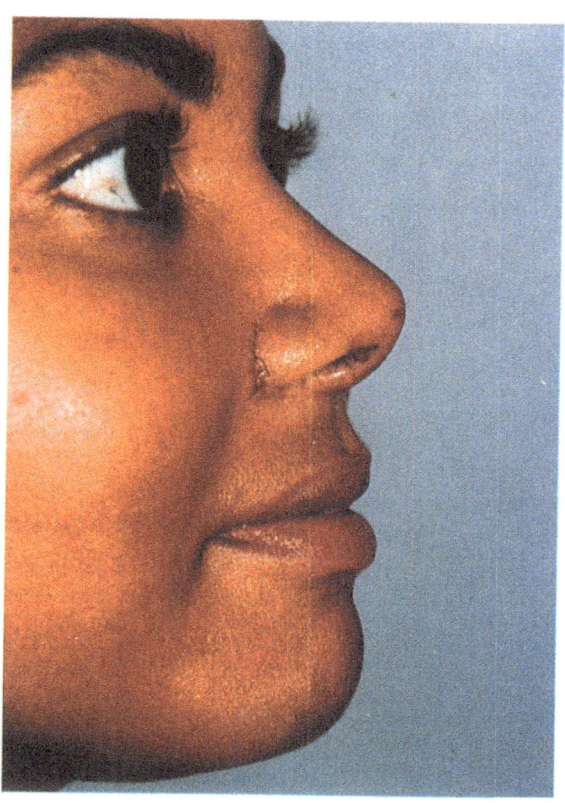

g

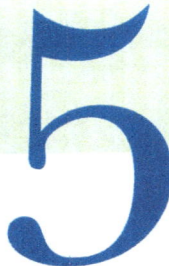

Postoperative Nasal Packing and Dressings

Nasal packing is sometimes feared by patients because discomfort can accompany its use and (especially) removal. Even so, packing may be important to avoid bleeding, stenosis, synechiae, and recurrent airway obstruction when performing septal reconstruction or turbinectomy. Discomfort can result from packing that is too tight, but more commonly results from a patient's inability to breathe through the nose with attendant pressure symptoms.

Merocel nasal tampons provide soft but adequate packing. They have a central airway that helps to equilibrate nasopharyngeal pressure. Tampon removal can be facilitated by soaking the tampon with local anesthetic prior to removal. For patients who cannot tolerate any discomfort, intravenous sedation brevital sodium (Brevital) can be administered prior to removal.

Gel-foam and other loose nasal packings do not provide the degree of pressure needed to stop the oozing or bleeding that occurs with major septal or turbinate work. But these lighter packings are ideal for smaller procedures.

Postoperative tape, splints, and dressings are helpful in several ways. First, they provide gentle pressure, which increases the patient's sense of security. Second, they aid in stabilizing osteotomies and grafts. Finally, they assist in decreasing edema. The author prefers a thin, well-padded, aluminum splint that "gives" with postoperative swelling.

The *appearance* of nasal dressings can also be important. Patients often equate the neatness and quality of the dressing with the quality of the surgery itself. A small, uniform, carefully placed dressing goes a long way toward alleviating patient postoperative anxiety about the surgery itself.

Packing Technique

Packing may be indicated after turbinate and/or septal surgery. The author uses a cannulated Merocel nasal tampon, cut to size and carefully wrapped in Telfa, trimmed so it does not extend past or occlude the ends of the central airway tube. The outer Telfa surface is then covered with antibiotic ointment and placed in the nasal cavity. Once inserted, a small amount of saline with bacitracin zinc (Bacitracin) is dripped onto the tampon to incite expansion, thus affording good intranasal pressure. Normal nasal secretions are trapped between the mucosa and the nonabsorbable surface of the Telfa, thus acting as a natural lubricant that facilitates subsequent removal.

Decongestant and antibiotic coverage continues until the packs are removed, anywhere from the 1st to 5th day postoperatively.

For patients who cannot tolerate the pain associated with packing removal, a properly monitored program of intravenous brevital sodium (Brevital) provides comfort for removing the nasal packs, and is very much appreciated.

Nasal Dressings

Benzoin, Steri-Strips, or brown paper adhesive tape, and an individually cut, form-fitting, aluminum splint are gently molded into place and covered with adhesive tape (Fig. 5-1 to 5-6). Heat-treated plastic or plaster splints are al-

Figures 5-1, 5-2, 5-3, 5-4, 5-5, 5-6
Proper postoperative nasal taping is important in stabilizing the nose, decreasing swelling, and expressing aesthetic creativity. It should be conservative in volume and gently compressive so tip circulation is not compromised. Leaving the tip apex uncovered affords an opportunity to inspect the skin color. Pinching the tip of the tape is a good way to apply controlled pressure. In addition, the tape supports the pull-out suture at the nasal tip, which contributes to the final positioning of the graft. These sutures will be removed in 5 days. To decrease crustiness and facilitate future suture removal, a small nonadhering dressing can be placed over the alar suture line, if indicated.

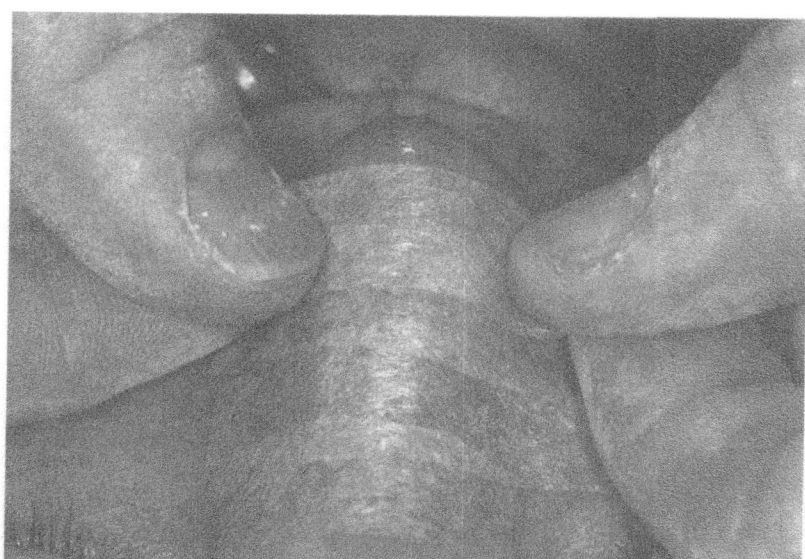

Figure 5-1

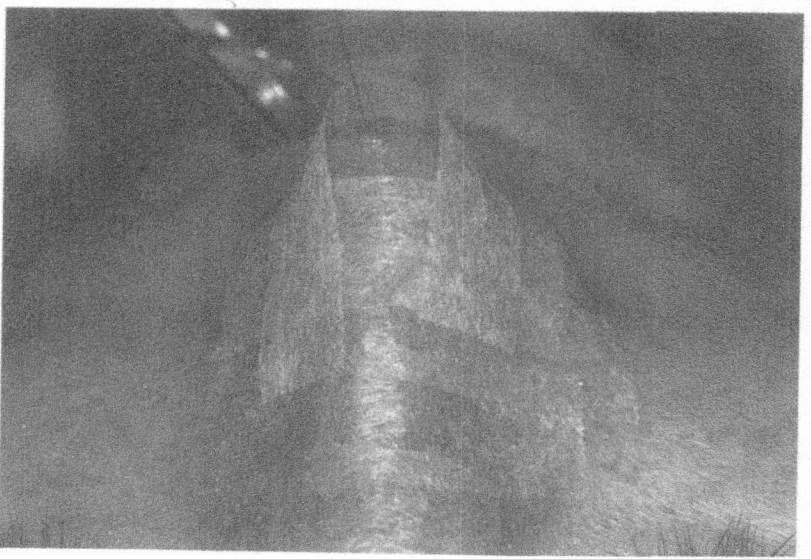

Figure 5-2

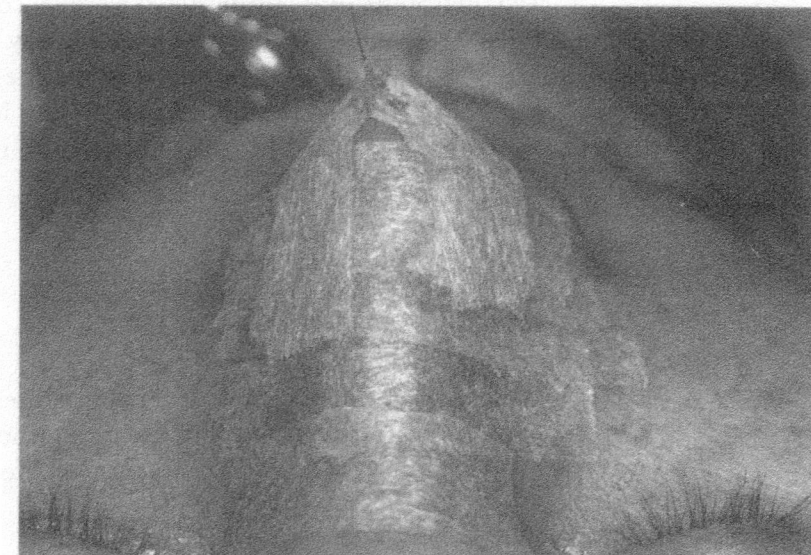

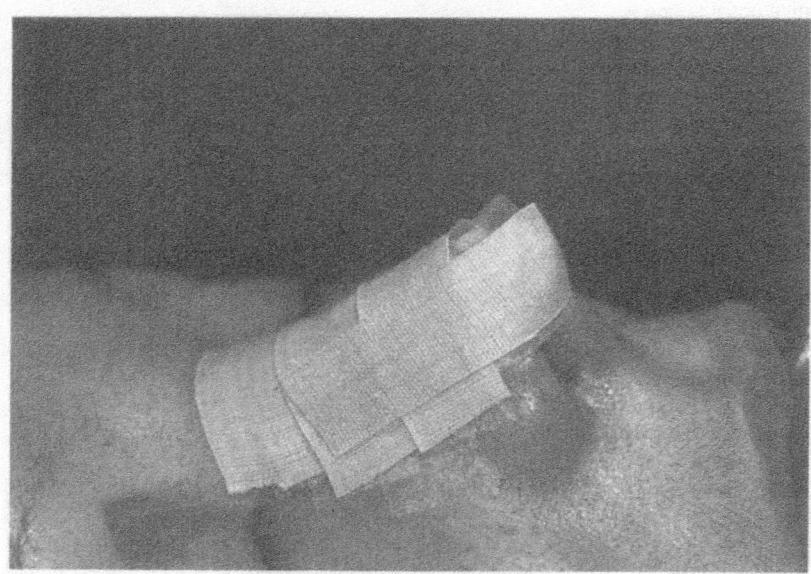

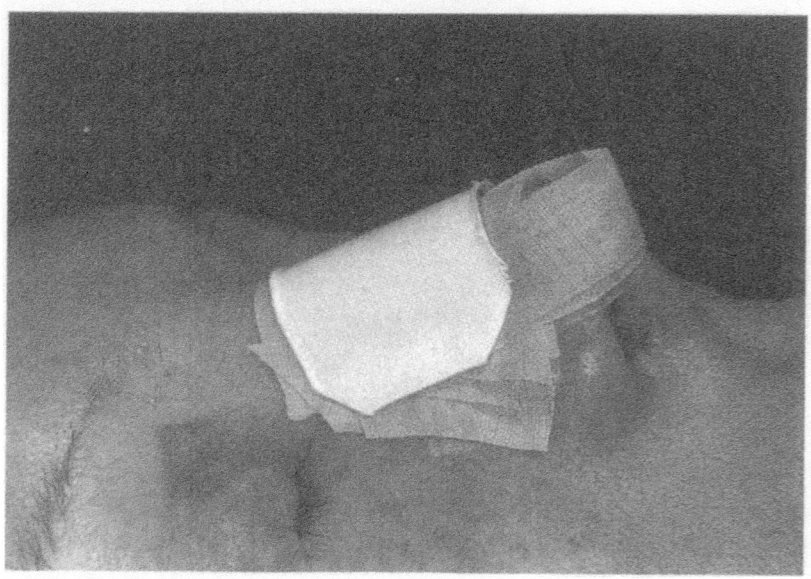

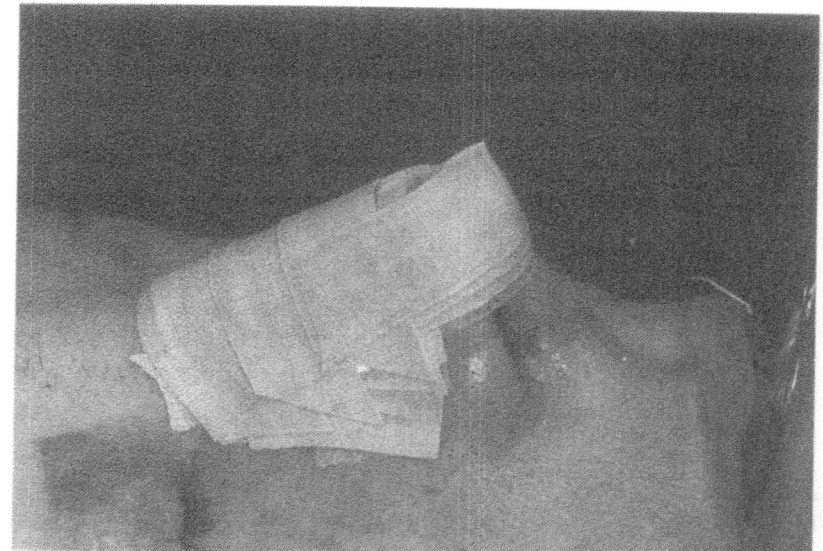

Figure 5-7
The conchal bowl is packed with Vaseline gauze to help maintain contour and to eliminate dead space. A greater auricular nerve block has been performed. The ear(s) are elevated twenty degrees to thirty degrees off the head by placing the gauze in the postauricular sulcus. In addition, a protective C-shaped arrangement of gauze may be placed around the ear prior to the application of a head dressing.

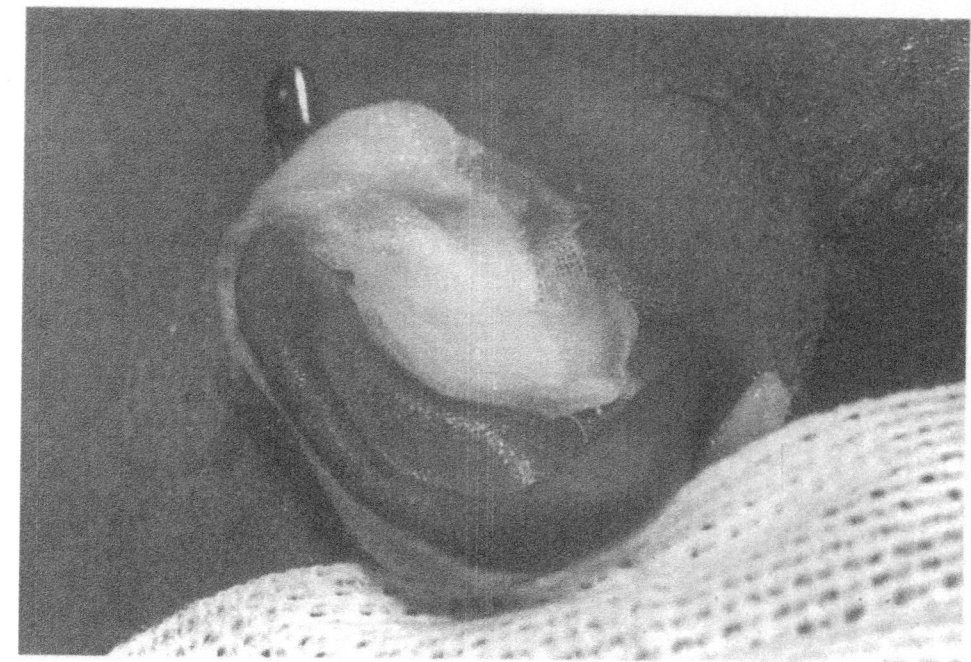

ternatives but are not as yielding. If tip vascularity needs monitoring, a small area is left untaped for easy viewing.

Conchal Cartilage Donor Site Dressings

The conchal cup is form-fitted with petroleum jelly (Vaseline) gauze. Molding the cup helps maintain soft-tissue shape and decreases dead space. The ear is elevated 20 degrees to 30 degrees off the head with the use of further gauze sponges (Fig. 5-7). 3-0 silk sutures can also be used as bolsters, or a gentle head dressing can be placed. All dressings are removed in 48 to 72 hours.

Postoperative Care

1. Appropriate nasal splints, taping, and dressings are applied.
2. Nasal pack dressings are removed in 1 to 5 days. The patient can be given a light brevital sodium (Brevital) anesthetic if necessary for comfort during removal. The Merocel packing is soaked with local topical anesthetic and easily slipped out.
3. Alar sutures are removed in 5 to 7 days.
4. The nasal tip is paper taped in a compression fashion each night for up to 6 weeks, when indicated.
5. Dilute triamcinolone acetonide injections (Kenalog 2.5–5 mg/cc) may be indicated after 6 weeks to decrease swelling in some cases. The solution is gently injected into the supratip or tip. The thick skin of the ethnic nose usually shows no atrophy with cautiously administered injections.
6. Additional procedures or revisions are not performed for at least 12 months.

6

Postoperative Patient Instructions

Complete written postoperative instructions are important for patients and those caring for them, and should be given to each patient after a complicated procedure like rhinoplasty. The following is a basic instruction list used in the author's office for rhinoplasty patients:

What to Expect Postoperatively

1. Some oozing from the nose is expected for a day or two, and a small gauze "mustache" dressing may be worn as a drip pad. You can change or remove it as necessary. Do NOT swallow blood because it can cause nausea.

2. Small amounts of dried mucus and blood may start to collect in the nose. On the 2nd day after surgery, the nostrils may be gently cleaned by carefully following these instructions:
   a. Mix equal amounts of lukewarm water and hydrogen peroxide in a small glass.
   b. Dip a cotton swap in this solution and very gently cleanse the edge of the nostrils and rim of your nose.
   c. Wait a few seconds for your nose to dry. Then using a different cotton swab, apply a thin coat of Vicks Vaporub, bacitracin, or Vaseline.

3. The inside of your nose may be moistened as often as you like with a balanced salt spray such as Ocean Spray (available from your pharmacy without prescription). The spray helps loosen any crusts. Be very gentle. Crusts should not be forcefully cleansed or pulled on. Allow the crusts to loosen on their own.

4. A pediatric suction bulb (available from any drug store) can be used to suction nasal secretions. After the splint is removed, you may blow your nose in a very gentle, nonforceful way. When blowing your nose, put light pressure on the top of the nose to decrease swelling.

5. It may be necessary to become a "mouth breather" for a short time. Avoid any activity that might induce sneezing, such as eyebrow plucking. When sneezing is unavoidable, sneeze with your mouth open.

6. Using a child's smaller toothbrush may be more comfortable during the early recovery stages.

7. If septal and/or turbinate surgery has been performed, there may be small sponge tampon packing inside your nose which has a small

breathing tube in the center. These packs are removed 4 to 5 days after surgery. Removal takes about an hour. A light-sleep anesthesia is used so you experience no pain. No food or drink is allowed for 6 hours prior to a visit for nasal tampon removal, and you must be accompanied to and from the doctor's office.

8. A form-fitting tape-splint dressing is also worn across the nose for 4 to 5 days. The packing is removed with the splint. The nose is then lightly taped for an additional day or two to decrease swelling.

9. As a result of taping, the skin of your nose may peel or may have developed clogged pores, whiteheads, or blackheads. Use a Cetaphil gentle cleansing bar three times per day to help clear up any such skin problems. If moderate irritation occurs, withhold nasal taping for 2 to 3 days until the skin irritation clears up.

10. A slight-to-moderate amount of bruising around the eyes is common. This usually disappears in 7 to 10 days. Slight oozing near the inner eye is due to a small puncture drain site which markedly decreases bruising and heals with an imperceptible scar. Only rarely, some bruising on the white of the eye may also occur and should disappear in 2 to 3 weeks. Numbness, especially at the tip of the nose, may be present, but will rapidly go away.

11. Use a couple of pillows to elevate your head when reclining or sleeping to help reduce swelling and bruising. Ice compresses will also help and are prepared as follows: fill a plastic bowl with ice cubes, water, and a shake of salt. Soak and wring out gauze pads, a small wash cloth, or the custom terrycloth pads provided by our office. Place them over the surgical site—10 minutes on, 5 minutes off. Never use ice bags directly against the skin, which may be numb due to local anesthetic and swelling.

12. Showers may be resumed on the 2nd day after surgery, but the splint and dressings should be covered with a towel or shower cap to keep them dry (it is acceptable if they get a bit damp from the ice-water compresses). If dressings become loose, cellophane (Scotch) tape or additional paper tape can be used to hold them in place. They should NOT be removed.

13. Dark rings infrequently occur around the eyes, especially if you are dark-complected. They will disappear with time. After your nasal splint is removed, you can use cover makeup around your eyes, if you desire.

14. Swelling, particularly at the nasal tip, may persist for several months, depending on the thickness of your skin. Our taping program is very helpful to eliminate any swelling, and you should closely follow the instructions for optimum results. In rare cases, swelling may not totally disappear for 1 to 2 years. Swelling is usually more apparent in the morning when you get up, and usually subsides as the day progresses (Figs. 6-1, 6-2).

15. To minimize swelling, avoid excessive bending and heavy lifting for at least 2 weeks. Also reduce salt and spices from your diet. Sunbathing, saunas, and extremely hot showers can also contribute to swelling and should be avoided for 6 to 12 weeks.

Figures 6-1, 6-2
This patient has not had surgery; her nasal tip swelling was a result of allergies. Nasal tip fullness was reduced within 2 weeks of nighttime tip taping. Although the results were only temporary in this patient, it is a helpful technique.

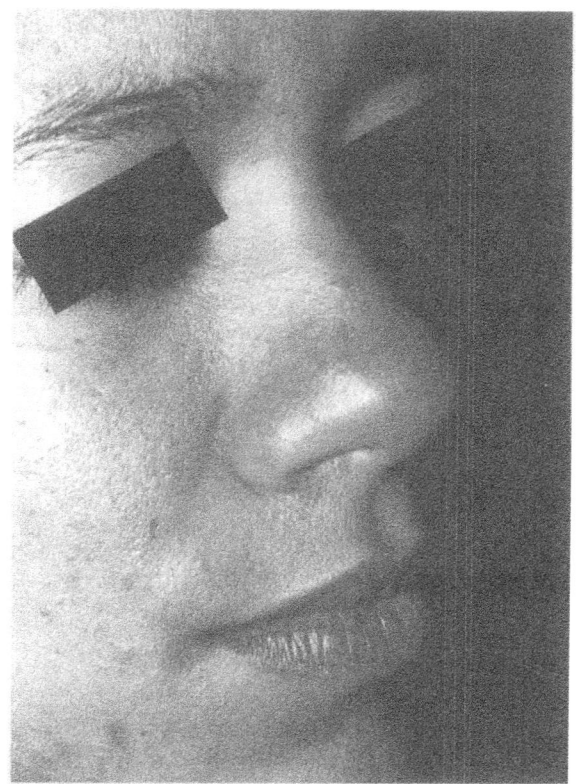

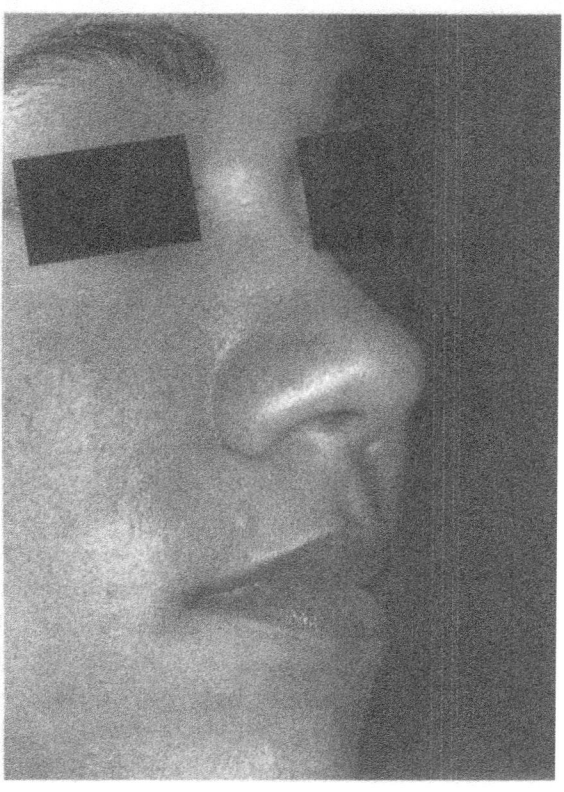

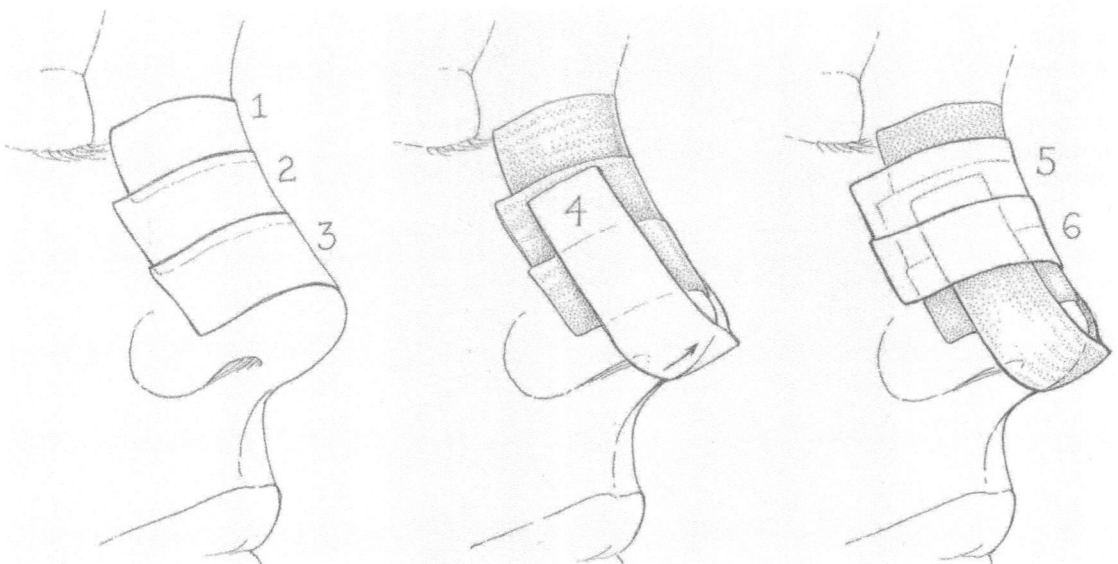

Figure 6-3
A most frequent complaint is nasal tip swelling after rhinoplasty. Despite attempts at intraoperative and early postoperative control, persistent induration and tip swelling can occur. It may last many months. Patients are generally quite pleased with the results of a nighttime taping program for 6–10 weeks postoperatively. Volumes of experience have been recorded about the successful use of compression garments for lymphedema, vascular incompetency, and early burn scar hypertrophy. The same principle applies to the nasal tip.

The following instructions are given to the patient: Gently "pressure taping" of the tip of your nose at night will help decrease swelling and improve the shape. Wash your nose with mild soap and water and dab dry. Wait 10 minutes. Cut six 2-inch strips of paper tape. Apply the first three strips as shown in the diagram, from the top of your nose to just in back of the tip, pressing down tightly. Place the fourth piece just underneath the tip, as shown, elevating the tip and pinching the end of the tape tightly but gently. Do not hurt yourself. If this causes any discomfort, apply in a more gentle fashion with less pressure. Apply the fifth and sixth pieces over the top for stabilization, as shown. This should be performed each night for the next several weeks. If your skin becomes irritated or breaks out, stop taping until irritation disappears.

16. Swelling normally disappears as follows: half in 2 to 3 weeks, another fourth over 8 to 12 weeks, and the last fourth in 6 to 12 months. After 2 or 3 weeks most patients find that, although some residual swelling may be noticeable to themselves, it is not noticeable to others.

17. Infrequently, a patient may feel (but rarely see) slight irregularities in the nose during the healing process. Bone, cartilage, and some layers of the skin have a propensity to develop small, temporary lumps under the surface while healing. These lumps occur most often near the inside of the eyes, near the bridge of the nose where bones join the cartilage, and just above, and to the sides of, the nose tip. The irregularities are usually callous tissue, enlarged glands, or thickened incision lines. They normally disappear with time. Swelling in these areas starts to subside about 10 days after surgery and usually disappears in 4 to 6 weeks. In addition to our regular taping program, light finger pressure can help reduce swelling. Gently use the tip of the index finger and press down for 10 seconds, once an hour.

18. You may notice some temporary nasal congestion or increased sensitivity to smoke or air conditioning for several weeks. If this stuffiness is bothersome to you, your surgeon can prescribe a nasal spray such as Nasalide. In cases where extensive structural work is to be performed inside the nose, your doctor may prescribe this spray for use *before* surgery to lessen postoperative swelling and stuffiness.

19. You can wear glasses over your splint. But after the splint is removed, glasses should not rest on the nose. Instead, they must be taped to your forehead or held in place by a special cheek-resting device (which can be supplied by the doctor) for the first 2 weeks.

20. Most patients say they feel better than expected after surgery and are able to return to work and social activities in 7 to 10 days.

21. Light exercise can be resumed at 2 weeks. But strenuous or contact sports, such as swimming, volleyball, football, basketball, and wrestling,

must be delayed for 6 to 12 weeks. Resumption of activities depends to a great extent on how you feel, how quickly your swelling subsides, and whether the activity is likely to increase your swelling, or even jeopardize the results of your surgery.

22. If you must travel by air within 6 weeks of your surgery, take a 30 mg pseudoephedrine decongestant tablet such as Sudafed 1 hour before landing. This will decrease the amount of air or fluid in your sinuses, thereby minimizing the discomfort that can result from changes in air pressure.

23. Contrary to old rumors, a properly performed nasal operation very rarely results in any detrimental voice change. Nasal surgery has been performed on many well-known singers with no detrimental change in their voices. In fact, many have noticed improvement.

24. Soft-tissue swelling can be markedly reduced during the first 3 to 6 weeks by gently pressure taping at night (Fig. 6-3). Gentle pressure taping also helps improve the nose's shape. In some cases, taping may be appropriate for longer periods.

Risks, Complications, and Revisions

Although we surgeons like to think of ourselves as perfectionists, none of us is perfect. The results of human enterprise cannot be guaranteed, and plastic surgery is certainly no exception. There are potential risks and complications involved with any surgical procedure. When patients are informed and aware of the risks as well as the standard procedures for managing those risks they are better able to understand, accept, and cope with a complication. A written explanation of all risks and potential complications should, therefore, be given to each patient and is not only very helpful to the patient but can be invaluable to the surgeon medically/legally. The following are the most frequently seen complications in ethnic rhinoplasty. Several are relatively more common than in Caucasian rhinoplasty.

Bleeding

Although some incisional oozing is expected for a few hours or days after surgery, heavy bleeding is unusual. Most cases of major bleeding result from some form of turbinate surgery. Cross-clamping, excising, and then cauterizing the anterior portion of the inferior turbinate is generally safe. But excising turbinate tissue deep in the nose that may not have been adequately cross-clamped can lead to bleeding. Adequately packing the deeper areas of the nose can also be difficult.

It is also important that patients avoid both aspirin and aspirinlike products. Hypertension must be adequately controlled (Fig. 7-1a, 7-1b). A thorough medical history and template bleeding time will uncover virtually any bleeding disorder.

Prolonged Bruising or Hyperpigmentation

When osteotomies are performed, infraorbital bruising is expected. In darker complexions with increased melanocytic activity and early hemosiderin deposition, prolonged bruising or pigmentation sometimes occurs. Patients who have a history of hyperpigmentation problems should be forewarned. Absolute protection from sun exposure is mandatory for as long

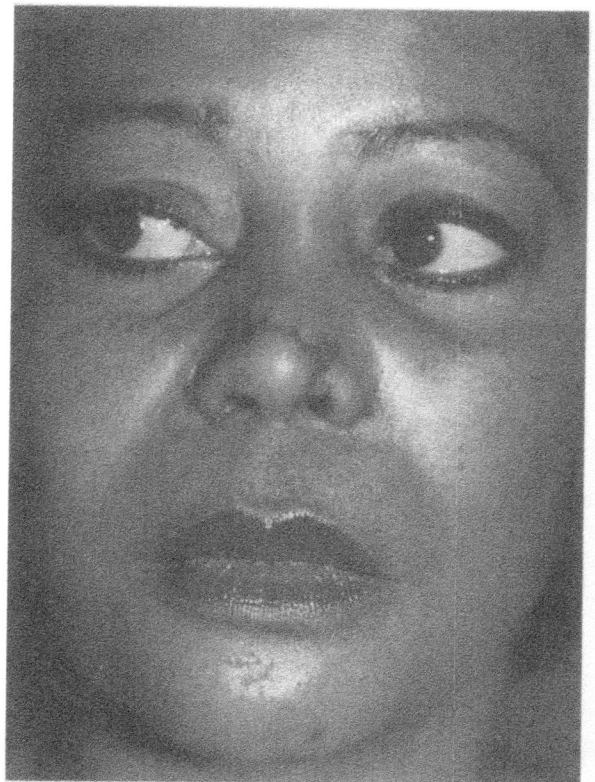 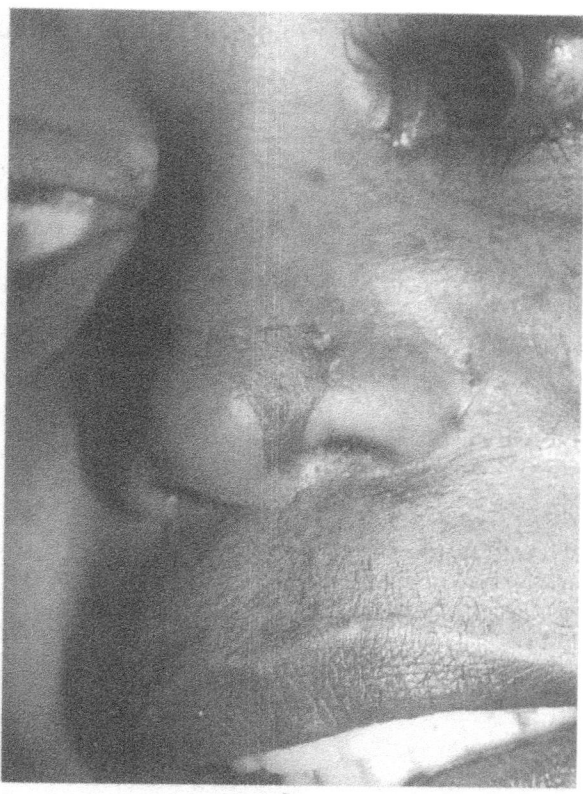

Figure 7-1a, 7-1b
This patient was hypertensive. Inadequate control of the hypertension led to nasal flap bleeding postoperatively. Dressings were removed 48 hours after surgery and the skin compromise noted. Secondary healing occurred, full-thickness skin grafting and multiple injections with dilute steroid followed.

as bruising and swelling persist. In severe cases total resolution of periorbital hyperpigmentation may take anywhere from 2 to 9 months.

Ethnic pigmentation irregularities and scarring in darker skin colors is frequently more noticeable at nasal incision lines. It is important to always discuss possible pigmentation changes and scarring with patients during the initial consultation and again immediately preoperatively. Hypopigmented scarring may be more easily remedied by tattooing that by revision procedures. If scarring is hypertrophic, judicious use of triamcinolone acetonide suspension 10 mg/ml (Kenalog) is beneficial. In any case, revisions or tattooing should wait at least 6 months to a year.

Infection

Postoperative sinus infections may be more common than previously thought. Factors leading to infection include temporary sinus blockade due to edema, presence of blood (acting as an excellent culture medium), or nasal bacterial colonization. Meticulous intranasal prepping, preoperative intravenous antibiotics, postoperative oral antibiotics, and decongestants are indicated. Cartilage graft infections can also occur. Frequent irrigation of the pocket with dilute povidine-iodine cleanser (Betadine) and thorough irrigation of the graft prior to placement are very helpful in reducing the likelihood of infection. Any obvious graft infection should be treated with immediately drainage, culture-specific antibiotics, and, if possible, frequent irrigation.

Prominent Alar or Postauricular Scarring

Significant alar scarring may result from many factors among which the most common are:

Excessive tension with subsequent wound separation

Suture reaction

Early epithelialization along large pores and/or suture tracts

Asymmetrical or misplaced incisions

Figure 7-2a, 7-2b
Overresection and improper matching of the alae to the cheek skin resulted in the unnatural appearance of the alar base. Unless there is an excess amount of alar tissue, correction is quite difficult. However, advancement of the cheek may sometimes provide sufficient tissue to help give a more natural appearance.

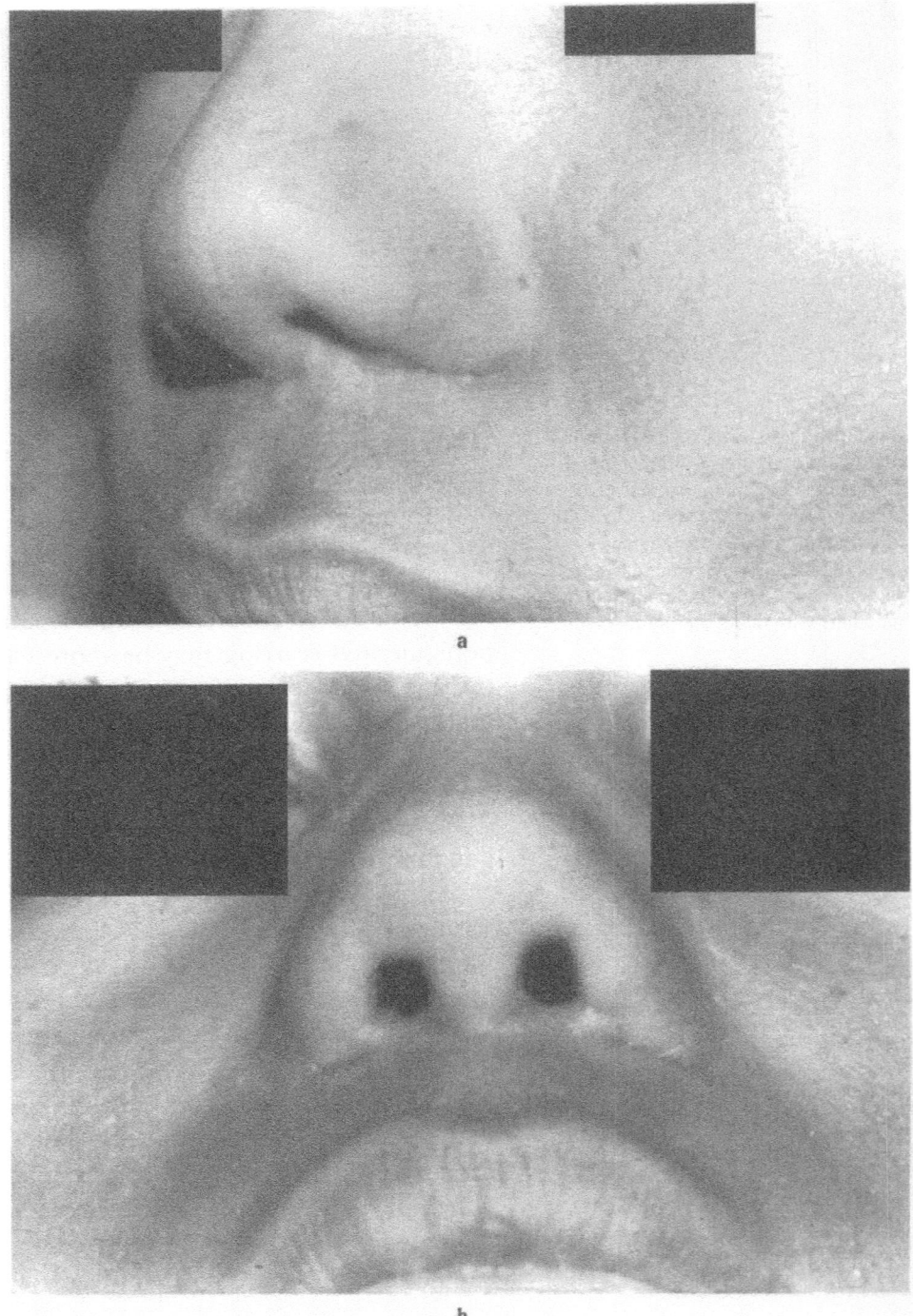

Hypertrophic scars or keloids in this area are extremely rare, in my experience. Secondary alar scar revisions should be performed cautiously, since it is easy to distort the shape of the alae and create a very unnatural appearance. During revision, the combination of excision of the scar and medial advancement and suturing of the cheek helps to prevent lateral pulling and subsequent straightening of the alar side wall (Fig. 7-2a, 7-2b). A minimum of 6 to 12 months should elapse prior to scar revision.

Excessive Alar Reduction

Erroneously removing too much tissue (Fig. 7-3a, 7-3b) or insufficiently undermining and advancing the cheek skin may result in flat alae with loss of natural base curves. After a period of 6 to 12 months, opening the incision and then undermining and advancing the cheek skin medially may provide improvement and stabilization.

Skin Reaction

Acne and other skin conditions are common in thick, sebaceous skin often seen in ethnic patients. Preoperative treatment with tretinoin (Retin-A) may be helpful. Reactions to tape applications may result in hyperpigmentation, which can be treated with a combination of Retin-A and hydroquinone.

Figure 7-3a, 7-3b
Excessively full, flaring alae present a significant contouring challenge. Intra-operative serial excisions and trial approximations may have to be performed in several attempts before a natural but adequately excised alar base results. To avoid asymmetry, very detailed measurements and exact excisions are important. It is wise to start with a limited alar excision before approximating the area. Further excision can easily be carried out as needed. But if too much alar tissue is excised, it is extremely difficult, if not impossible, to correct. This patient's early postoperative result shows probable overresection of the left ala. Notice the horizontally shaped right nostril and the vertrically shaped left nostril. Preserving a triangular base with slight convexity of the lateral alar wall is desirable.

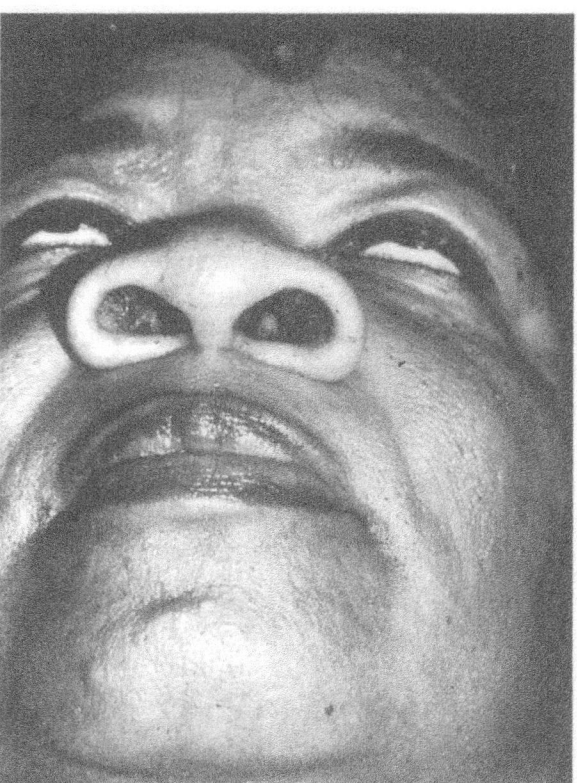
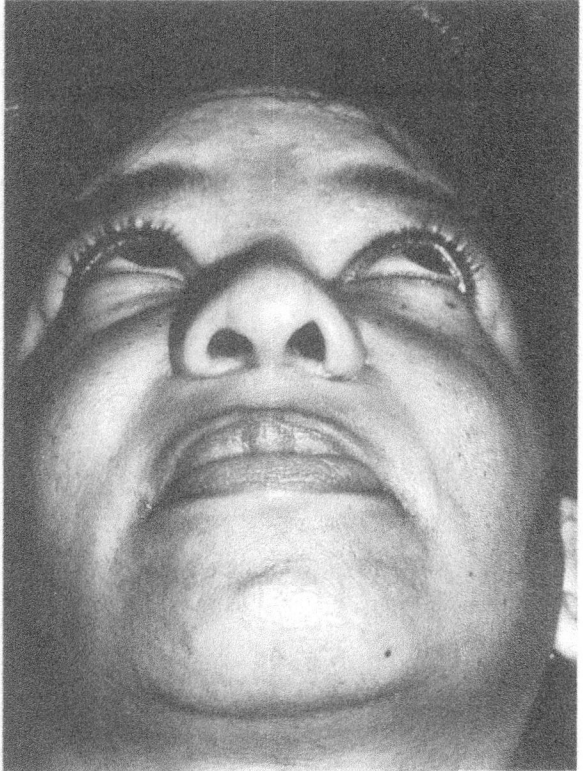

a   b

Airway Obstruction

The most frequent source of postoperative airway obstruction is turbinate hypertrophy. Conservative treatments such as topical cortisone, nasal sprays, or dilute steroid injections may help resolve postoperative swelling. Temporary reactive turbinate swelling can occur for a number of reasons, such as:

1. Osteotomies just adjacent to the turbinates may cause bleeding into the turbinate area. The prominent vascularity of the turbinates can result in secondary swelling. If airway obstruction still persists 3 to 6 months postoperatively, further turbinate reduction may be warranted.
2. After septal or turbinate surgery, synechiae may form and require revision.
3. Overreduction of the alae or collapse of the internal valve can result in a compromised airway.

Nasal Asymmetry, Graft Irregularity, Displacement, and Extrusion

When combining osteocartilaginous augmentation with soft-tissue reduction, irregularities and asymmetry can be quite common. But slight irregularities and asymmetries are very common, even in nonoperated noses. Patients should be forewarned that slight, palpable irregularities and visible asymmetries will be found after most nasal procedures. Asymmetries may or may not be more common during the period of swelling. Dorsal grafts and tip grafts are rarely perfectly smooth and symmetric. Nostril asymmetry, particularly from the worm's eye view, may be more noticeable when alar reduction is combined with tip grafting. Care must be taken to measure precisely and to excise a balanced amount of tissue from each side of the alar base. During the early postoperative period, slight-to-moderate asymmetries may be correctable with injections of triamcinolone acetonide suspension 10 mg/ml (Kenalog) further diluted. If graft distortion is detected during the first few days after surgery, the percutaneous stabilization sutures can be readjusted to reposition the graft. But when distortion is noted later, surgical revision is usually required. Significant asymmetries and/or irregularities may require *major* revision of both soft tissue and grafts (Fig. 7-4a, 7-4b, 7-4c, 7-4d). However, revisions should be delayed until healing is complete, sometimes as late as 18 months postoperatively.

Graft Resorption

Hematoma, graft mobility, infection, and a poorly vascularized bed are the most common reasons for graft resorption. With a scarred bed, particularly when a result of previous Silastic grafts, significant cartilage or bone resorption is not uncommon. Capsulectomy, although often quite difficult to accomplish, is sometimes necessary to create a more vascular bed. On the dorsum, a new subperiosteal dissection may be of benefit to create a more

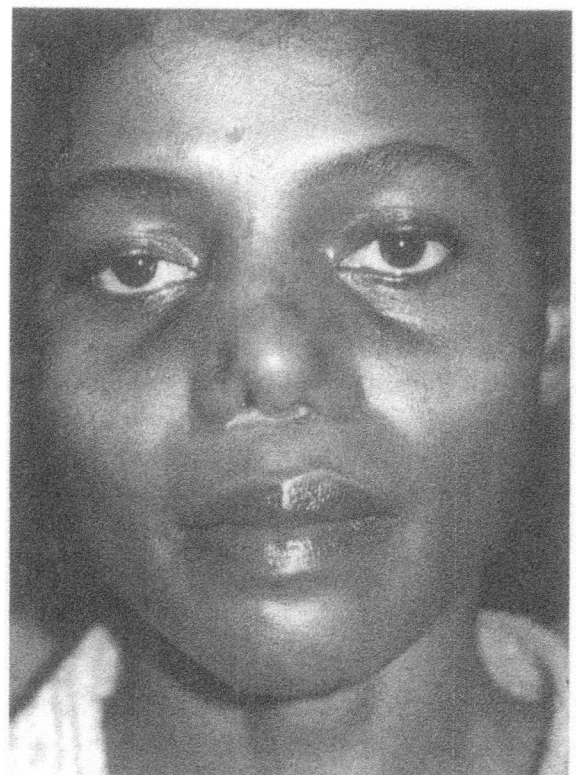 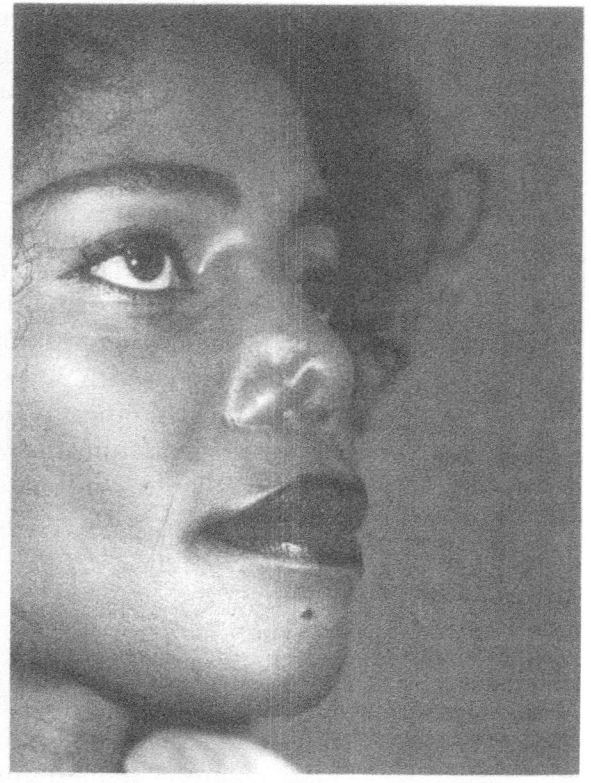

a   b

Figure 7-4a, 7-4b
This complication resulted from the work of an inexperienced surgeon who performed overresection of alar cartilage, excised excessive soft tissue, and overused Silastic grafts. Subsequent infection, Silastic extrusion, and predictable tissue contraction followed. This patient's personal preoperative photograph revealed that a very conservative rhinoplasty should have been the surgeon's plan. Ten months later, when the patient's tissue had softened, auricular cartilage grafting was performed. Numerous infectious foreign body fragments were removed from this patient's nose. Dorsal Silastic grafts and Dacron fragments were in the dorsum. Cotton fragments had been inadvertently forced up into the body of the nasal vault. These were lodged between the nasal bones when the surgeon performed the osteotomies.

vascular base. Likewise, a separate, deeper plane created in the tip may provide a more vascularized bed than the previous scar capsule. Patients should be forewarned that secondary autografting after removal of an alloplastic prosthesis has a significantly higher rate of resorption.

Prolonged Swelling and/or Erythema

When multiple nasal incisions and grafts are made on thick skin, long-term swelling is common. Permanent edema (longer than 2 years) or fibrosis can occur. Minimizing intraoperative bleeding and swelling through the use of head elevation, safe hypotensive anesthesia techniques, compression, and ice application significantly decreases the degree and duration of postoperative swelling. A 4 to 6-week nighttime taping program definitely results in a more rapid resolution of edema. I have found that very dilute steroid injections (though controversial), followed by a few nights per week of nighttime taping, are very helpful in refractory cases.

Postoperative fibrosis in the Asian nasal tip and alae has been less responsive to triamcinolone acetonide (Kenalog) than with other ethnic groups. This may be due to the thicker fibrous dermis. Adding the calcium channel blocker verapamil hydrochloride and/or 5FU is generally beneficial. Edema is usually reduced and resultant fibrosis minimized in Asian (as well as other) "pea-pod" tip graft patients with nighttime nasal taping for a minimum of 6 to 12 weeks, and often longer. Minimizing postoperative fibrosis results in a more tapered nose and smaller nasal tip.

Many of my Asian patients have had extraordinary skills in applying makeup and shadowing to give greater nasal definition to an otherwise flat, thick nose. These same makeup skills often result in exquisitely attractive eye and eyelid makeup.

Ethnic patients requesting nasal surgery have a high propensity toward (at least initial) dissatisfaction due to the following: (1) unrealistic expectations as to the degree of sculpturing, thinness, and nasal shapeliness possible, (2) sometimes persistent postoperative swelling, (3) the likelihood of need for two procedures, with proper interval, especially involving the nasal tip, and (4) reactions of others regarding improvements to their appearance. There are tip-offs to identify the overly optimistic or perfectionistic patients, those who bring to the consultation large volumes of ads or photographs that depict unrealistic nasal goals.

Revision Surgery

It is the author's opinion that difficult rhinoplastic surgeries may well result in a greater number of both requested and performed revisions. The most common request concerns a thickened tip, which has not been reduced or sculptured to the patient's satisfaction. Temporizing a request with

Figure 7-4c, 7-4d
In managing this complication, both ears were used to create new alar cartilages and a "pea-pod" tip graft. Four months later, the alar scars were revised and the lateral cheek skin undermined 2 cm. The dermal base was then sutured to the vestibular periosteum to create a narrower base. Caution must be exercised in applying postoperative taping. The combination of a long-acting anesthetic to eliminate pain as a warning sign, excessive swelling, alar resections, and constricting taping can result in possible vascular compromise. The full-thickness skin graft became slightly hyperpigmented.

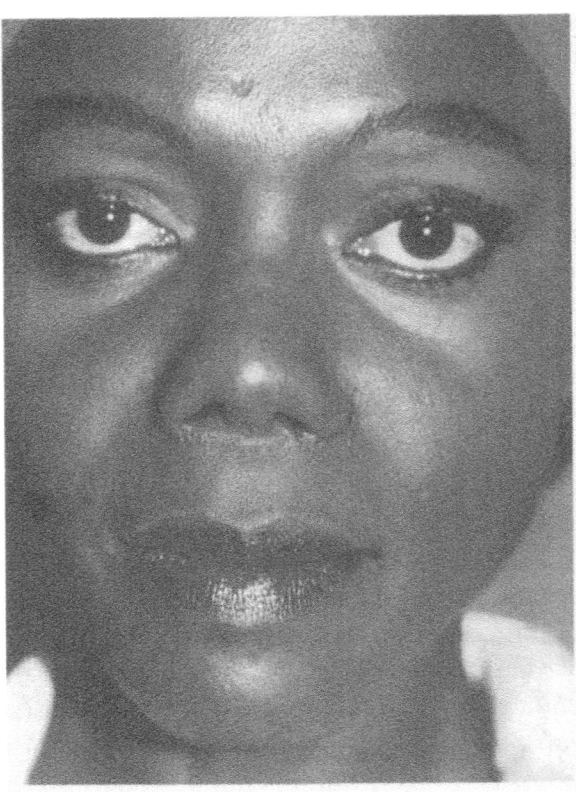

c

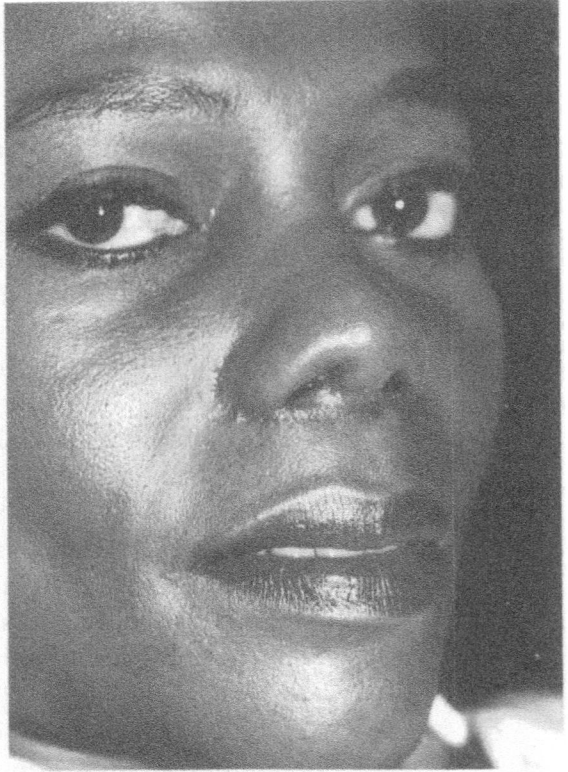

d

use of dilute 2–5 cc Kenalog (triamcinolone acetonide suspension 10 mg/ml) injections every 6 to 8 weeks, pressure taping, possible use of limited small-probe ultrasound, and gentle pressure molding may provide both physically AND emotionally comforting temporized improvement. The author has found that the program above, under conservative management, provides sufficient visible benefit to most patients over a period of several weeks to several months. Significant tip revisions should wait at least 1 year. Patients with thicker nose induration and scar formation propensities may require even longer between initial surgery and any follow-up revision. Such a wait may be distressing to a patient, but thorough preoperative counseling, coupled with visible progress and the techniques above, usually proves at least grudgingly acceptable. When extensive tip work has already been done and the surgeon feels as much improvement as possible has already been attained, and the remaining tissues are fibrous and scarred, performing further surgery may not only be of no benefit but may actually be detrimental.

Ethnic patients should be counseled that a prolonged period of healing is normal and that compressive nighttime taping and intermittent injections of triamcinolone acetonide suspension 10 mg/ml (Kenalog) further diluted may be required to decrease persistent swelling. Salt intake should be minimized, and sun exposure and very hot environments eliminated. The overly optimistic or overly perfectionistic patient should be adequately counseled toward more realistic expectations. All patients should be consistently counseled that no revision surgery will be performed for at least 6, and usually 12, months.

Planning for any anticipated revisions starts with clear, candid communication between patient and surgeon at the initial consultation. Realistic expectations for the results from each surgical procedure must be formulated, discussed, and agreed upon by both. When more than one procedure is anticipated, the nature of the additional procedure(s), the waiting period(s) between procedures, the costs of the additional procedure(s), etc., should be discussed at the initial consultation. Such physician candor helps to prevent unrealistic expectations, which, when unfulfilled, often result in requests for early or impossible revisions.

Patients should be further advised that revision surgery may offer very little in terms of significant improvement if the primary operation has been optimally performed. In any case, elective revisions should wait 6 to 12 months.

While routine Caucasian rhinoplasties may carry a patient-requested revision rate of only 5% to 10%, ethnic rhinoplasties probably carry a 10% to 20% patient-requested revision rate. For ethnic rhinoplasties, the most common revision requests include:

1. Persistent fullness of the tip and base
2. Graft asymmetry or irregularity
3. Insufficient augmentation of dorsum or tip
4. Airway obstruction
5. External scarring

Persistent Fullness of the Tip and Base

Although the desire for a thin, tapered tip is common, simple reduction of soft tissue and/or cartilage will generally not achieve the desired result in a tip having thick skin with minimal alar cartilaginous support. An ultra-supportive and projecting tip graft will be necessary to give the illusion of a thinner tip. The patient must be willing to accept the increased projection in order to have a thinner-appearing tip. Although the amount of tip projection needed to create adequate definition may initially appear excessive to a patient, in the author's experience, there are far fewer complaints from patients with overprojecting tips than from those with underprojecting tips. Even a Pinocchio-type tip is preferred if it will achieve greater definition. Caucasians conversely rarely desire overprojection.

Persistent nasal tip swelling is one of the most common postoperative complaints. When the surgeon is satisfied with the width and projection of the tip, the patient should be counseled that, when the swelling resolves, the appearance of the tip should improve significantly. Conservative management with nighttime taping, patient reassurance, and, occasionally, very dilute steroid injections into the supratip and tip area, usually suffices (Fig. 7-5). It may be psychologically beneficial to have patients participate in the swelling resolution process with a nighttime taping regimen and regular follow-up visits.

The nasal tip, with its dependent position and thick soft tissue envelope, requires the longest time for total edema resolution, sometimes as long as 18 to 24 months. The process takes especially long when major soft-tissue reduction and cartilage grafting have been performed.

Figure 7-5
Site of dilute steroid injection for supratip swelling. The supratip and the junction of intranasal mucosal closure (i.e., intercartilaginous and septal incisions) can form increased thickness postoperatively. Good mucosal edge approximation is paramount to avoid overlap and mucosal in-growth, sometimes resulting in mucosal cysts in the supratip area. When indicated, a series of dilute steroid injections is used to help decrease nasal tip thickness. A series of four injections over a 2 to 4-week period is usually sufficient.

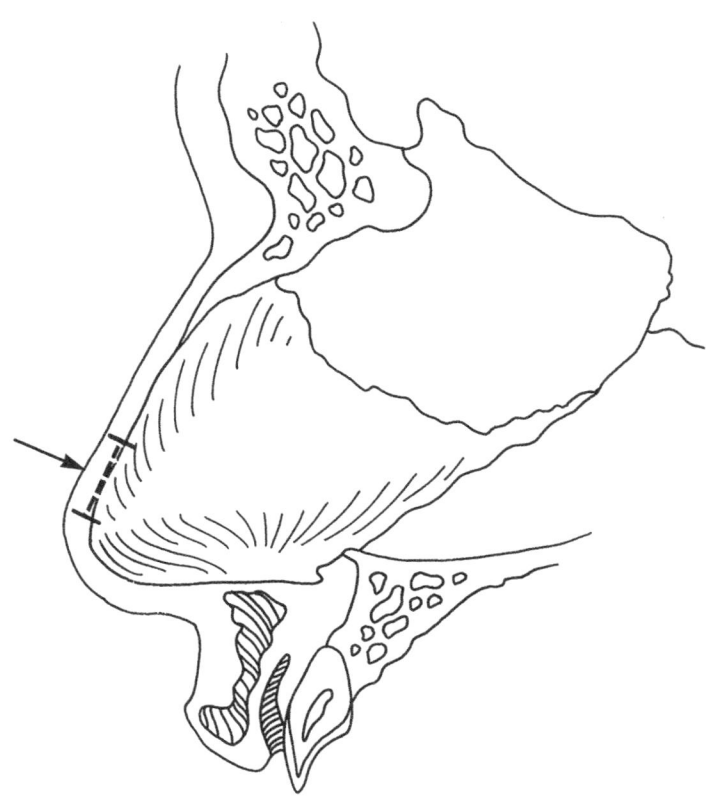

The characteristic wide, thick, flaring nostrils of the ethnic nose pose a significant challenge to the surgeon. Overresection results in a flattened, stenotic appearance to the nostrils, while underresection may lead to patient dissatisfaction and requests for further reduction. The ethnic nose may require internal thinning or narrowing, or anterior segmental reduction. When revising an overresected nostril, a successful strategy includes incising the original scar, undermining and advancing the cheek skin medially with stabilization to the piriform soft tissue or periosteum, and curvilinear suturing.

Graft Irregularity or Asymmetry

The adage "what you see is what you (will) get" is all too often the case with dorsal or tip grafting. "Minor" irregularities visible at the time of the original nasal operation may turn out to be major when the edema resolves. Every attempt should be made to correct graft irregularity at the time of the original operation. Irregularities rarely straighten themselves out with time.

A cartilage graft must be smooth and symmetrical for a "natural" result and the graft must be placed in the pocket under symmetrical stresses. Because cartilage has "memory," grafts eventually spring back to their original contour, unless prevented by scoring or crushing.

Thick skin can provide good postoperative camouflage. Tip skin is characteristically thicker than dorsal skin. *Fine* irregularities in dorsal or tip grafts can be corrected with additional small, crushed-cartilage grafts. Early postoperative irregularities may be temporarily treated with collagen injections. *Gross* irregularities may require graft repositioning or replacement. Conservative longitudinal incisions or total crushing with the JOST crusher have been useful to eliminate much of the spring in dorsal grafts. Crushing has not resulted in significant graft resorption. When maximum projection is desired, tip grafts should not be crushed. Visible graft edges and slight irregularities can be improved by adding a layer of mastoid or temporalis fascia.

Again, if the primary operation gave satisfactory results, revisions should not be performed hastily—even if the patient is dissatisfied. Before undertaking any revisions, the surgeon must be confident that any potential improvement warrants the risk of reoperation. "Minor" revisions of the tip can frequently reveal surprises that become major.

If additional cartilage is necessary to perform a revision, the virgin ear should be used. Any scarring that resulted from graft harvesting would limit the flexibility and, to some degree, the viability of cartilage in the original ear.

Insufficient Augmentation of Dorsum or Tip

Where the basic dorsal graft has good shape and position, adding another cartilage graft on top of the original may provide sufficient additional augmentation. Depending on the condition and thickness of the skin coverage, conservative overgrafting can usually be performed 6 to 12 months after surgery. If only a small amount of additional tip projection is desired, an onlay graft placed on top of a graft already in place *may* be sufficient (Fig. 7-6). But if more substantial projection is desired, the old graft must be removed and replaced by a longer, more supportive "pea-pod" graft. It is my experience that, even in minor tip revision, surprises may occur that will force the entire earlier graft to be replaced. The surgeon and patient must be prepared for total graft removal and replacement with a new, larger graft.

Airway Obstruction

Enlarged turbinates are the most frequent cause of persistent nasal obstruction. Even though turbinate reduction may appear to be adequate intraoperatively, it may be insufficient as a result of long-term postoperative swelling or reactive hypertrophy. Osteotomies can result in bleeding into the turbinates with resultant fibrosis and enlargement. Obstruction may improve over time with aid of hydration, antihistamines, and topical or injectable steroids. Conservative outfracturing under local anesthesia can provide relief in some cases. But if the obstruction persists despite conservative management, further surgical reduction may be warranted.

Septal perforations, sometimes seen with large septal graft excisions, may result in crusting and, if the perforation is small, whistling. This whistling can be managed by flap reconstruction or by enlarging the perforation.

Substantial septal deviation which persists despite an adequately performed septoplasty should be treated by submucous resection of the deviated portion. The resection also provides a source of graft material.

Another frequent source of airway obstruction is a vomerine ledge, which requires excision. Great care must be exercised in its resection to avoid resecting mucosa, which could lead to stenosis.

External Scarring

Prominent alar scarring may be due to a number of technical factors such as an imprecise closure or excessive tension on the closure with resultant

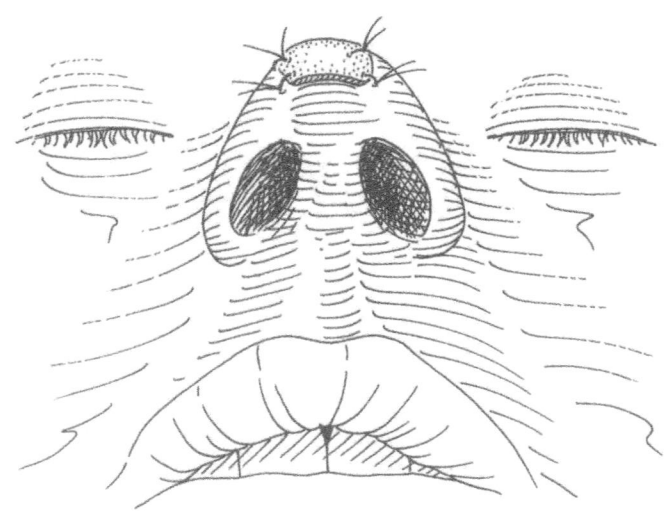

Figure 7-6
Corrections of 1 to 2 mm can often be made with the use of a small onlay cartilage graft or small piece of fascia. Pull-out sutures are used for positioning just as with the larger tip and dorsal grafts. The surgeon, however, must be prepared to replace the existing graft with an entirely new one.

wide scars, suture-line or pore epithelialization, increased width and irregularities, etc. If secondary scar revision is required, one must avoid creating an unnatural shape to the alae. Scar excision combined with medial cheek advancement often decreases the capacity for lateral pulling and straightening to the normal convexity of the alar side walls. Alar scarring or asymmetry may be repaired or revised after 6 to 12 months, while only cases of substantial deformity warrant a more rapid revision.

The sample "Nuisances/Risks" handout (Fig. 7-7) is representative of informational handouts we provide our patients on various preoperative regimens, surgical procedures, and postoperative care.

A WORD ABOUT NUISANCES, INCONVENIENCES, AND SIDE EFFECTS, VERSUS TRUE RISKS AND COMPLICATIONS FROM AESTHETIC SURGERY

Although we all (including plastic surgeons) would like to think of ourselves as perfectionists, we do not live in a perfect world. The results of no human enterprise can be guaranteed with absolute certainty. There are certain variances in the outcome of any activity which have to be accepted by all involved. A ballplayer enters a ball game knowing that he is doing his best, but the outcome of his performance is only statistically predictable. This is true of any athlete who engages in a sport or runs a race, a student who attempts to take a test, a business attempting to make a certain number of sales, etc. The fact that we are human beings with certain biological variances ensures that the outcome of any of our activities is unpredictable. We cannot totally predict the sexual outcome or timing of a birth, the duration of someone's life, etc. Therefore, it is reasonable to assume that the postoperative course and potential results of a well-planned plastic surgical operation cannot come out perfect each time. Fortunately, excellent results occur upwards of 95% of the time, but there is the potential 5% (one out of twenty) of patients who experience a true complication. Fortunately, the vast majority of these complications are correctable with time, as in the case of asymmetrical or distorted results due to surgical technique or healing processes. The very serious complications in aesthetic surgery, such as paralysis or death from either a local of general anesthesia, blindness or blepharoplasty, significant deformity after surgery, etc., are so rare as to be almost negligible compared to the risks we take from daily activities such as driving or sporting activities such as bicycling, scuba diving, etc. To put this in perspective, aesthetic surgery is extremely safe in relation to the many other unsafe things that we engage in on a daily basis.

Much more frequently bothersome are the nuisances and side effects caused by surgery. These are treatable and rapidly resolvable and should not be thought of as being serious complications. An example would be a stitch reaction (redness and festering at the incision line) which, when removed and treated properly with topical antibiotics, normally heals quite satisfactorily. This is not a serious problem. This is only a nuisance and a side effect. A true complication may be one entailing a permanent problem requiring surgical intervention. As you requested, I have given you a list of what, in my opinion, are complications which are possible, although usually uncommon or extremely rare in their occurrence.

The following in an alphabetical list of the majority of known risks involved with plastic surgery. This is *not* an all-inclusive list. This has been prepared at the request of patients who desire to know the majority of possible, common, or extremely rare complications that can occur from surgery. Although some of these may be categorized as side effects and happen not infrequently, most are extremely rare or unusual.

(continued)

Figure 7-7

RISKS

A

Airway Problems
Allergic Reaction
Amnesia
Anesthesia Reaction
Asymmetry
Atrophy of Skin

B

Back Ache/Orthopedic Injuries
Bandage Constriction or Irritation
Bleeding
Excessive Bleeding, Requiring Transfusion
Blindness
Blood Test Abnormalities
Breakdown or Malfunction of Equipment
Bruising/Broken Blood Vessels

C

Cautery Burns or Malfunction
Collapse of Tissue Supports
Constipation, Acute or Chronic
Cyst Formation

D

Death
Deformity or Distortion of Tissues
Delayed Healing
Discharge
Discoloration of Tissues, Acute or Prolonged
Division of Anatomical Structures
Dressing Reactions
Dryness of Skin

(continued)

E

Early Discharge from Hospital/Insurance Requirements
Edema, Acute or Chronic
Emboli or Blood Clots
Emotional Problems
Excessive Tissue Left or Excised
Exposure of Vital Structures, Acute or Chronic

F

Fainting, With or Without Injuries
Financial Problems/Surgery Risks, Complications
Firmness
Fluid Build-Up/Seroma or Hematoma Formation
Fluid Leaks
Foreign Body Retention
Fractures of Bones or Cartilage
Functional Interference

G

H

Health Problems/Risks & Complications, Acute or Chronic
Heart Abnormalities
Heart Attacks
Heart Infections
Heartbeat Irregularities
Hives, Acute or Chronic
Hospitalization Requirements after Surgery

I

Inconvenience/Personal-Professional Lifestyle/Risks & Complications
Infection, Acute or Chronic
Infections, Secondary/Yeast, Fungi, etc.
Infections, Unusual, Acute/Chronic, Short/Long Term
Inflammation of Tissues, Acute or Chronic
Itching, Acute or Chronic

J

(continued)

K

L

Loss of Hair or Teeth

Lymph Node Enlargement, Acute or Chronic (biopsy may be required)

M

Medication Requirements Due to Complications, Acute/Long Term

Menstrual Cycle Abnormalities

Movement Problems of Body Parts

N

Nausea

Need for Further Surgery

Nerve Damage, Motor/Sensory, Temporary/Permanent

O

Organ Dysfunction

Overdose of Medications

P

Pain, Acute/Chronic, Short/Long Term

Pneumonia or Other Lung Abnormalities

Pneumothorax or Collapsed Lung

Pregnancy due to Birth Control Dysfunction

Pregnancy & Fetal Abnormalities if Pregnancy at Time of Surgery

Q

R

Redness or Erthema of Skin or Operative Site or Associated Area,
    Acute/Chronic, Short/Long Term

Rejection of Implants/Suture Material

Relationship Problems Pre- or Postoperatively

Revision Surgery Needs, One or Multiple

(continued)

S

Scars
Sensitivity to Heat, Cold, Sun, Wind, etc.
Sensory Loss
Skin Breakout, Before or After Surgery
    Requiring Treatment and/or Resulting in Chronic Acne or Scarring
Skin Irregularity or Depressions
Skin, Nail, or Hair Loss/Abnormalities, Acute/Chronic, Short/Long Term
Sore Throat
Stitch or Suture Reaction, Requirements for Additional Removal,
    Possible Retention
Structure Abnormalities
Structural Deformity
Swelling

T

Thrombophlebitis
Tissue Loss

U

Unknown Complications
Unnatural Results
Unpredictable Future
Unrelaxed Body

V

W

Weight Gain/Loss
Worse Wrinkles
Worse Appearance
Wrong Operation

X

Y

Z

8

The Ten Commandments of Ethnic Rhinoplasty

Because a basic, well-organized surgical plan is important whether one is dealing with a simple or a very complicated rhinoplasty, I have established and always try to follow these Ten Commandments of Ethnic Rhinoplasty:

I. *Carefully evaluate the individual's anatomy, physiology, and psychology.*

II. *Establish realistic goals for the patient and for yourself.*

III. *Prepare a detailed preoperative evaluation and surgical plan.*

IV. *Consider the use of preoperative "BASICS" (**B**enadryl, **A**ntibiotics, **S**teroids, **I**ce, **C**ompression, and **S**tandard Surgical Preparations).*

V. *Mix your own fresh local anesthetic with epinephrine.*

VI. *Maintain nasal airway function.*

VII. *Use only autologous grafts whenever possible.*

VIII. *Control swelling and bleeding intraoperatively with "ICE" (**I**ce, **C**ompression, and **E**levation).*

IX. *Prepare a postoperative care plan such as "DAMP" (**D**ietary and **A**ctivity restrictions, **M**edication, and **P**ressure).*

X. *Perform revision procedures only when truly warranted.*

I. Carefully Evaluate the Individual's Anatomy, Physiology, and Psychology.

Anatomical, physiological, and psychological issues should be clearly and candidly discussed with the patient. It has proven very helpful to sit with patients in front of a mirror or projection screen to discuss and evaluate their anatomy with them. Some preexisting medical conditions, apparent or occult, can affect the final outcome of the surgery. For example, if the patient has a history of hypertension, diabetes, collagen-vascular disease, etc., preoperative medical evaluation and treatment may be indicated. Proper assessment of the patient's psychology avoids any possible postoperative anger, depression, etc. For particularly difficult noses, more than one preoperative office visit may be necessary to establish a confident relationship with the patient, together with a sound surgical plan.

II. Establish Realistic Goals for the Patient and for Yourself.

The average patient appreciates an honest aesthetic prognosis, even if it falls below his or her desires or initial expectations. Always listen to the patient's point of view. Encourage patients to bring in photographs demonstrating examples of their likes and dislikes. The downsides of surgery must always be discussed. It is very difficult for patients to accept the period of prolonged swelling unless they have been thoroughly prepared for it prior to surgery. Establishing realistic and honest goals usually decreases requests for unnecessary revisions.

III. Prepare a Detailed Preoperative Evaluation and Surgical Plan.

Detailed preoperative evaluations should be mandatory in order to avoid intraoperative surprises. It is also useful to complete a detailed preoperative *diagrammatic* plan, especially for complicated cases (see Fig. 2-1). Areas requiring special consideration are:

A. The size and source of graft material available. All available potential sources should be noted:
   1. Septum vs. ear vs. cranial area
   2. Mastoid vs. temporalis fascia
B. The type and size of alar reduction anticipated.
C. The type and size of tip graft anticipated.
D. The amount and type of septal and turbinate surgery required. Corrective surgery of the septum should not be performed until the need for septal graft material has been determined, as septal scoring may negate its use as a stable graft.

IV. Consider the Use of Preoperative "BASICS" (Benadryl, Antibiotics, Steroids, Ice, Compression, and Standard Surgical Preparations).

These "BASICS" help to decrease intraoperative and postoperative swelling. As with any surgical procedure, but particularly rhinoplasty, there will be cellular disruption with attendant third space swelling. The intranasal area and the large sebaceous glands will be colonized with bacteria. This combination can result in prolonged swelling, subclinical infection, and possible long-term edema. Because these controllable, nonsurgical factors do have a very real impact on surgical results and patient satisfaction, the following regimen is recommended:

A. Preoperatively administer Benadryl 50 mg IV, dexamethasone phosphate (Decadron) 6–10 mg IV, and cephalosporin 0.5–1.0 g IV (in penicillin-sensitive patients, I use vancomycin hydrochloride 500 mg IV).
B. Place crushed ice in a sterile glove and apply to the nose before and after injecting the local anesthetic.
C. Standard surgical preparation with special attention to cleansing the intranasal area of dried mucous, etc., is very important when placing grafts. Dry mucus can harbor significant amounts of bacteria.

V. Mix Your Own Fresh Local Anesthetic with Epinephrine.

I use bupivacaine hydrochloride (Marcaine) 0.5% with epinephrine 1:100,000 by adding 0.5 cc of 1:1000 epinephrine to a 50-cc bottle of 0.5% plain bupivacaine hydrochloride (Marcaine). Standard local anesthetics with epinephrine may lose substantial potency with long storage, elevated environmental temperature, light exposure, etc. A small dose of 5–7.5 cc of the local solution mixed with 150 units of hyaluronidase (Wydase) minimizes tissue distortion and maximizes hemostasis. You can inject prior to prepping. The delay allows for adequate vasoconstriction.

In order to see the contour definition of the dorsum and bridge, do not inject either. A ring block from the medial canthus to the alar base, columellar base, and dorsal mucosal septum provides a good block and adequate hemostasis.

VI. Maintain Nasal Airway Function.

Reducing the size of the nose may compromise the airway unless precautions are taken. Straightening the septum, narrowing an enlarged vomer ledge, reducing enlarged turbinates, and *conservatively* resecting the dorsal vault or the alae will help to maintain an adequate airway.

VII. Use Only Autologous Grafts Whenever Possible.

I prefer autologous cartilage grafts from the septum or the ear. When using autologous cartilage, substantial pressure can be cautiously placed on the nasal tip without subsequent erosion. Although Silastic grafts have been used successfully in primary ethnic rhinoplasties, late erosion of the tip skin or late extrusion or mobility of the dorsal grafts can occur. This is especially problematic in revision rhinoplasties.

VIII. Control Swelling and Bleeding Intraoperatively with "ICE" (Ice, Compression, and Elevation).

Excessive intraoperative swelling can distort the patient's anatomy. A sterile glove can be filled with crushed ice, placed over the nose, and then gently compressed for a few seconds. If used intermittently during the surgery, the ice can help decrease swelling. Gentle compression with or without the ice glove helps decrease bleeding and swelling, especially after osteotomies. Elevation of the head helps decrease oozing and swelling as well. General anesthesia has the advantage of not only ensuring a motionless patient but also helping to provide controlled hypotension. Excessive bleeding during surgery can distort anatomy and prolong the procedure.

IX. Prepare a Postoperative Care Plan such as "DAMP" (Dietary and Activity Restrictions, Medications, and Pressure).

A. **Dietary Restriction:** Patients should be advised to decrease or eliminate salt and spice intake. They are also told to decrease or eliminate alcohol intake and tobacco use.

B. **Activity Restriction:** There must be no sun exposure, heavy exercise, or elevated heat exposure for 6 to 12 weeks.

C. **Medications:** Patients often benefit from a short course of an antihistamine such as terfenadine (Seldane) if swelling is significant. Intranasal topical cortisone sprays can also be helpful. Oral cortisone has not been of significant benefit.

D. **Pressure:** Postoperative nighttime nasal taping is of substantial benefit in decreasing tip swelling.

X. Perform Revision Procedures Only When Truly Warranted.

Revisions should be directly correlated to the mutual expectations of the patient and surgeon. Establishing realistic expectations prior to surgery will usually decrease the demand for unrealistic additional procedures. It is very important that an honest appraisal of expected results be formed and candidly discussed with the patient well in advance of surgery. If necessary, minor revision procedures such as alar base scar revision and small additional cartilage grafts can usually be performed 6 to 12 months after surgery. Major revision procedures such as replacement of large dorsal or tip grafts may require a 12 to 24-month wait.

Revision procedures should not be attempted unless a reasonable degree of success is foreseeable. The usual pressures from a patient must not take precedence over good surgical judgment. In certain cases, such as when a very large reduction of soft tissue is necessary, revisions are warranted and to be expected. Foreseeable revision requirements should be determined and discussed with the patient preoperatively to avoid any disappointment after the initial major surgery.

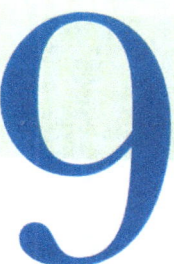

Detailed Representative Case Studies

This 22-year-old black male complained of his wide, nonprojecting, undefined and ptotic nasal tip. He was also concerned about his dorsal bump and the "droopy" appearance of his nose.

On examination the patient had a slight nasion depression located at midpupil level. There was a slight deficiency of nasal bone projection, but moderate width, giving the nose a broad and tented appearance. The patient had prominent dorsal septocartilage and relatively flimsy upper lateral cartilages. The nasal tip was flat, nondefined, and poorly projected. The alae cartilages were broad and of moderate thickness, but flimsy. The nasal spine and maxilla were slightly hypoplastic and the columella was hanging.

In assessing the patient's overall facial features and discussing his desires, using both representative examples and photographs, the patient wanted only relatively conservative changes made to the bony nasal bridge. He desired a straight or very slightly curved nasal dorsum. The patient's large lips precluded significantly reducing the nose and he was against enlarging the nose, particularly the dorsum. The patient did not desire lip reduction or chin augmentation. He sought moderate alar reduction.

The intranasal examination revealed a septum moderately deviated to the right with a full vomer deflection. The turbinates were moderately hypertrophic. The upper lateral valvular mechanism was almost closing upon deep inspiration.

The patient and I did not reach agreement on acceptable and achievable surgical goals in the first consultation. The patient was seen twice preoperatively. For the second consultation, the patient brought in photographs of noses smaller and more defined than I felt I could meet. I discussed in detail the limitations in the degree of definition and overall reduction possible. I explained to him that to balance the nose with the face, a slight supratip dorsal cartilaginous reduction with nasion and nasal tip/spine augmentation and a "pea-pod" tip graft would give an overall definition improvement. The patient reluctantly agreed to a dorsal and "pea-pod" tip augmentation after we reviewed and discussed the balance of facial features in the photographic noses he had selected. The patient understood that his postsurgical nose would not be smaller, but would be better defined and more balanced. Obtaining good airway function was also a goal (another reason to not overreduce the nose and upper lateral carti-

125

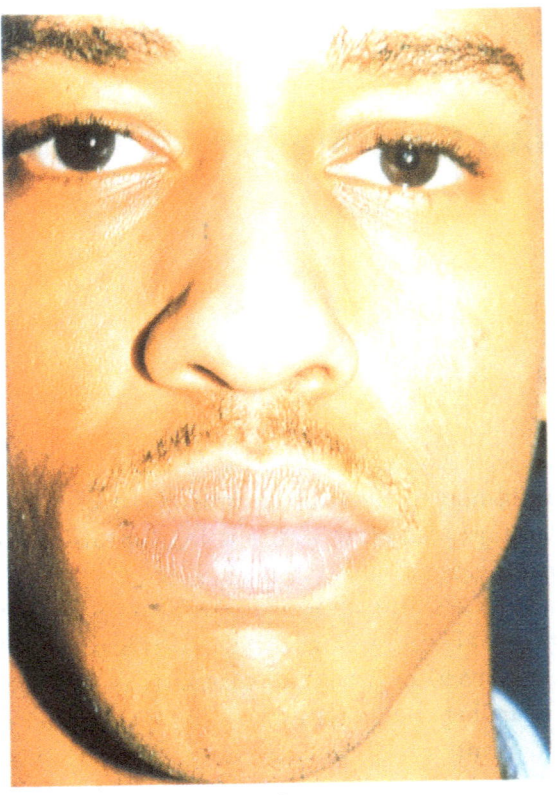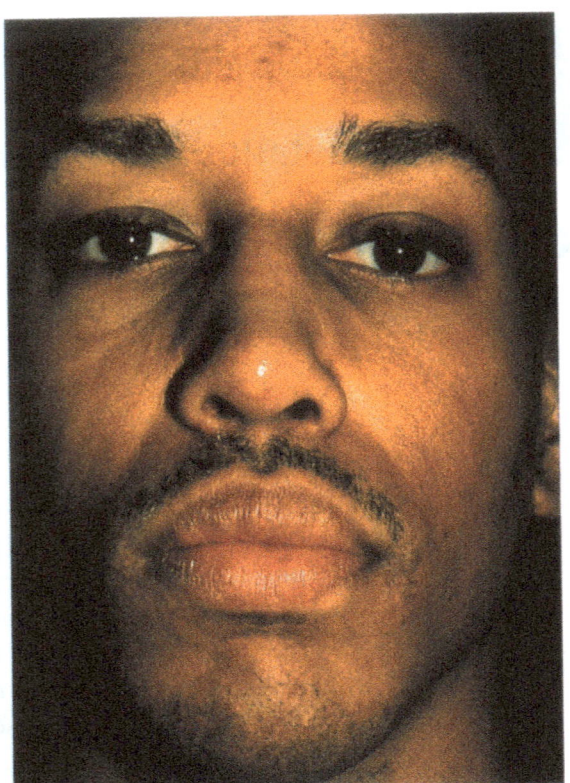

Figure 9-1a, 9-1b
This black male had a very thick, bulbous, and undefined nasal tip.

lages). To improve the airway the surgical plan was to excise the deflected septum and vomer, to reduce the anterior portion of the turbinates, and to leave adequately closed mucosa to decrease rhinorrhea.

The five-page Preoperative Nasal Checklist was used for the patient's consultative evaluation (Fig. 9-2).

Operative Procedure

1. The procedures were performed under general anesthesia. 0.5% Bupivacaine hydrochloride (Marcaine) with epinephrine was used to infiltrate the nose, left ear, septum, and turbinates. Eight milligrams of intravenous Decadron and 25 mg of intravenous diphenhydramine hydrochloride (Benadryl) with 1 g of cephalosporin was administered.

2. A left curvilinear postauricular incision was made and conchal cup cartilage was excised and placed into a saline-moistened sponge. After bleeding was controlled, 0.5% bupivacaine hydrochloride (Marcaine) with 1:100,000 epinephrine and dilute 5 mg/cc Kenalog (10 mg/ml suspension of triamcinolone acetonide) was sprayed into the wound. It was then closed over a .25" Penrose drain. Petroleum ribbon packing was molded into the anterior conchal cup and postauricular sulcus for compression.

3. A moistened orolpharyngeal pack was placed and petroleum jelly packing was placed deep within the posterior nasal vault to decrease any

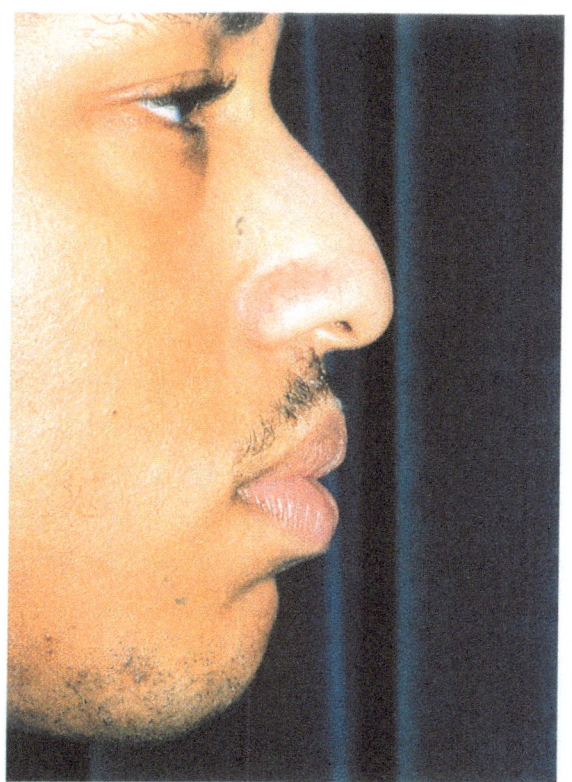

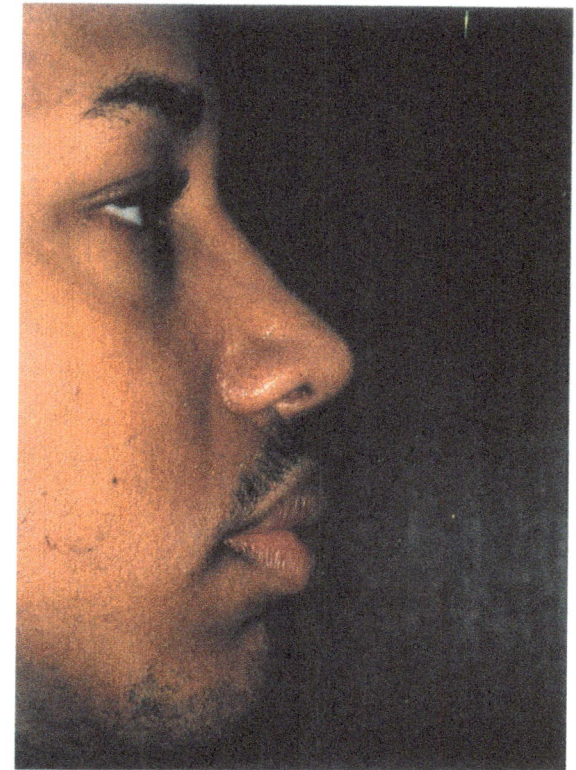

c

d

Figure 9-1c, 9-1d
During surgery, the superior three-fourths of the alar cartilages were excised, the alar base was reduced, and a 2.8 cm × 0.8 cm "pea-pod" tip graft was placed.

flow of blood below the posterior pharynx to minimize coughing and nausea postoperatively.

4. Afrin-soaked cotton pledgets were used to shrink nasal mucosa. Septal excision was performed through the left nasi aperture with excision of the obstructing septal segment and vomer ridge. A modified submucous resection of the interior turbinate was performed. After infiltration, a Bovie cutting current was used to incise the turbinate down to bone. The mucosal leaves were elevated, the obstructed bony segment was excised, and the turbinate mucosa sutured over the open wound. Further cauterization and outfracturing were performed, and 5 mg/cc Kenalog (10 mg/ml suspension triamcinolone acetonide) was injected into the area. At that point a secondary set of petroleum jelly gauze packets was utilized to compress the operative area. 4-0 catgut and plain mattress sutures were used in the septum and in closing the turbinate mucosa.

5. Intercartilaginous incisions were made and the dorsum, superior third of the lateral nasal wall (including the bone), and upper lateral cartilage segments were freed. Soft tissue was left attached to the bottom two-thirds of the nasal bones to provide good support after infracturing.

6. Through limited refractors, a broken-tip #11 blade was utilized to carefully excise the excessive projecting cartilaginous dorsum. Great care was taken to leave intact the mucosa between the septum and upper lateral cartilages. It was not necessary to trim the upper lateral carti-

PREOPERATIVE NASAL EVALUATION AND CHECKLIST

I use a checklist when preoperatively assessing patients. It assists me in obtaining a history, assessing the aesthetic goals of the patient, and performing a complete nasal examination. In addition, a complete medical history and physical examination should be performed prior to surgery.

NASAL CHECKLIST

Name: __Patient Z_____ Date:_____

Previous History Of:

Childhood or adulthood injuries?   Yes_____ No__X__ If yes, explain:_____

Nasal Surgery?   Yes_____ No__X__
  Date and Specifics?   _____
  X-Rays?   Yes_____ No_____

_____Nasal Airway Obstruction: Left_____ Right_____ Both__X__ Consistent__X__
                                                                          Intermittent_____

_____Sinus Infections: Yes_____ No__X__ When:_____

_____Nasal Allergy Symptoms: Yes_____ No__X__
                                          _____Stuffiness _____Sneezing _____Postnasal Drip

_____Nasal Spray Use: Yes_____ No__X__
                                          Type:_____ Frequency:_____

_____Nasal Bleeding: Yes_____ No__X__

_____Smoking: Yes_____ No__X__ How much_____PPD

_____Aspirin or Aspirin-like Medication Use:_____

_____Hypertension: Yes_____ No__X__

_____Previous History of Troublesome Scarring: Yes_____ No__X__
                                          Where_____ Specifics_____

Additional Comments: _____

                                         _____

Figure 9-2
Preoperative Nasal Evaluation and Checklist.

Patient's Aesthetic Goals:

I. Dorsum/Bridge
   ___Retain Convexity
   ___Retain Width
   _X_ Reduce Bridge Width
   _X_ Reduce Dorsum To:
      ___Straight   _X_ Slight Concavity
      ___Moderate Concavity
   ___Graft Dorsum   _X_ Graft Nasion   ___Graft Frontal Bone
   ___Other: _____

II. Tip
   ___No Change
   _X_ Reduce Width
   _X_ More Tip Projection
   ___No Angle Change
   ___Elevate Angle To _____

III. Alar Base
   ___No Change
   _X_ Narrow
   ___Graft Nasal Base

Additional Comments/Procedures: _____

_____

_____

Nasal Examination:

A basic general physical examination should be performed.

I. Skin: ___Normal ___Medium _X_Thick ___Hypopigmented
_X_Sebaceous ___Normal Pigment
___Scars _X_Hyperpigmented

II. Septum: ___Straight _X_Deviated ___Left _X_Right
___% Obstruction ___Left ___Right
___Sufficient For Use As Graft ___Yes ___No

III. Vomer: ___Straight
_X_Deflected: ___Left _X_Right
___Spurred: ___Left ___Right

IV. Nasal Valve: ___Open
_X_Narrow
___Compromised

V. Turbinates: ___Small ___Right ___Left ___Both
___Deep ___Normal ___Right ___Left ___Both
___Flat _X_Enlarged ___Right ___Left _X_Both

VI. Nasion: Angle: ___DEPRESSED___

VII. Dorsum/Bridge: _X_Convex ___Straight ___Concave
___Narrow _X_Wide ___Normal Width
___Regular ___Irregular

VIII. Upper Lateral Cartilage: ___Narrow _X_Medium ___Wide

IV. Tip: ___Narrow ___Normal _X_Wide
___Adequate Projection
_X_Insufficient Projection

X. Columella: ___Normal ___Retracted _X_Hanging
___Angle: _____ ___Narrow _X_Wide

XI. Nasal Spine: _X_Small ___Normal ___Large

XII. Alar Base: ___Normal ___Moderate Width _X_Excessive Width

Surgical Plan:

Grafting To Be Performed: _X_ Yes   ___No

Source Of Graft: ___Cranial Bone
           _X_ Auricular
           ___Septum
           ___Other: _____

I. Nasion
     ___No Change
     ___Ostectomy
     _X_ Graft

II. Septum
     ___Septectomy
     _X_ Septoplasty
     ___Vomer Spur Ostectomy
     _X_ Packing   ___Yes   ___No — Left ___   Right ___   Both _X_

III. Turbinates
     _X_ Inject   Left ___   Right ___   Both _X_
     _X_ Cauterization   Left ___   Right ___   Both _X_
     ___Clamping/Excis.   Left ___   Right ___   Both ___
     _X_ S.M. Resections   Left ___   Right ___   Both ___

IV. Dorsum/Bridge
     ___Ostectomies
     _X_ Rasp
     _X_ Osteotomy
     ___Graft
           ___Septum
           ___Auricular
           ___Cranial
           ___Other

V. Columella
     ___No Change
     _X_ Raise To _open_ Angle

Additional Comments/Procedures: _____

_____

_____

Surgical Plan: (continued)

VI. Tip

    ____No Change

    __X__Reduce Alar Cartilages

        Approach: __X__Cartilage Splitting Incisions

                    ____Rim Incisions

                    ____Open Technique

`single intercarti-laginous`

    __X__Tip Grafting: Yes _X_   No ____

        ____Septum

        __X__Auricular

        ____Other:_____

VII. Base

    ____No Change

    ____Reduce Spine

    __X__Augment Spine

    __X__Augment Maxilla

VIII. Alae

    ____No Change

    __X__Reduce

        ____Small

        __X__Medium

        __X__Large

Additional Comments/Procedures: _____

_____

_____

lages. Small spreader grafts were necessary to maintain the valvular mechanism.

7. Two millimeter-osteotomes were used to punch through the piriform aperture, and a stepwise fracturing was performed from the interior nasal-maxillary junction upward to the medial canthal area.

8. Infracturing was performed, and 7 minutes of moderate nasal sponge compression was performed to decrease any osteotomy bleeding and subsequent bruising.

9. Right alar rim incisions were connected from the lateral dorsum and incised to medial crus and down to the nasal spine. The depressor nasi musculature was divided and a pocket over the nasal spine developed. The distal septal cartilage was excised in a small triangular fashion to assist in tip elevation. The alar base was incised a fraction of a millimeter above the alar crease. This gave better access to the nose.

10. A fine rasp smoothed the dorsum. The alar cartilages were not delivered, but a very small reduction of the upper third through the single intercartilaginous posterior cartilage delivery technique was performed to provide a slight increase in alar definition at this site. The salvaged septal cartilage was crushed and a nasion graft placed securely with a 5-0 Dexon pull-out suture. The auricular cartilage was excised and formed into a concave-to-concave "pea-pod" tip graft with 4-0 and 5-0 Dexon.

11. The right alar-to-columella incision just behind the medial footplate was opened and the entire alar cartilage and soft tip conservatively degloved. The lateral and frontal view of the nose was evaluated and a methylene blue mark placed at the desired tip projection point. A "pea-pod" tip graft and a small quantity of right postauricular fascia were placed over the tip of the graft to decrease "pointing."

12. The "pea-pod" tip graft measured 2.8 cm $\times$ 0.8 cm. 4-0 Dexon pull-out sutures were placed at each end of the graft. The deeper nasal spine end was placed and secured with a pull-out 4-0 Dexon suture. The tip was elevated with a double-hook and the tip of the "pea-pod" tip graft placed within the nasal tip, guided by the pull-out suture. The graft's position was adjusted two or three times to ensure the optimum midline and projecting position of the graft. Two 4-0 plain catgut mattress sutures were placed through the graft and columella. The right columellar incision was then closed. A left columellar and left tip incision was not performed to ensure a proper envelope of circumferential vascularized tissue.

13. The incised alar base was retracted and a subdermal dissection on the cheek side was performed for approximately 1 cm. This allowed good mobility of the base of the flap medially toward the piriform aperture, narrowing the base. The alae were then reduced by excising a triangular segment of tissue from each alar edge. After hemostasis was ensured a single 5-0 PDS suture was passed through the base and through the alae. This resulted in a more convex alar appearance than the normally seen flat alar triangularity. When the base is moved medially, the springy alar cartilage ensures proper convexity and curvature of the alar walls. The alar base was then closed with 6-0 interrupted nylon su-

tures. The petroleum jelly packing was removed and Merocel nasal tampons soaked in 0.5% bupivacaine hydrochloride (Marcaine) with epinephrine were placed inside the nose. Additional intranasal wounds were closed with 5-0 plain catgut. Benzoin form-fitting tape and a thin formed-aluminum splint were placed.

The patient was instructed in the use of postoperative ice compresses to the eyes. The patient will be using Arnica tablets and the homeopathic program mentioned in the patient postoperative instructions (see Chapter 5, "Postoperative Nasal Packing and Dressings").

The dressing was changed and pull-out sutures clipped at 4 days. Retaping was applied for an additional 2 days. Thereafter, the patient's nose was left untaped during the day, but pressure taped at night for 2 to 4 weeks to ensure tip edema resolution. At 48 hours, the intranasal Merocel packing was soaked with 1% Xylocaine with epinephrine and gently removed. The internal Merocel tube equalized nasopharyngeal pressure and the patient had not felt stuffy or that he had nasal packs in place.

Postoperative Comments

One year postoperatively, the patient had a straight, normally projecting dorsum. There was a very slight dorsal nasal curve, as the patient desired. The tip was well projecting with a normal, open nasolabial angle. The tip had a much more defined apex located slightly above the dorsal line and incorporated a very slight supratip break. The thickness of the alae was reduced. The width of the nose was slightly decreased, but balanced. The upper lateral cartilages were untouched and nasal valving upon inspiration was minimal. The tip graft and tip elevation improved the patient's airway flow subjectively and objectively. Alar aperture and side walls were narrowed and rotated medially. The scars were very inconspicuous and acceptable.

Patient Y (Fig. 9-3a, 9-3b, 9-3c, 9-3d)

This 40-year-old Black female complained of thickness and poor definition of her nose. Intranasal examination revealed a nasal septum deflected to the right and moderate hypertrophy of the turbinates. Her nasal dorsum was wide, but the projection satisfactory. The tip was broad, thick, and ill defined. The alae were broad. The patient had a slightly hanging columella and retraction of the nasal spine. She desired a smaller, more refined nose. Surgical limits due to thick skin were discussed in detail with her. The patient understood that the size and bulkiness of the tip could not be significantly reduced, but definition and refinement could be improved. She accepted more tip projection if it improved the definition. The patient was happy with her other facial features and did not desire other changes. One aspect of the patient's emotional/psychological makeup was impatience, which made it difficult for her to complete the necessary waiting time to achieve optimal results. It was explained to the patient that postoperatively she would require both nighttime taping and dilute intermittent Kenalog

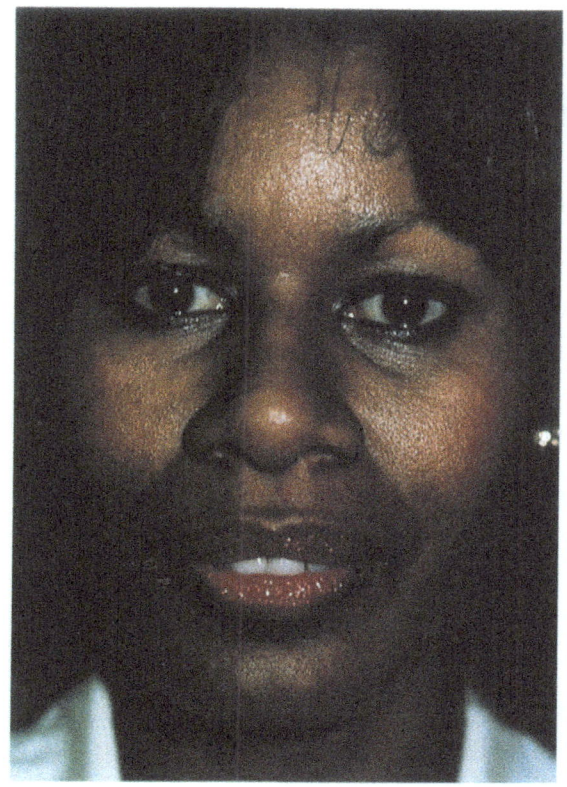 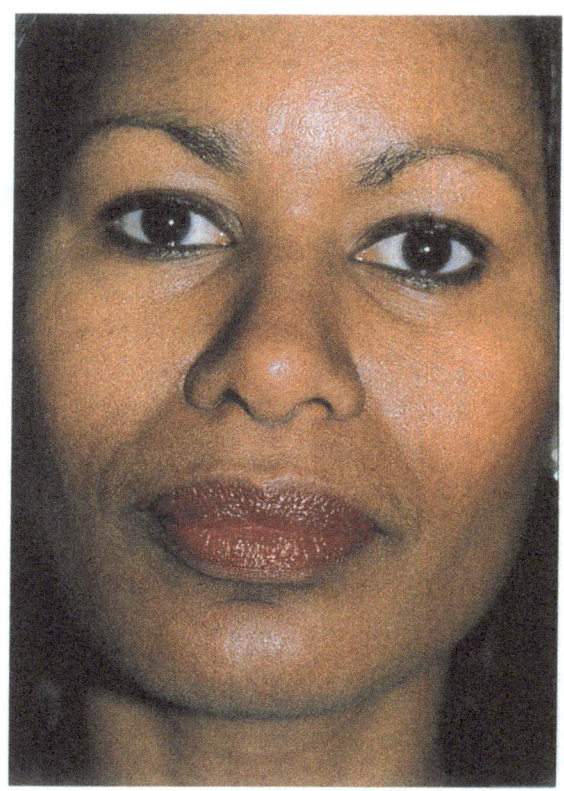

Figure 9-3a, 9-3b
This black female has already undergone two unsuccessful rhinoplasties. A previously placed, small tip graft failed to provide adequate projection.

(10 mg/ml suspension triamcinolone acetonide) injections to improve the resolution of tip swelling.

The five-page Preoperative Nasal Checklist was used for the patient's consultative evaluation (Fig. 9-4).

Operative Procedure

1. The operation was performed under general anesthesia. Eight milligrams of intravenous dexamethasone sodium phosphate (Decadron) and 25 mg of intravenous diphenhydramine hydrochloride (Benadryl) with 1 g of cephalosporin was administered.
2. 0.5% bupivacaine hydrochloride (Marcaine) with epinephrine was used to infiltrate the right ear, septum, turbinates, and entire nose.
3. Septal cartilage was excised and the obstructing vomer segment fractured with an osteotome and excised.
4. The turbinates were infiltrated, with bupivacaine hydrochloride (Marcaine) and then with 5 mg/cc Kenalog (10 mg/ml suspension triamcinolone acetonide). The left turbinate was more enlarged than the right. A flap was elevated, the protuberant turbinate bone was excised, and the flap was cauterized and sutured back over the bare area. Petroleum jelly packing was initially placed deep within the nasal vault to decrease blood in the posterior pharynx. The packing was removed

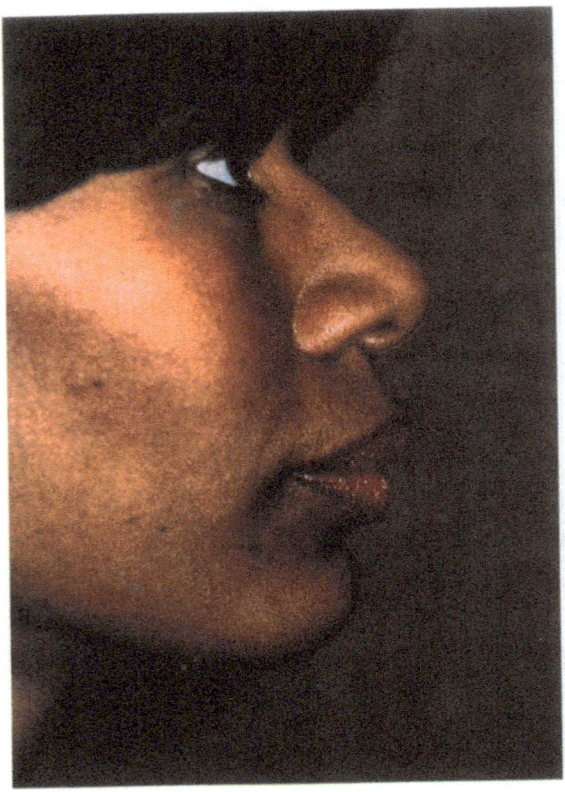

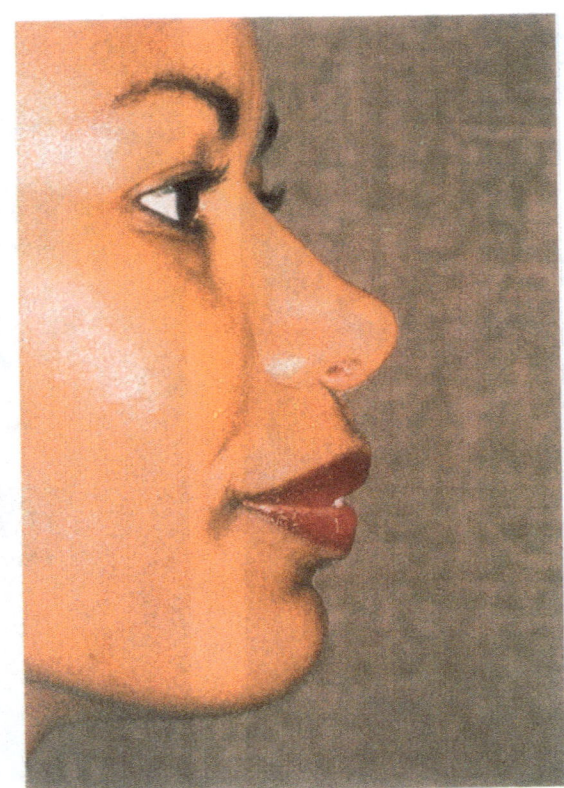

Figure 9-3c, 9-3d
The nose has greater projection due to the placement of a 3.5 cm × 1 cm "pea-pod" graft. No tip defatting was possible, because of scarring, but the amount of projection gives the illusion of a thinner lip.

and a Merocel nasal tampon soaked in local anesthetic and coated with bacitracin zinc was placed within the nasal area.

5. The left helical cartilage cup was excised through a waving postauricular incision. The area was then closed with 4-0 Dexon and 4-0 Prolene and petroleum jelly packing form-fitted into the area. The cartilage was taken and placed into a saline-moistened 4 × 4 and placed over an ice bag. The ice bag was placed under a sterile waterproof drape to keep the cartilage cooled.

6. A chromic catgut mattress suture to decrease bleeding in the closure of the septum was performed. This suture is especially helpful when excised bone or cartilage is replaced in the septal pocket.

7. The dorsum was freed. The lateral walls were kept attached and not undermined to ensure good support of the nasal bones with infracturing.

8. A dorsal irregularity was lightly rasped. Approximately 1–2 mm of irregular dorsal cartilaginous septum was excised.

9. Osteotomies were performed through the piriform aperture. This was done early and not later. The rougher parts of the procedure should be done early so as to not disrupt fine distal cartilage grafting that may be done later on in the procedure. Bilateral "bucket handle" alar rim incisions were made and the right side carried down to just below the medial cartilaginous footplate to gain access to the tip. The cartilages were dissected. As much fibrofatty tissue as possible was dissected and left on the alar cartilages. A plane was chosen to leave just a slight amount of subdermal soft tissue on the skin with most of it on the car-

PREOPERATIVE NASAL EVALUATION AND CHECKLIST

I use a checklist when preoperatively assessing patients. It assists me in obtaining a history, assessing the aesthetic goals of the patient, and performing a complete nasal examination. In addition, a complete medical history and physical examination should be performed prior to surgery.

NASAL CHECKLIST

Name:___Patient Y_____ Date:_____

Previous History Of:

Childhood or adulthood injuries?   Yes_____ No___X___ If yes, explain:_____

Nasal Surgery?   Yes_____ No___X___
  Date and Specifics?   _____
  X-rays?   Yes_____ No_____

_____Nasal Airway Obstruction: Left_____ Right_____ Both___X___ Consistent___X___
                                                                                    Intermittent_____

_____Sinus Infections: Yes_____ No___X___ When:_____

_____Nasal Allergy Symptoms: Yes_____ No___X___
                                               _____Stuffiness _____Sneezing _____Postnasal Drip

_____Nasal Spray Use: Yes_____ No___X___
                                               Type:_____ Frequency:_____

_____Nasal Bleeding: Yes_____ No___X___

_____Smoking: Yes___X___ No_____ How much_____PPD

_____Aspirin or Aspirin-like Medication Use:_____

_____Hypertension: Yes_____ No___X___

_____Previous History of Troublesome Scarring: Yes_____ No___X___
                                               Where_____ Specifics_____

Additional Comments: _____
                                               _____

Figure 9-4
Preoperative Nasal Evaluation and Checklist.

Patient's Aesthetic Goals:

I. Dorsum/Bridge
    ___Retain Convexity
    _X_Retain Width
    ___Reduce Bridge Width
    _X_Reduce Dorsum To:
        ___Straight   _X_Slight Concavity
        ___Moderate Concavity
    ___Graft Dorsum   ___Graft Nasion   ___Graft Frontal Bone
    ___Other: _____

II. Tip
    ___No Change
    _X_Reduce Width
    _X_More Tip Projection
    ___No Angle Change
    ___Elevate Angle To _____

III. Alar Base
    ___No Change
    _X_Narrow
    ___Graft Nasal Base

Additional Comments/Procedures: _____
_____
_____

Nasal Examination:

A basic general physical examination should be performed.

I. Skin: ___Normal ___Medium _X_Thick ___Hypopigmented
_X_Sebaceous ___Normal Pigment
___Scars _X_Hyperpigmented

II. Septum: ___Straight _X_Deviated ___Left _X_Right
___% Obstruction ___Left ___Right
___Sufficient For Use As Graft ___Yes ___No

III. Vomer: ___Straight
_X_Deflected: ___Left _X_Right
___Spurred: ___Left ___Right

IV. Nasal Valve: ___Open
_X_Narrow
___Compromised

V. Turbinates: ___Small ___Right ___Left ___Both
___Deep ___Normal ___Right ___Left ___Both
___Flat _X_Enlarged ___Right ___Left _X_Both

VI. Nasion: Angle: _____

VII. Dorsum/Bridge: ___Convex _X_Straight ___Concave
___Narrow _X_Wide ___Normal Width
___Regular ___Irregular

VIII. Upper Lateral Cartilage: _X_Narrow ___Medium ___Wide

IV. Tip: ___Narrow ___Normal _X_Wide
___Adequate Projection
_X_Insufficient Projection

X. Columella: ___Normal ___Retracted _X_Hanging
___Angle: ___closed___ ___Narrow ___Wide

XI. Nasal Spine: ___Small _X_Normal ___Large

XII. Alar Base: ___Normal ___Moderate Width _X_Excessive Width

Surgical Plan:

Grafting To Be Performed: _X_ Yes   ___ No

Source Of Graft: ___ Cranial Bone
                    _X_ Auricular
                    ___ Septum
                    ___ Other: _____

I. Nasion
    _X_ No Change
    ___ Ostectomy
    ___ Graft

II. Septum
    ___ Septectomy
    _X_ Septoplasty
    ___ Vomer Spur Ostectomy
    ___ Packing   ___ Yes   ___ No — Left ___   Right ___   Both ___

III. Turbinates
    _X_ Inject   Left ___   Right ___   Both _X_
    ___ Cauterization   Left ___   Right ___   Both ___
    _X_ Clamping/Excis.   Left _X_   Right ___   Both ___
    ___ S.M. Resections   Left ___   Right ___   Both ___

IV. Dorsum/Bridge
    ___ Ostectomies
    _X_ Rasp
    ___ Osteotomy
    ___ Graft
        ___ Septum
        ___ Auricular
        ___ Cranial
        ___ Other

V. Columella
    ___ No Change
    _X_ Raise To _open_ Angle

Additional Comments/Procedures: _____

_____

_____

VI. Tip
    ____No Change
    _X_Reduce Alar Cartilages
       Approach: ____Cartilage Splitting Incisions
                       _X_Rim Incisions
                       ____Open Technique

    _X_Tip Grafting: Yes _X_   No ____
       ____Septum
       _X_Auricular
       ____Other:_____

VII. Base
    ____No Change
    ____Reduce Spine
    ____Augment Spine
    _X_Augment Maxilla

VIII. Alae
    ____No Change
    _X_Reduce
       ____Small
       _X_Medium
       ____Large

Additional Comments/Procedures:

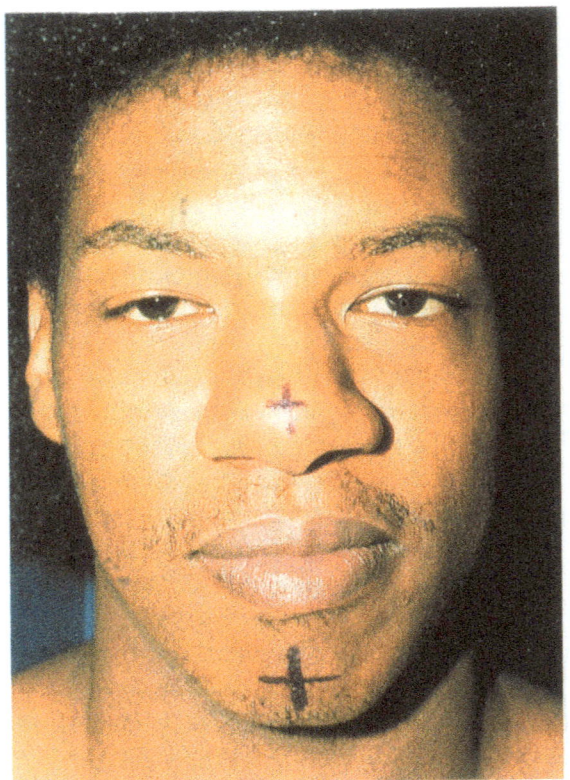

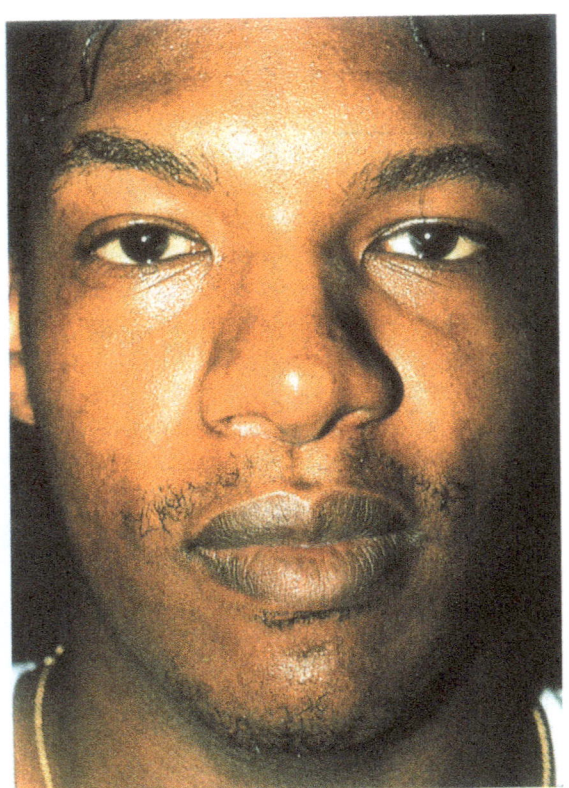

Figure 9-5a, 9-5b
This black male had a very thick, bulbous nasal tip.

tilage. These dissections are done very cautiously so as not to devascularize the area. The patient had bulky, thicker-than-normal alar cartilages.

10. The superior three-fifths of the lateral cartilages and mucosa were left intact.

11. Conchal cartilage from the right ear was used to construct a "pea-pod" graft of 3.5 cm × 1 cm. The graft extended from the nasal spine to nasal tip. 4-0 Dexon pull-out sutures were used.

12. Excess auricular and septal cartilage was used to augment the maxilla.

13. The alae were incised 1 mm along the crease.

14. Four millimeters of the alae was excised. The wounds were approximated with placed 5-0 PDS and 6-0 nylon.

15. The mucosa were closed with 5-0 plain catgut.

16. Nasal tape and an aluminum splint were used.

Postoperative Comments

Postoperatively, the patient has an attractive, minimally sloped dorsum, good tip projection, and a narrower tip. Her airway was also improved.

Patient X (Fig. 9-5a, 9-5b, 9-5c, 9-5d)

This young black male was concerned about his excessively large nose. The patient complained about the width of the nose, the prominence of the alae, and the nondefined bulky nasal tip. He requested a particularly well

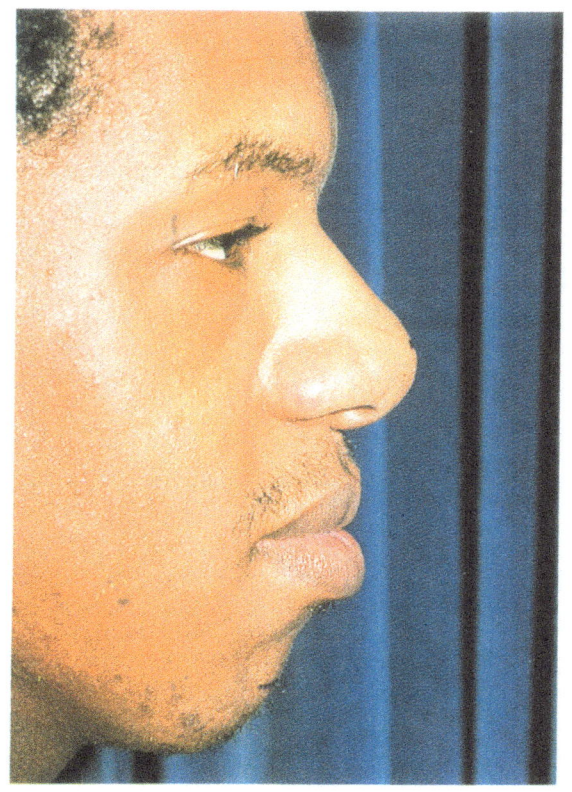
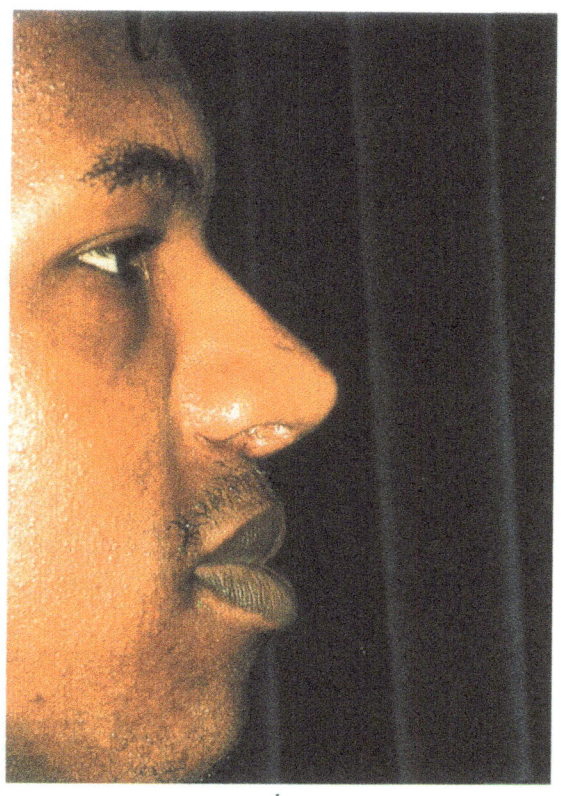

c

d

Figure 9-5c, 9-5d
To correct this, a very stiff, double-layered 3.5 cm × 1 cm conchal cartilage graft was utilized, and minimal tip thinning was performed. Again, this demonstrates the ability of this graft to give the illusion of thinner tip skin.

defined nasal tip. The patient was rather large and did not want an excessively small nose, but desired improved balance with his facial features. He additionally desired a chin implant. The patient's nasion and dorsal bridge projection was adequate. He had maxillary retrusion and onlay cartilage grafts were planned along with a nasal spine graft. The patient was told that due to the size of his nose, he might require more than one procedure.

The five-page Preoperative Nasal Checklist was used for the patient's consultative evaluation (Fig. 9-6).

Operative Procedure

1. The procedure was performed under general anesthesia. Eight milligrams of intravenous dexamethasone sodium phosphate (Decadron) and 25 mg of intravenous diphenhydramine hydrochloride (Benadryl) with 1 g of cephalosporin was administered.
2. 0.5% Bupivacaine hydrochloride (Marcaine) with epinephrine was utilized to infiltrate the nose, left ear, septum, and turbinates.
3. A left curvilinear postauricular incision was made and the conchal cup cartilage was excised and placed into a saline-moistened sponge. After bleeding was controlled, 0.5% bupivacaine hydrochloride (Marcaine) with 1:100,000 epinephrine and dilute Kenalog (10 mg/ml suspension triamcinolone acetonide) was sprayed into the wound. It was then closed over a .25" Penrose drain. Petroleum ribbon packing was molded into the anterior conchal cup and postauricular sulcus for compression.

PREOPERATIVE NASAL EVALUATION AND CHECKLIST

I use a checklist when preoperatively assessing patients. It assists me in obtaining a history, assessing the aesthetic goals of the patient, and performing a complete nasal examination. In addition, a complete medical history and physical examination should be performed prior to surgery.

NASAL CHECKLIST

Name: _Patient X_____   Date:_____

Previous History Of:

Childhood or adulthood injuries?   Yes_____ No__X__ If yes, explain:_____

Nasal Surgery?   Yes_____ No_____
    Date and Specifics?   _____
    X-rays?   Yes_____ No_____

_____Nasal Airway Obstruction: Left_____ Right_____ Both__X__ Consistent__X__
    Intermittent_____

_____Sinus Infections: Yes_____ No__X__ When:_____

_____Nasal Allergy Symptoms: Yes_____ No__X__
    _____Stuffiness   _____Sneezing   _____Postnasal Drip

_____Nasal Spray Use: Yes_____ No__X__
    Type:_____   Frequency:_____

_____Nasal Bleeding: Yes_____ No__X__

_____Smoking: Yes_____ No__X__ How much_____PPD

_____Aspirin or Aspirin-like Medication Use:_____

_____Hypertension: Yes_____ No__X__

_____Previous History of Troublesome Scarring: Yes_____ No__X__
    Where_____ Specifics_____

Additional Comments: _____

_____

Figure 9-6
Preoperative Nasal Evaluation and Checklist.

Patient's Aesthetic Goals:

I. Dorsum/Bridge
_____Retain Convexity
_____Retain Width
__X__Reduce Bridge Width
__X__Reduce Dorsum To:
       _____Straight   __X__Slight Concavity
       _____Moderate Concavity
_____Graft Dorsum   _____Graft Nasion   _____Graft Frontal Bone
_____Other: _____

II. Tip
_____No Change
__X__Reduce Width
__X__More Tip Projection
_____No Angle Change
_____Elevate Angle To _____

III. Alar Base
_____No Change
__X__Narrow
_____Graft Nasal Base

Additional Comments/Procedures: _____
_____
_____
_____

Nasal Examination:

A basic general physical examination should be performed.

I. Skin: ___Normal ___Medium _X_Thick ___Hypopigmented
_X_Sebaceous ___Normal Pigment
___Scars _X_Hyperpigmented

II. Septum: ___Straight _X_Deviated _X_Left ___Right
___% Obstruction ___Left ___Right
___Sufficient For Use As Graft ___Yes _X_No

III. Vomer: ___Straight
_X_Deflected: _X_Left ___Right
___Spurred: ___Left ___Right

IV. Nasal Valve: ___Open
_X_Narrow
___Compromised

V. Turbinates: ___Small ___Right ___Left ___Both
___Deep ___Normal ___Right ___Left ___Both
___Flat _X_Enlarged ___Right ___Left _X_Both

VI. Nasion: Angle: ___Closed___

VII. Dorsum/Bridge: ___Convex _X_Straight ___Concave
___Narrow _X_Wide ___Normal Width
___Regular ___Irregular

VIII. Upper Lateral Cartilage: _X_Narrow ___Medium ___Wide

IV. Tip: ___Narrow ___Normal _X_Wide
___Adequate Projection
_X_Insufficient Projection

X. Columella: ___Normal ___Retracted _X_Hanging
_X_Angle: ___Closed___ ___Narrow ___Wide

XI. Nasal Spine: _X_Small ___Normal ___Large

XII. Alar Base: ___Normal ___Moderate Width _X_Excessive Width

Surgical Plan:

Grafting To Be Performed: _X_ Yes   ___ No

Source Of Graft: ___ Cranial Bone
                    ___ Auricular
                    _X_ Septum
                    ___ Other: _____

I. Nasion
___ No Change
___ Ostectomy
_X_ Graft

II. Septum
___ Septectomy
_X_ Septoplasty
___ Vomer Spur Ostectomy
_X_ Packing   _X_ Yes   ___ No — Left ___   Right ___   Both _X_

III. Turbinates
_X_ Inject   Left ___   Right ___   Both _X_
___ Cauterization   Left ___   Right ___   Both ___
___ Clamping/Excis.   Left ___   Right ___   Both ___
___ S.M. Resections   Left ___   Right ___   Both ___

IV. Dorsum/Bridge
___ Ostectomies
_X_ Rasp
_X_ Osteotomy
___ Graft
    ___ Septum
    ___ Auricular
    ___ Cranial
    ___ Other

V. Columella
___ No Change
_X_ Raise To _open_ Angle

Additional Comments/Procedures: _____

_____

_____

Surgical Plan: (continued)

VI. Tip
___No Change
__X__ Reduce Alar Cartilages
    Approach: ___Cartilage Splitting Incisions
                   __X__ Rim Incisions
                   ___Open Technique

__X__ Tip Grafting: Yes __X__   No ___
    ___Septum
    __X__ Auricular
    ___Other:_____

VII. Base
___No Change
___Reduce Spine
__X__ Augment Spine
___Augment Maxilla

VIII. Alae
___No Change
__X__ Reduce
    ___Small
    __X__ Medium
    ___Large

Additional Comments/Procedures: _____
_____
_____

4. A moistened oralpharyngeal pack was placed and petroleum jelly packing was placed deep within the posterior nasal vault to decrease any flow of blood below the posterior pharynx to minimize coughing and nausea postoperatively.

5. Oxymetazoline hydrochloride–soaked (Afrin) cotton pledgets were used to shrink nasal mucosa. Septal excision was performed through the left nasi aperture with excision of the obstructing septal segment, and excision of the vomer ridge. A modified submucous resection of the interior turbinate was performed. The mucosal leaves were elevated and the obstructed bony segment was excised and the turbinate mucosa sutured over the open wound. Further cauterization, outfracturing, and 5 mg/cc Kenalog (10 mg/ml suspension triamcinolone acetonide) was injected into the area. At that point a secondary set of petroleum jelly gauze packets was utilized to compress the operative area. 4-0 catgut and plain mattress sutures were used in the septum and in closing the turbinate mucosa.

6. Intercartilaginous incisions were made and the dorsum was freed. The superior half of the lateral nasal wall, including the bone and upper lateral cartilage segments, was freed. Soft tissue was left attached to the bottom half of the nasal bones to provide good support after infracturing.

7. Through lighted refractors, a #11 broken-tip blade was used to carefully excise the excessively projecting cartilaginous dorsum. Great care was taken to leave the mucosa between the septum and upper lateral cartilages intact. It was not necessary to trim the upper lateral cartilages. Spreader grafts were not necessary to maintain the valvular mechanism.

8. Two millimeter-osteotomes were used to punch through the piriform aperture and a stepwise fracturing was performed from the inferior nasal-maxillary junction upward to the medial canthal area.

9. Infracturing and 5 minutes of moderate nasal compression were performed to decrease any osteotomy bleeding and subsequent bruising.

10. Intercartilaginous incisions were connected over the dorsum and incised down to the nasal spine. The depressor nasi musculature was divided and a pocket over the nasal spine developed. The distal septal cartilage was excised in a small triangular fashion to assist in tip elevation. The alar base was incised a fraction of a millimeter above the alar crease to give better access to the nose.

11. A fine rasp smoothed the dorsum. The upper third of the alar cartilages were reduced through the single intercartilaginous posterior cartilage delivery technique to provide a slight increase in alar definition at the site. The salvaged septal cartilage was crushed and a nasion graft placed securely with a 5-0 Dexon pull-out suture. The auricular cartilage was excised and formed into a concave-to-concave "pea-pod" tip graft with 4-0 and 5-0 Dexon.

12. A right alar-to-columella incision just behind the medial footplate was performed and the entire alar cartilage and soft tip conservatively degloved. The lateral and frontal view of the nose was evaluated and a bupivacaine hydrochloride (Marcaine) injection placed at the desired

tip projection point. A "pea-pod" tip graft was constructed and a small quantity of right postauricular fascia was used over the tip of the graft to decrease "pointing."

13. The "pea-pod" tip graft measured 3.5 cm × 1 cm. 4-0 Dexon pull-out sutures were placed at each end of the graft. The deeper nasal spine end was placed and secured with a pull-out 4-0 Dexon suture. The tip was elevated with a double-hook and the tip of the needle followed by the "pea-pod" tip graft placed within the nasal tip. Two 4-0 plain catgut mattress sutures were placed through the columella and then the right columellar incision was closed. No left columellar or left tip incision was performed to ensure an envelope of properly vascularized tissue.

14. The incised alar base was subdermally dissected on the cheek side for approximately 1 cm to allow good mobility of the flap base medially toward the piriform aperture. The alae were then reduced by excising a 4-mm segment of tissue from each alar edge. After hemostasis was ensured, a single 5-0 PDS suture was passed through the base and through the alae. The alar base was then closed with 6-0 interrupted nylon sutures. The petroleum jelly packing was removed and Merocel nasal tampons soaked in 0.5% bupivacaine hydrochloride (Marcaine) with epinephrine were placed inside the nose. Additional intranasal wounds were closed with 5-0 plain catgut. Benzoin, form-fitting tape and a thin formed-aluminum splint were placed.

The patient was instructed in the use of postoperative ice compresses to the eyes. The patient used Arnica tablets and the homeopathic program mentioned in the patient postoperative instructions (see Chapter 6, "Postoperative Patient Instruction").

At 48 hours, the intranasal Merocel packing was soaked with 1% Xylocaine with epinephrine and gently removed. The inner Merocel tube equalized nasopharyngeal pressure and the patient did not feel that he had nasal packs in place. The dressing was changed and pull-out sutures clipped at 4 days. Retaping was applied for an additional 2 days. Thereafter, the patient was left with the nose untaped during the day, but pressure taped at night for 2 to 4 weeks to ensure tip edema resolution.

Postoperative Comments

Fourteen months postoperatively, the patient had a straight, normally projecting dorsum. There was a very well projecting tip with a normal nasolabial angle. The tip had a "tented" effect which gave the appearance of a thinner tip. The thickness of the alae was reduced. The width of the nose was decreased, but balanced. Upper lateral cartilages were untouched, and nasal valving upon inspiration was minimal. The tip graft improved the patient's airway flow. It was subjectively and objectively improved. Alar aperture and side walls were narrowed and rotated medially. The alar scars were very inconspicuous and acceptable. The patient was very pleased with the improved balance of his nose. Minimal tip soft-tissue thinning and a very stiff, double-layered 3 cm × 1 cm conchal cartilage "pea-pod" tip graft provided greater definition and gives the illusion of thinner tip skin.

This patient desired a revision rhinoplasty. She had two previous nasal operations and desired further refinement of the nose, especially the nasal tip. The patient felt that her nasal tip drooped and that she had a hanging columella and a depressed nasion. The dorsum contained a Silastic graft. Functionally, the patient complained of left nasal airway obstruction and some valvular collapse with deep inspiration. On speculum examination, the patient had a septum deflected to the left, with a right hypertrophic turbinate and polyp. She was treated for 1 week preoperatively with topical cortisone spray. Long-acting, nonsedating antihistamines were also of benefit.

The surgical plan was as follows:

1. Replacement of the Silastic dorsal graft with crushed septal cartilage.
2. An open approach to the tip was planned. The graft would be placed through a stepped columellar incision.
3. An auricular cartilage graft would be used to construct a "pea-pod" tip graft.
4. The alar bases were to be conservatively reduced and medially rotated.

The five-page Preoperative Nasal Checklist was used for the patient's consultative evaluation (Fig. 9-8).

Figure 9-7a, 9-7b
This Asian female had a scarred, thick, undefined nasal tip.

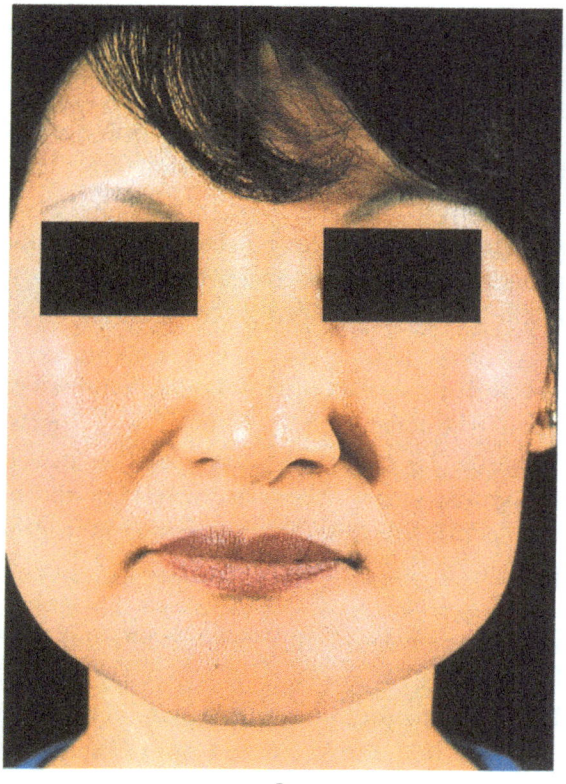

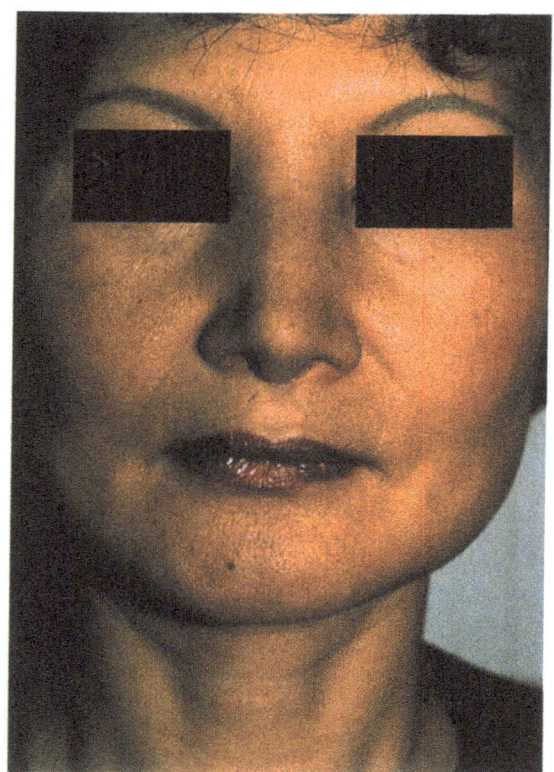

a

b

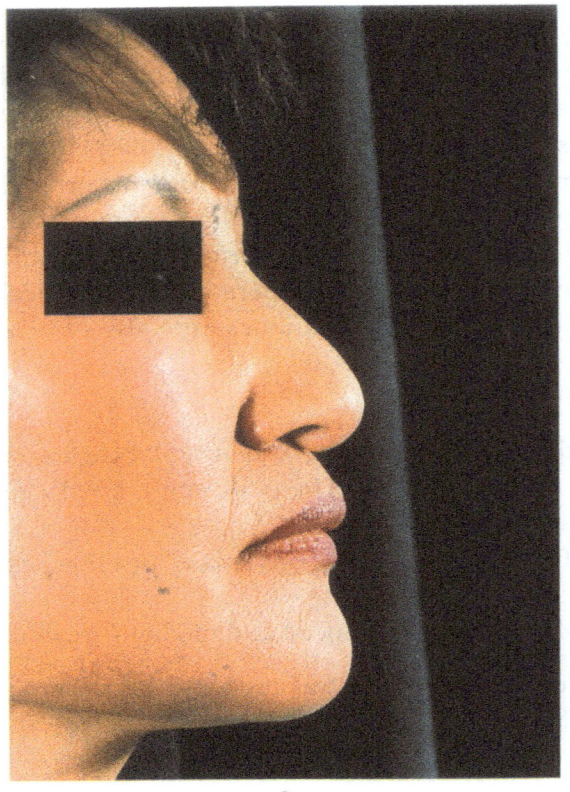

Figure 9-7c, 9-7d
A midline, open rhinoplasty was performed, and a 3 cm × 1.25 cm "peapod" graft was placed.

Operative Procedure

1. A general anesthetic was administered. Eight milligrams of intravenous dexamethasone sodium phosphate (Decadron) and 25 mg of intravenous diphenhydramine hydrochloride (Benadryl) with 1 g of cephalosporin was administered.

2. 0.5% Bupivacaine hydrochloride (Marcaine) with epinephrine 1:100,000 was used to infiltrate the internal and external nose. Care was taken to avoid dorsal nasal infiltration in order to better judge the degree of dorsal correction with grafting. The left ear was infiltrated.

3. The posterior nasal vault was packed with petroleum jelly gauze and the pharynx packed with saline-moistened sponge to decrease blood accumulation in the posterior pharynx.

4. After slight blanching was seen due to epinephrine effect, 5 mg/cc Kenalog (10 mg/ml suspension triamcinolone acetonide) was injected into the nasal tip and turbinates. To ensure retention of this steroid, it was injected after the vasoconstrictive effect was noted. In the author's opinion, dilute Kenalog (10 mg/ml suspension triamcinolone acetonide) administered prior to surgery markedly decreases acute and chronic edema.

5. Due to the associated columellar incision, very limited alar incisions were planned. A stepped columella incision was made. Very cautious dissection was performed anterior to the medial footplate. The entire anterior nose was dissected up to the lateral crus and upper lateral cartilages. The dorsal Silastic graft was removed and the dorsal capsule

PREOPERATIVE NASAL EVALUATION AND CHECKLIST

I use a checklist when preoperatively assessing patients. It assists me in obtaining a history, assessing the aesthetic goals of the patient, and performing a complete nasal examination. In addition, a complete medical history and physical examination should be performed prior to surgery.

NASAL CHECKLIST

Name:_Patient W_____ Date:_____

Previous History Of:

Childhood or adulthood injuries?   Yes_____ No__X___ If yes, explain:_____

Nasal Surgery?   Yes__X__ No_____
  Date and Specifics?
  X-rays?   Yes_____ No_____

_____Nasal Airway Obstruction: Left_____ Right_____ Both__X__ Consistent___X___
                                                                 Intermittent_____

_____Sinus Infections: Yes_____ No__X__ When:_____

_____Nasal Allergy Symptoms: Yes_____ No__X__
               _____Stuffiness _____Sneezing _____Postnasal Drip

_____Nasal Spray Use: Yes_____ No__X__
               Type:_____ Frequency:_____

_____Nasal Bleeding: Yes_____ No__X__

_____Smoking: Yes_____ No__X__ How much_____PPD

_____Aspirin or Aspirin-like Medication Use:_____

_____Hypertension: Yes_____ No__X__

_____Previous History of Troublesome Scarring: Yes_____ No__X__
                                           Where_____ Specifics_____

Additional Comments: _____

                                            _____

Figure 9-8
Preoperative Nasal Evaluation and Checklist.

Patient's Aesthetic Goals:

I. Dorsum/Bridge
____Retain Convexity
____Retain Width
__X__Reduce Bridge Width
__X__Reduce Dorsum To:
     ____Straight   ____Slight Concavity
    __X__Moderate Concavity
____Graft Dorsum   __X__Graft Nasion   ____Graft Frontal Bone
____Other: _____

II. Tip
____No Change
__X__Reduce Width
__X__More Tip Projection
____No Angle Change
____Elevate Angle To _____

III. Alar Base
____No Change
__X__Narrow
____Graft Nasal Base

Additional Comments/Procedures: _____
_____
_____

Nasal Examination:

A basic general physical examination should be performed.

I. **Skin:** ___Normal ___Medium _X_Thick ___Hypopigmented
___Sebaceous ___Normal Pigment
___Scars ___Hyperpigmented

II. **Septum:** ___Straight _X_Deviated _X_Left ___Right
___% Obstruction ___Left ___Right
___Sufficient For Use As Graft ___Yes ___No

III. **Vomer:** ___Straight
_X_Deflected: _X_Left ___Right
___Spurred: ___Left ___Right

IV. **Nasal Valve:** ___Open
_X_Narrow
___Compromised

V. **Turbinates:** ___Small ___Right ___Left ___Both
___Deep ___Normal ___Right ___Left ___Both
___Flat _X_Enlarged _X_Right ___Left ___Both

VI. **Nasion:** Angle: _____

VII. **Dorsum/Bridge:** _X_Convex ___Straight ___Concave
___Narrow _X_Wide ___Normal Width
___Regular ___Irregular

VIII. **Upper Lateral Cartilage:** _X_Narrow ___Medium ___Wide

IV. **Tip:** ___Narrow _X_Normal ___Wide
___Adequate Projection
_X_Insufficient Projection

X. **Columella:** ___Normal ___Retracted _X_Hanging
___Angle: _closed_ ___Narrow ___Wide

XI. **Nasal Spine:** _X_Small ___Normal ___Large

XII. **Alar Base:** ___Normal _X_Moderate Width ___Excessive Width

Surgical Plan:

Grafting To Be Performed: X Yes   ___No

Source Of Graft: ___Cranial Bone
                    X Auricular
                    ___Septum
                    ___Other: _____

I. Nasion
    ___No Change
    ___Ostectomy
    X Graft

X

II. Septum
    ___Septectomy
    X Septoplasty
    ___Vomer Spur Ostectomy
    X Packing   ___Yes   ___No — Left ___   Right ___   Both X

III. Turbinates
    X Inject   Left ___   Right ___   Both X
    ___Cauterization   Left ___   Right ___   Both ___
    ___Clamping/Excis. Left ___   Right ___   Both ___
    ___S.M. Resections Left ___   Right ___   Both ___

IV. Dorsum/Bridge
    ___Ostectomies
    ___Rasp
    X Osteotomy
    X Graft
        ___Septum
        X Auricular
        ___Cranial
        ___Other

V. Columella
    ___No Change
    X Raise To_open_Angle

Additional Comments/Procedures: _____

_____

_____

VI. Tip
    <u>X</u> No Change
    ___ Reduce Alar Cartilages
        Approach: ___ Cartilage Splitting Incisions
                       ___ Rim Incisions
                       ___ Open Technique

    <u>X</u> Tip Grafting: Yes <u>X</u>   No ___
        ___ Septum
        <u>X</u> Auricular
        ___ Other:_____

VII. Base
    ___ No Change
    ___ Reduce Spine
    <u>X</u> Augment Spine
    ___ Augment Maxilla

VIII. Alae
    ___ No Change
    <u>X</u> Reduce
        ___ Small
        <u>X</u> Medium
        ___ Large

Additional Comments/Procedures: _____

was subperiosteally dissected. Layered septal cartilage secured together with 5-0 Vicryl was used to graft the dorsum and nasion.

6. A 3 cm × 1.25 cm "pea-pod" tip graft was constructed. The tip pocket was deepened over the nasal spine and the right alar cartilage freed from the medial footplate to the lateral extent of the cartilage. The concave-to-concave side of the graft was sutured together with 5-0 Dexon. Dexon was then wrapped around the graft to provide a stiffer, more supportive strut.

7. Piriform osteotomies were performed. In darker-complected patients, piriform osteotomies are preferable to external stab skin incisions. Even though small 1–2-mm nicks may not be seen in fair skin, in the black patient, they may look like a dark mole or scar. Once the periosteum is elevated, the osteotome can be placed against the nasomaxillary junction, a subperiosteal tunnel can be created, and the osteotomies then performed. Five to 7 minutes of pressure is applied in order to markedly decrease swelling and bruising.

8. A premeasured excision of the alar base is performed. Undermining of the wound defect at the vestibular border-cheek junction is performed, and, utilizing 5-0 PDS sutures, a medial approximation is performed to create a smaller, more medially positioned base.

9. A curved mosquito clamp is placed through the columellar-tip incision and the tip is projected where the apex is located. Frontal, lateral, and oblique viewing is performed. The apex is then measured and marked. A "pea-pod" graft is positioned into the nasal tip, utilizing forceps. The "pea-pod" tip graft base suture is then placed deep within the nasal spine and brought out at the columellar-labial angle. The graft is then appropriately positioned. The position and projection is then checked very carefully. A French knot is then tied at both apex and base, and a 4-0 chromic catgut mattress suture is placed through the columella and graft to secure the position.

10. The alar and columellar wounds are closed with 5-0 chromic catgut. A 4-0 or 5-0 PDS is then used to approximate the alae to the repositioned vestibular-cheek alar base defect. The sutures are placed bilaterally and viewed from various perspectives to ensure symmetry and proper positioning.

11. The open wounds are irrigated with 0.5% bupivacaine hydrochloride (Marcaine) with epinephrine and 5 mg/cc Kenalog (10 mg/ml suspension triamcinolone acetonide). All mucosa wounds are closed with 5-0 plain catgut.

12. The intranasal Merocel nasal packing is checked for position.

13. Benzoin tape dressing is applied to the nose and form-fitting brown paper tape, brown adhesive tape, a form-fitting aluminum splint, and an additional covering of brown paper tape is applied. Xeroform dressing is applied to the alar suture-line to decrease dry blood and crustiness and to ensure a clean wound at time of suture removal (5 days postoperatively).

14. Ice compresses are applied to the patient's eyes. The head is elevated and the patient is carefully and gently extubated and returned to the recovery area. The moistened pharyngeal pack has prevented blood

from going into the posterior nasal pharynx. Great care is taken to suction all blood and mucus to prevent coughing.

Postoperative Comments

Postoperatively, the patient's nasion and dorsum are balanced with good projection. The tip is well defined and its projection has eliminated the top ptosis. The alar base is narrowed. This patient was particularly pleased with her new profile.

Patient V (Fig. 9-9a, 9-9b, 9-9c, 9-9d)

This 42-year-old black male complained of a nondefined, bulbous nasal tip and wide, flaring nostrils. His tip was depressed, especially when he smiled.

On examination, the patient had a depressed nasion. Although it appeared that the patient had a dorsal nasal bump, in reality there was a lack of dorsal septal and tip support. The alar walls were thick. The alar cartilages felt thin and were nonsupportive. The nostrils flared significantly and there was a relative maxillary retrusion. The patient's septum was midline, but the turbinates were hypertrophic.

The five-page Preoperative Nasal Checklist was used for the patient's consultative evaluation (Fig. 9-10).

Figure 9-9a, 9-9b
This black male had a moderately thick, flattened tip.

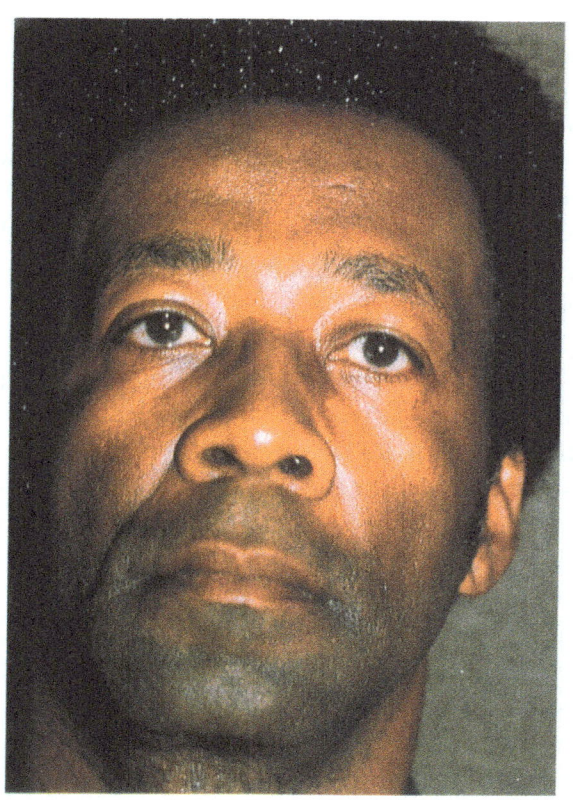 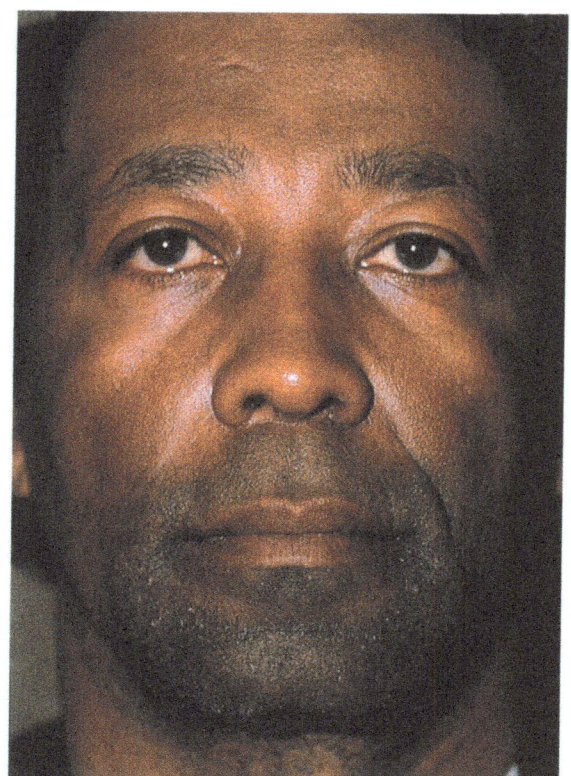

a

b

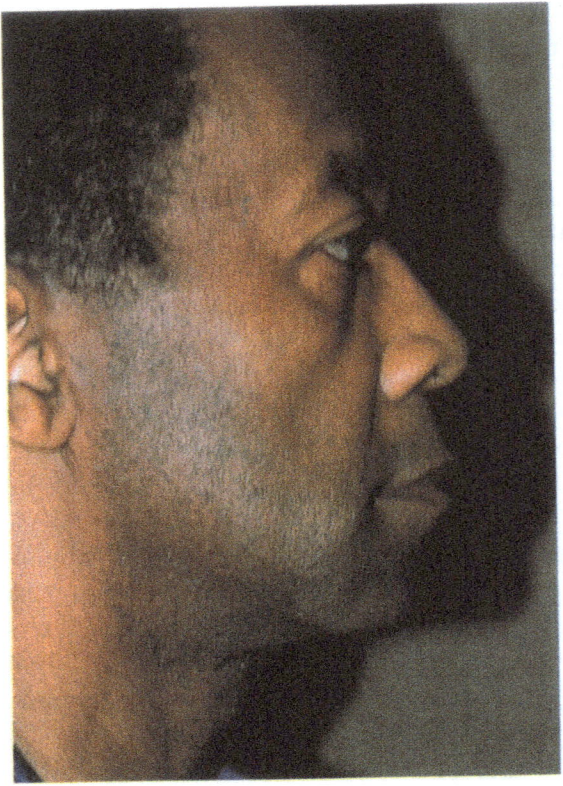
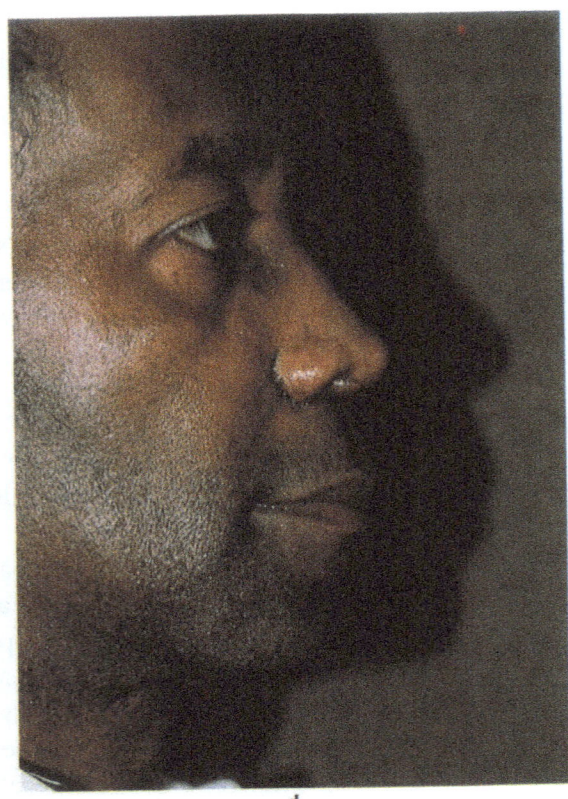

c   d

Figure 9-9c, 9-9d
Insertion of a 2.75 cm × 1 cm "pea-pod" graft was performed and tip projection was improved. With adequate projection in mind, the concave side was sutured to the convex side of the cartilage. Alar base reduction provided a less bulky, thinner margin.

Operative Procedure

1. The procedure was performed under general anesthesia. Eight milligrams of intravenous dexamethasone sodium phosphate (Decadron) and 25 mg of intravenous diphenhydramine hydrochloride (Benadryl) with 1 g of cephalosporin was administered.
2. 0.5% Bupivacaine hydrochloride (Marcaine) with epinephrine was used to infiltrate the left ear, septum, turbinates, and entire nose.
3. Petroleum jelly packing was deeply placed within the nasal vault and a saline-moistened sponge placed in the oral pharynx to decrease post-pharyngeal blood collection.
4. The helical cartilage conchal cup was excised through a waving postauricular incision. Bupivacaine hydrochloride (Marcaine) and Kenalog (10 mg/ml suspension triamcinolone acetonide) was sprayed into the wound. The area was then closed with 4-0 Dexon and Prolene and petroleum jelly packing was form-fitted into the area. The cartilage was taken and placed onto a saline-moistened 4 × 4 and placed over an ice bag. The ice bag was placed under a sterile waterproof drape so that the cartilage was kept cooled.
5. An approximately 2.75 cm × 1 cm "pea-pod" graft was carved and constructed utilizing several sutures of 5-0 Dexon. The apex and base had a stabilization suture placed.
6. Intracartilaginous incisions were made. The dorsum was skeletonized.
7. Piriform osteotomies were performed and digital pressure was applied for at least 5 minutes to decrease bruising.

PREOPERATIVE NASAL EVALUATION AND CHECKLIST

I use a checklist when preoperatively assessing patients. It assists me in obtaining a history, assessing the aesthetic goals of the patient, and performing a complete nasal examination. In addition, a complete medical history and physical examination should be performed prior to surgery.

NASAL CHECKLIST

Name: _Patient V_____ Date:_____

Previous History Of:

Childhood or adulthood injuries?   Yes_____ No__X__ If yes, explain:_____

Nasal Surgery?   Yes_____ No__X__
  Date and Specifics?   _____
  X-rays?   Yes_____ No__X__

_____Nasal Airway Obstruction: Left_____ Right_____ Both__X__ Consistent_____X___
                                                                          Intermittent_____

_____Sinus Infections: Yes_____ No_____ When:_____

_____Nasal Allergy Symptoms: Yes_____ No__X__
                                         _____Stuffiness _____Sneezing _____Postnasal Drip

_____Nasal Spray Use: Yes__X__ No_____
                                         Type:_____ Frequency:_____

_____Nasal Bleeding: Yes_____ No__X__

_____Smoking: Yes_____ No__X__ How much_____PPD

_____Aspirin or Aspirin-like Medication Use:_____

_____Hypertension: Yes_____ No__X__

_____Previous History of Troublesome Scarring: Yes_____ No_____
                                         Where_____ Specifics_____

Additional Comments: _____
                                         _____

Figure 9-10
Preoperative Nasal Evaluation and Checklist.

Patient's Aesthetic Goals:

I. Dorsum/Bridge
    ___Retain Convexity
    ___Retain Width
    _X_Reduce Bridge Width
    ___Reduce Dorsum To:
        ___Straight   ___Slight Concavity
        ___Moderate Concavity
    ___Graft Dorsum   _X_Graft Nasion   ___Graft Frontal Bone
    ___Other: _____

II. Tip
    ___No Change
    ___Reduce Width
    _X_More Tip Projection
    ___No Angle Change
    ___Elevate Angle To _____

III. Alar Base
    ___No Change
    _X_Narrow
    ___Graft Nasal Base

Additional Comments/Procedures: _____
    _____
    _____

Nasal Examination:

A basic general physical examination should be performed.

I. Skin: ___Normal ___Medium _X_ Thick ___Hypopigmented
___Sebaceous ___Normal Pigment
___Scars _X_ Hyperpigmented

II. Septum: _X_ Straight ___Deviated ___Left ___Right
___% Obstruction ___Left ___Right
___Sufficient For Use As Graft ___Yes _X_ No

III. Vomer: _X_ Straight
___Deflected: ___Left ___Right
___Spurred: ___Left ___Right

IV. Nasal Valve: _X_ Open
___Narrow
___Compromised

V. Turbinates: ___Small ___Right ___Left ___Both
___Deep ___Normal ___Right ___Left ___Both
___Flat _X_ Enlarged ___Right ___Left _X_ Both

VI. Nasion: Angle: ____deep____

VII. Dorsum/Bridge: ___Convex ___Straight ___Concave
___Narrow ___Wide ___Normal Width
_X_ Regular ___Irregular

VIII. Upper Lateral Cartilage: ___Narrow ___Medium _X_ Wide

IV. Tip: ___Narrow ___Normal _X_ Wide
___Adequate Projection
_X_ Insufficient Projection

X. Columella: _X_ Normal ___Retracted ___Hanging
_X_ Angle: ___closed___ ___Narrow ___Wide

XI. Nasal Spine: _X_ Small ___Normal ___Large

XII. Alar Base: ___Normal ___Moderate Width _X_ Excessive Width

Surgical Plan:

Grafting To Be Performed: _X_ Yes   ___ No

Source Of Graft: ___ Cranial Bone
                     _X_ Auricular
                     ___ Septum
                     ___ Other: _____

I. Nasion
   ___ No Change
   ___ Ostectomy
   _X_ Graft

II. Septum
   ___ Septectomy
   ___ Septoplasty
   ___ Vomer Spur Ostectomy
   ___ Packing   ___ Yes   ___ No — Left ___   Right ___   Both ___

III. Turbinates
   _X_ Inject   Left ___   Right ___   Both _X_
   ___ Cauterization   Left ___   Right ___   Both ___
   ___ Clamping/Excis. Left ___   Right ___   Both ___
   _X_ S.M. Resections Left ___   Right ___   Both _X_

IV. Dorsum/Bridge
   ___ Ostectomies
   ___ Rasp
   _X_ Osteotomy
   ___ Graft
       ___ Septum
       ___ Auricular
       ___ Cranial
       ___ Other

V. Columella
   ___ No Change
   _X_ Raise To _open_ Angle

Additional Comments/Procedures: _____
_____
_____

VI. Tip
   _X_ No Change
   ___ Reduce Alar Cartilages
      Approach: ___ Cartilage Splitting Incisions
                   ___ Rim Incisions
                   ___ Open Technique

   _X_ Tip Grafting: Yes _X_   No ___
   ___ Septum
   _X_ Auricular
   ___ Other:_____

VII. Base
   ___ No Change
   ___ Reduce Spine
   _X_ Augment Spine
   _X_ Augment Maxilla

VIII. Alae
   ___ No Change
   _X_ Reduce
      ___ Small
      _X_ Medium
      ___ Large

Additional Comments/Procedures: _____
                                   _____
                                   _____

8. The turbinates were infiltrated with 10 mg/cc Kenalog (10 mg/ml suspension triamcinolone acetonide) and submucously resected with the Colorado tip.

9. The alar cartilages were not reduced. A "pea-pod" pocket was dissected by a rim incision from the lateral footplate down to inferior and just posterior to the medial footplate.

10. A lateral and frontal view of the optimum tip projection was noted and painted with a dot of methylene blue.

11. A dissection was carried out over onto the maxilla, and excess crushed septal and conchal cartilage was used to augment the maxilla and nasal spine.

12. The "pea-pod" tip graft was placed and secured into place. 4-0 plain catgut sutures were placed through the columella to stabilize the graft. The wounds were then closed with 5-0 plain catgut and 5-0 Dexon.

13. The alar base was incised with resection of approximately 3 mm.

14. The base was dissected and freed for 1.5 cm onto the cheek and advanced toward the nose with 5-0 PDS.

15. The depressor nasi muscle was excised.

16. The alar "wing" was then reapproximated medially to the base with 5-0 PDS and the wound closed with 6-0 nylon.

17. The dorsal "pea-pod" tip graft suture was pulled tight and tape-pinched around the tip to provide maximum superior and anterior projection.

18. Brown paper tape and a form-fitted aluminum splint were placed.

Postoperative Comments

On frontal view, the patient has a narrower, more pleasing contour to the alar base. The nostrils still maintain their curvature due to the medial advancement of the alar base toward the piriform aperture. On lateral view, the improved tip projection and definition are apparent. Quite frequently, even a thick tip can appear thin due to the "tenting" of the "pea-pod" tip graft. If less "pointing" is desired, the "pea-pod" tip graft can be either shortened or bolstered distally with fascia.

Patient U (Fig. 9-11a, 9-11b, 9-11c, 9-11d)

This Asian female complained of a "parrot's beak" appearance of her nose. She desired dorsum nasal improvement and more definition to the depressed tip. On frontal view, the patient was concerned about the width of her bridge and alar base.

On examination, the patient had a depressed and high-riding nasion. She had small but palpable nasal bones with a prominent septal cartilage hump. The tip was depressed with tethering of the columella. The upper lateral alar cartilages were flimsy. Intranasal examination revealed a good airway, but some valving upon deep inspiration was noted.

The surgical plan was limited to:

1. Skeletonization and piriform osteotomies to narrow the bridge.

2. The dorsal and caudal septum would be slightly reduced with minimal dorsal rasping of the nasal bone.

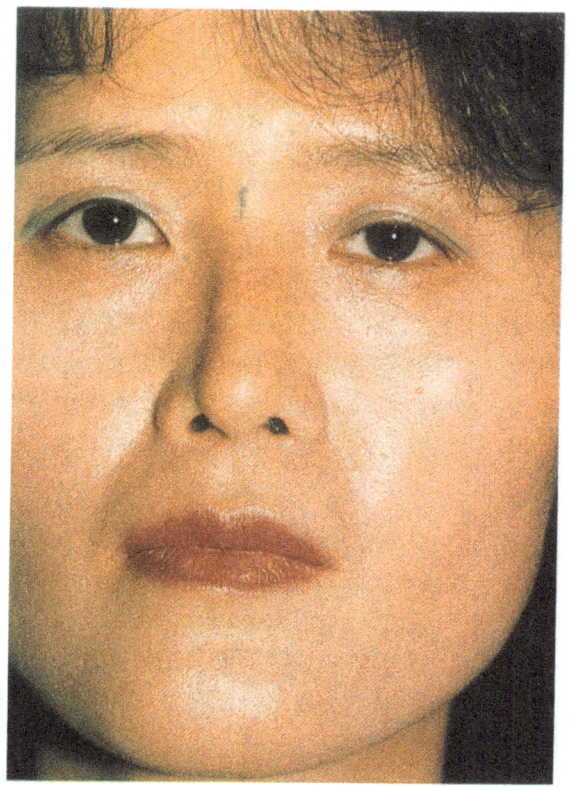 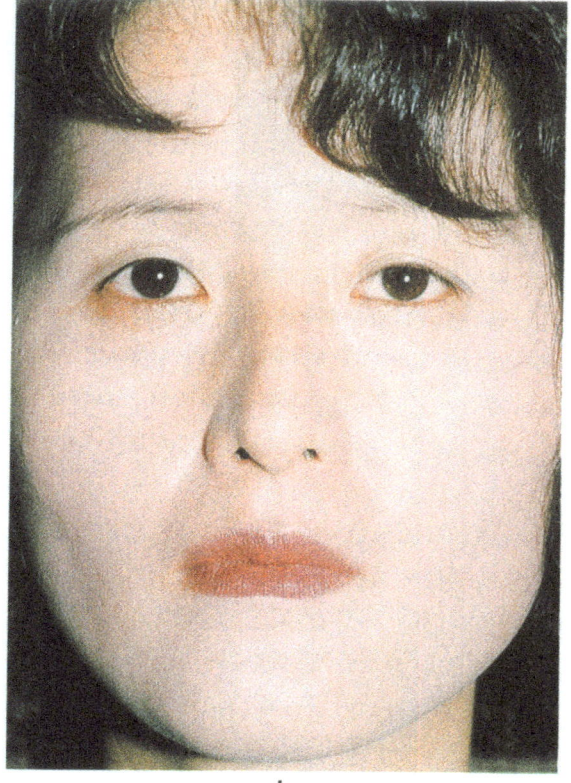

Figure 9-11a, 9-11b
This Asian female also had a moderately thick, flattened tip.

3. A nasion-dorsal crushed-cartilage graft would be placed, along with minor alar reductions with medial cheek advancement.
4. Insertion of a "pea-pod" nasal tip graft.
5. Small spreader grafts would be placed to decrease nasal valving.

The five-page Preoperative Nasal Checklist was used for the patient's consultative evaluation (Fig. 9-12).

Operative Procedure

1. The procedure was performed under general anesthesia. Eight milligrams of intravenous dexamethasone sodium phosphate (Decadron) and 25 mg of intravenous diphenhydramine hydrochloride (Benadryl) with 1 g of cephalosporin was administered to decrease swelling.
2. 0.5% Bupivacaine hydrochloride (Marcaine) with epinephrine was used to infiltrate the left ear, septum, turbinates, and entire nose.
3. Petroleum jelly packing was placed deep within the nasal area.
4. Alar base incisions were made to slightly narrow the base. They were performed at this time to improve visualization.
5. A small septal cartilage segment measuring 2 cm × 0.5 cm was excised and utilized for spreader graft insertions.
6. 5 mg/cc Kenalog (10 mg/ml suspension triamcinolone acetonide) was injected into the turbinates.
7. 4-0 plain catgut mattress sutures were placed through the septal leaves.

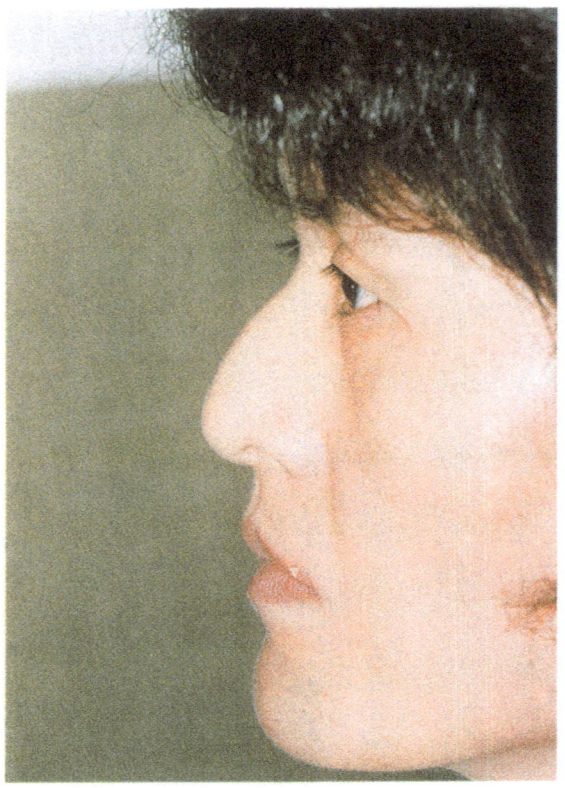

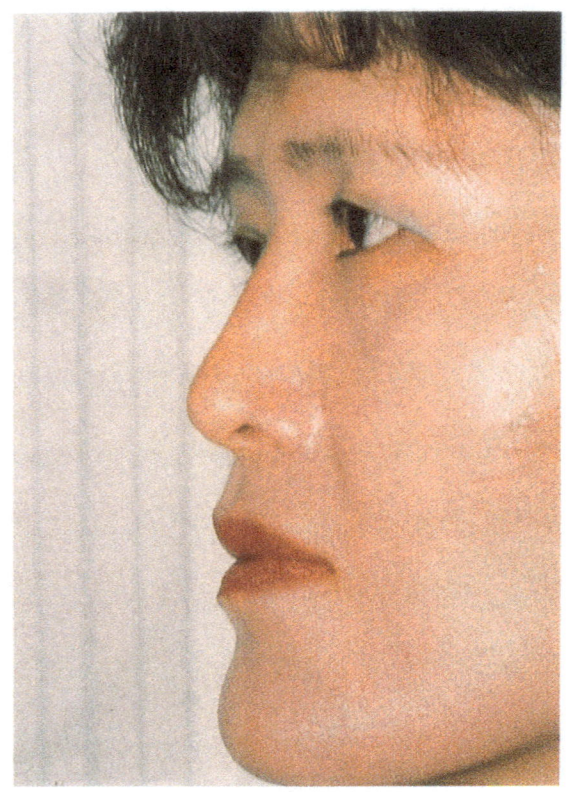

c   d

Figure 9-11c, 9-11d
Again, tip projection was improved after the insertion of a 2.75 cm × 1 cm "pea-pod" graft. The nasal spine was also grafted to give additional fullness.

8. Additional petroleum jelly packing was placed against the septum. It was later replaced with Merocel nasal tampons.

9. Intercartilaginous incisions were made and limited dorsal skeletonization was performed.

10. Excessive dorsal septocartilage was excised and the bony hump rasped smooth.

11. Piriform osteotomies were performed with a 2-mm osteotome and digital pressure was applied for at least 5 minutes to decrease bruising.

12. The left helical cartilage cup was excised through a waving postauricular incision. The wound was sprayed with bupivacaine hydrochloride (Marcaine) and Kenalog (10 mg/ml suspension triamcinolone acetonide). The area was then closed with 4-0 Dexon and 4-0 Prolene and petroleum jelly packing form-fitted into the area. A .25" Penrose drain was utilized to drain the inferior aspect of the wound.

13. The cartilage was taken and placed into a saline-moistened 4 × 4.

14. An approximately 2.75 cm × 1 cm "pea-pod" graft was carved and constructed utilizing several sutures of 5-0 Dexon. The apex and base had a pull-out stabilization suture placed.

15. The tip cartilages were small and flimsy and only the superior fourth was excised. No upper lateral cartilage was excised.

16. A 2-mm excision was made from the caudal septum for a small degree of elevation.

17. A rim incision was carried from the dorsal nostril down just posterior and inferior to the columella medial footplate.

PREOPERATIVE NASAL EVALUATION AND CHECKLIST

I use a checklist when preoperatively assessing patients. It assists me in obtaining a history, assessing the aesthetic goals of the patient, and performing a complete nasal examination. In addition, a complete medical history and physical examination should be performed prior to surgery.

NASAL CHECKLIST

Name:___Patient U_____ Date:_____

Previous History Of:

Childhood or adulthood injuries?   Yes_____ No__X__ If yes, explain:_____

Nasal Surgery?   Yes_____ No__X__
    Date and Specifics?   _____
    X-rays?   Yes_____ No__X__

_____Nasal Airway Obstruction: Left_____ Right_____ Both__X__ Consistent__X__
                                                                          Intermittent_____

_____Sinus Infections: Yes_____ No__X__ When:_____

_____Nasal Allergy Symptoms: Yes_____ No__X__
                                         _____Stuffiness _____Sneezing _____Postnasal Drip

_____Nasal Spray Use: Yes_____ No__X__
                                         Type:_____ Frequency:_____

_____Nasal Bleeding: Yes_____ No__X__

_____Smoking: Yes_____ No__X__ How much_____PPD

_____Aspirin or Aspirin-like Medication Use:_____

_____Hypertension: Yes_____ No__X__

_____Previous History of Troublesome Scarring: Yes_____ No__X__
                                         Where_____ Specifics_____

Additional Comments: _____
                                         _____

Figure 9-12
Preoperative Nasal Evaluation and Checklist.

Patient's Aesthetic Goals:

I. Dorsum/Bridge
____Retain Convexity
____Retain Width
_X_Reduce Bridge Width
_X_Reduce Dorsum To:
____Straight   _X_Slight Concavity
____Moderate Concavity
_X_Graft Dorsum   _X_Graft Nasion   ____Graft Frontal Bone
____Other: _____

II. Tip
____No Change
_X_Reduce Width
_X_More Tip Projection
____No Angle Change
____Elevate Angle To _____

III. Alar Base
____No Change
_X_Narrow
____Graft Nasal Base

Additional Comments/Procedures: _____
_____
_____

Nasal Examination:

A basic general physical examination should be performed.

I. Skin: ___Normal   _X_Medium   ___Thick   ___Hypopigmented
           ___Sebaceous   _X_Normal Pigment
           ___Scars   ___Hyperpigmented

II. Septum: _X_Straight   ___Deviated   ___Left   ___Right
                            ___% Obstruction   ___Left   ___Right
              _X_Sufficient For Use As Graft   _X_Yes   ___No

III. Vomer: _X_Straight
              ___Deflected: ___Left   ___Right
              ___Spurred: ___Left   ___Right

IV. Nasal Valve: ___Open
                   ___Narrow
                   _X_Compromised

V. Turbinates: ___Small   ___Right   ___Left   ___Both
     ___Deep   ___Normal   ___Right   ___Left   ___Both
     ___Flat   _X_Enlarged   ___Right   ___Left   ___Both

VI. Nasion: Angle: _____deep_____

VII. Dorsum/Bridge: _X_Convex   ___Straight   ___Concave
                      ___Narrow   _X_Wide   ___Normal Width
                      ___Regular   ___Irregular

VIII. Upper Lateral Cartilage: _X_Narrow   ___Medium   ___Wide

IV. Tip: _X_Narrow   ___Normal   ___Wide
           ___Adequate Projection
           _X_Insufficient Projection

X. Columella: ___Normal   _X_Retracted   ___Hanging
                _X_Angle: _____normal_____   ___Narrow   ___Wide

XI. Nasal Spine: _X_Small   ___Normal   ___Large

XII. Alar Base: _X_Normal   ___Moderate Width   ___Excessive Width

Surgical Plan:

Grafting To Be Performed: _X_ Yes   ___ No

Source Of Graft: ___ Cranial Bone
                     _X_ Auricular
                     ___ Septum
                     ___ Other: _____

I. Nasion
    ___ No Change
    ___ Ostectomy
    _X_ Graft

II. Septum
    ___ Septectomy
    _X_ Septoplasty
    ___ Vomer Spur Ostectomy
    _X_ Packing   _X_ Yes   ___ No — Left ___   Right ___   Both _X_

III. Turbinates
    _X_ Inject   Left ___   Right ___   Both _X_
    ___ Cauterization   Left ___   Right ___   Both ___
    ___ Clamping/Excis. Left ___   Right ___   Both ___
    ___ S.M. Resections Left ___   Right ___   Both ___

IV. Dorsum/Bridge
    ___ Ostectomies
    _X_ Rasp
    _X_ Osteotomy
    _X_ Graft
        ___ Septum
        _X_ Auricular
        ___ Cranial
        ___ Other

V. Columella
    ___ No Change
    _X_ Raise To _open_ Angle

Additional Comments/Procedures: _____
_____
_____
_____

Surgical Plan: (continued)

VI. Tip

    ___No Change
    _X_ Reduce Alar Cartilages

        Approach: ___Cartilage Splitting Incisions
                     _X_ Rim Incisions
                     ___Open Technique

    _X_ Tip Grafting: Yes _X_   No ___
        ___Septum
        _X_ Auricular
        ___Other:_____

VII. Base

    ___No Change
    ___Reduce Spine
    _X_ Augment Spine
    _X_ Augment Maxilla

VIII. Alae

    ___No Change
    _X_ Reduce
        ___Small
        _X_ Medium
        ___Large

Additional Comments/Procedures: _____

_____

_____

18. A dissection was carried out over the nasal spine up to the nasal tip and a pocket was created.
19. A lateral and frontal view of the optimum tip projection was noted and painted with a dot of methylene blue.
20. Small dorsal/septal pockets were placed just underneath the upper lateral cartilages and two spreader grafts placed and closed with 5-0 plain catgut.
21. The depressor nasi muscle was incised and a segment removed to decrease tip droopiness when she smiled.
22. The "pea-pod" tip graft was placed and secured into place with superior and inferior pull-out Dexon sutures. 4-0 plain catgut sutures were placed through the columella to stabilize the graft. The wounds were then closed with 5-0 plain catgut.
23. The alar base wound was then undermined for 1–1.5 cm out onto the cheek, and after hemostasis was ensured, advanced toward the nostril with 5-0 PDS.
24. Two millimeters of excessive alae were then taken and the alae advanced medially and inferiorly. This gave a slight width reduction without compromising the base or airway.
25. The wounds were then closed with 6-0 nylon. All intranasal wounds were closed.
26. A form-fitting tape-aluminum splint was placed.
27. Excess septal and conchal cartilage was used to augment the nasal spine and maxilla. This was crushed and placed through an intraoral incision.
28. The tip dorsal pull-out suture was pulled out tightly and compressed taped so that the graft would stay distal and superior within its pocket.

Postoperative Comments

Eleven months postoperatively, tip projection was improved after insertion of the "pea-pod" tip graft. After the dorsal and nasion grafts, the nasion had a much less depressed appearance. The patient's nose was much more balanced and pleasing to her in both frontal and profile views.

Patient T (Fig. 9-13a, 9-13b, 9-13c, 9-13d)

This Hispanic male has had four previous rhinoplasties in an attempt to reduce his nose. Family photographs revealed an inherited thick, bulky nose with a large, thick-skinned envelope. The patient had a large oval face and would not have a balanced appearance with an overly reduced nose. His desire was to have more reduction and refinement than would be recommended.

Upon examination externally, his nasion was excessively full, and the bridge was flattened and slightly depressed. Despite an extended discussion, the patient did not want a prominent bridge, and, in fact, desired some degree of concavity. No reduction or augmentation was planned. The nasal bridge was wide and previous osteotomies were high. The patient had a very full supratip. Manually pulling the soft tissue nasal tip down revealed a

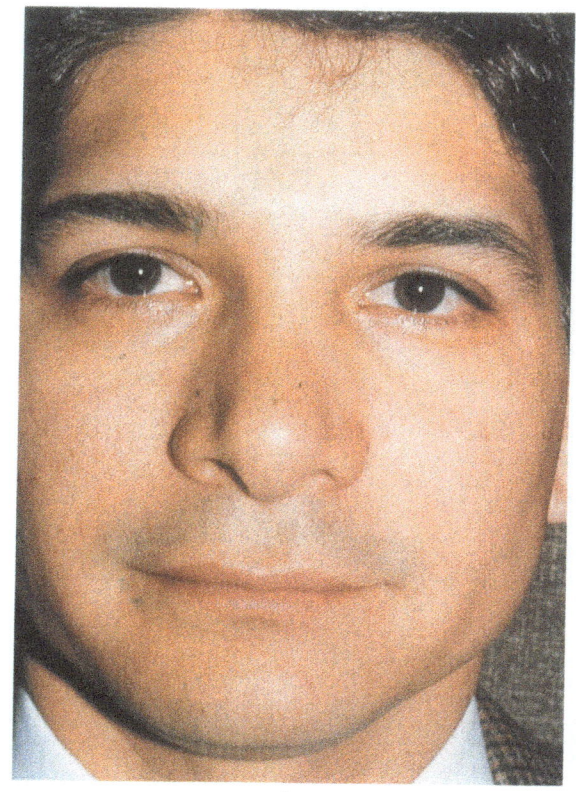
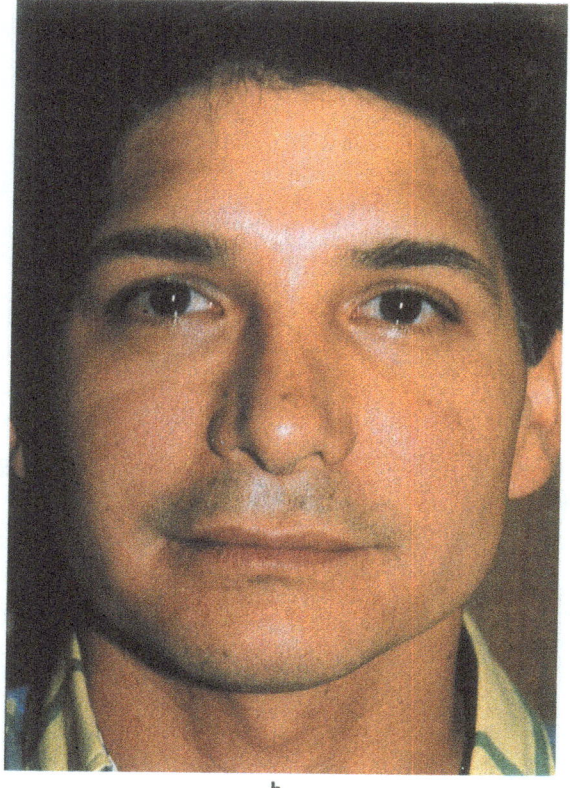

Figure 9-13a, 9-13b
This Hispanic male patient had received four previous reduction rhinoplasties without graft support.

prominent caudal septal projection. The tip was flimsy, unsupported, thick, and fibrous. The columella was hanging. The patient had a small degree of maxillary retrusion. The alae were full and, with smiling and animation, revealed a ptotic nasal tip due to a hyperactive depressor nasi muscle.

The intranasal examination revealed a previously resected septum, with prominent scarred turbinates. There was a deep vomer obstruction in the left side of the nose.

The five-page Preoperative Nasal Checklist was used for the patient's consultative evaluation (Fig. 9-14).

Operative Procedure

1. A general anesthetic was administered. Eight milligrams of intravenous dexamethasone sodium phosphate (Decadron) and 25 mg of intravenous diphenhydramine hydrochloride (Benadryl) with 1 g of cephalosproin was administered.
2. 0.5% Bupivacaine hydrochloride (Marcaine) with epinephrine was infiltrated into the nasal area, and supratrochlear, infraorbital, and interior palatine nerve blocks were performed.
3. After vasoconstrictive effect was noted, 5 mg/cc Kenalog (10 mg/ml suspension triamcinolone acetonide) was injected into the nasomaxillary osteotomy sites and nasal tip.
4. The left vomer area and turbinate were also injected with bupivacaine

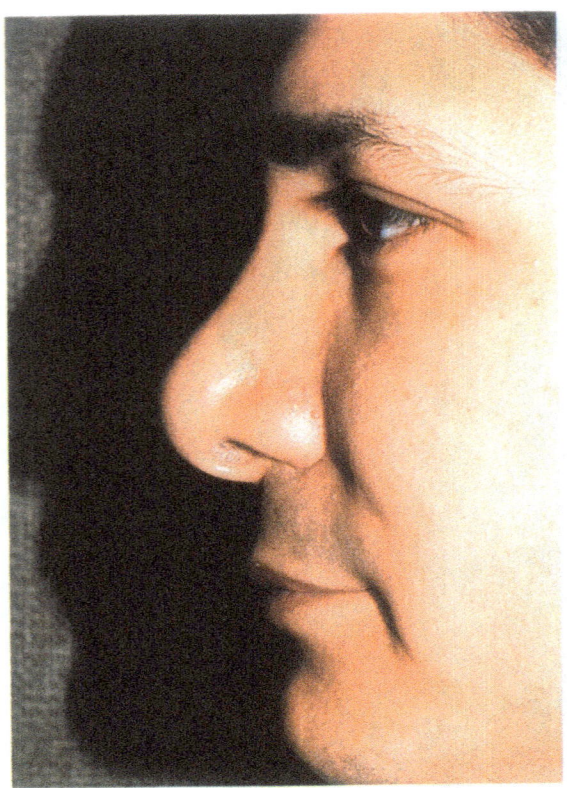
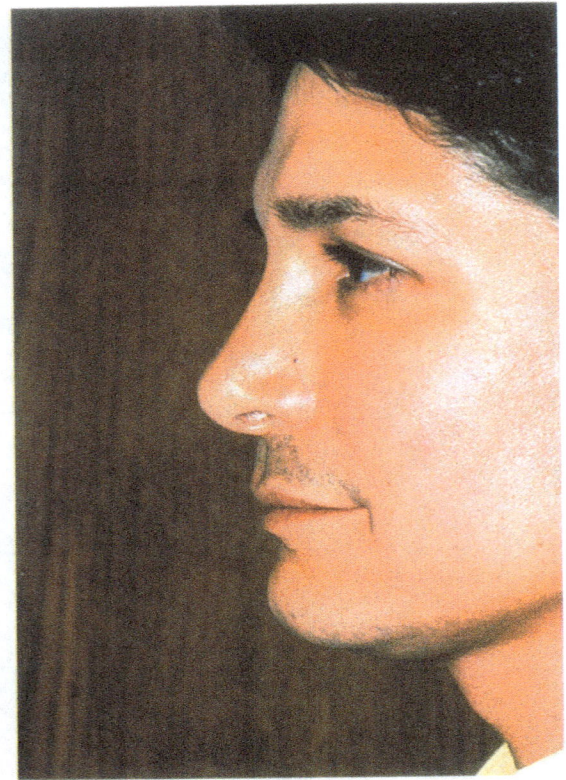

c

d

Figure 9-13c, 9-13d
A combination of alar base reduction, geometric soft-tissue reduction, and the insertion of the "pea-pod" graft gave the improved result.

hydrochloride (Marcaine) and Kenalog (10 mg/ml suspension triamcinolone acetonide).

5. The left ear was infiltrated with bupivacaine hydrochloride (Marcaine).

6. Skeletonization was performed through an intercartilaginous incision.

7. The dorsum was exposed.

8. The caudal septal prominence was excised with a broken #11 blade.

9. The alae were incised to allow better access to the intranasal area.

10. A left septal incision was made and a submucous resection of the deep vomer obstruction was performed. The right turbinate was injected and the left inferior turbinate excised in a submucous fashion and the scarred mucosa sutured over the defect utilizing 5-0 plain catgut.

11. The previously placed petroleum jelly packs were removed and Merocel nasal tampons were placed.

12. Through the piriform-alar base wound, a 2-mm osteotome was utilized and a subperiosteal pocket was developed. Stepped osteotomies were performed at a site lower than the previous osteotomies.

13. Digital pressure was used to infracture the nasal bones.

14. Digital pressure was applied for 5 minutes to decrease bruising.

15. At the right tip, an incision was made and carried down to the medial crus. The tip was exposed. There was a very small width of alar cartilage, and only minimal resection was performed.

16. The left postauricular area was prepped with a separate sterile set-up. The conchal cartilage was excised. Bupivacaine hydrochloride (Marcaine) and dilute Kenalog (10 mg/ml suspension triamcinolone ace-

PREOPERATIVE NASAL EVALUATION AND CHECKLIST

I use a checklist when preoperatively assessing patients. It assists me in obtaining a history, assessing the aesthetic goals of the patient, and performing a complete nasal examination. In addition, a complete medical history and physical examination should be performed prior to surgery.

NASAL CHECKLIST

Name:_Patient T_____ Date:_____

Previous History Of:

Childhood or adulthood injuries? Yes_____ No_____ If yes, explain:_____

Nasal Surgery? Yes__X__ No_____
 Date and Specifics?
 X-rays? Yes_____ No_____
_____

_____Nasal Airway Obstruction: Left_____ Right_____ Both__X__ Consistent__X__
                   Intermittent_____

_____Sinus Infections: Yes_____ No__X__ When:_____

_____Nasal Allergy Symptoms: Yes_____ No__X__
        _____Stuffiness _____Sneezing _____Postnasal Drip

_____Nasal Spray Use: Yes_____ No__X__
      Type:_____ Frequency:_____

_____Nasal Bleeding: Yes_____ No__X__

_____Smoking: Yes_____ No__X__ How much_____PPD

_____Aspirin or Aspirin-like Medication Use:_____

_____Hypertension: Yes_____ No__X__

_____Previous History of Troublesome Scarring: Yes__X__ No_____
                Where_____ Specifics_____

Additional Comments: _____
            _____

Figure 9-14
Preoperative Nasal Evaluation and Checklist.

Patient's Aesthetic Goals:

I. Dorsum/Bridge
   ___Retain Convexity
   ___Retain Width
   _X_Reduce Bridge Width
   _X_Reduce Dorsum To:
        ___Straight   _X_Slight Concavity
        ___Moderate Concavity
   ___Graft Dorsum   ___Graft Nasion   ___Graft Frontal Bone
   ___Other: _____

II. Tip
   ___No Change
   _X_Reduce Width
   _X_More Tip Projection
   ___No Angle Change
   ___Elevate Angle To _____

III. Alar Base
   ___No Change
   _X_Narrow
   ___Graft Nasal Base

Additional Comments/Procedures: _____
_____
_____

Nasal Examination:

A basic general physical examination should be performed.

I. Skin: ___Normal   ___Medium   _X_Thick   ___Hypopigmented
_X_Sebaceous   _X_Normal Pigment
___Scars   ___Hyperpigmented

II. Septum: ___Straight   _X_Deviated   _X_Left   ___Right
___% Obstruction   ___Left   ___Right
___Sufficient For Use As Graft   ___Yes   ___No

III. Vomer: ___Straight
_X_Deflected: _X_Left   ___Right
___Spurred: ___Left   ___Right

IV. Nasal Valve: ___Open
_X_Narrow
___Compromised

V. Turbinates: ___Small   ___Right   ___Left   ___Both
___Deep   ___Normal   ___Right   ___Left   ___Both
___Flat   _X_Enlarged   ___Right   ___Left   _X_Both

VI. Nasion: Angle: ___normal___

VII. Dorsum/Bridge: ___Convex   ___Straight   _X_Concave
___Narrow   _X_Wide   ___Normal Width
___Regular   ___Irregular

VIII. Upper Lateral Cartilage: _X_Narrow   ___Medium   ___Wide

IV. Tip: ___Narrow   ___Normal   _X_Wide
___Adequate Projection
_X_Insufficient Projection

X. Columella: ___Normal   ___Retracted   _X_Hanging
_X_Angle: ___closed___   ___Narrow   _X_Wide

XI. Nasal Spine: _X_Small   ___Normal   ___Large

XII. Alar Base: ___Normal   ___Moderate Width   _X_Excessive Width

Surgical Plan:

Grafting To Be Performed: __X__ Yes ____ No

Source Of Graft: ____ Cranial Bone
                __X__ Auricular
                ____ Septum
                ____ Other: _____

I. Nasion
    __X__ No Change
    ____ Ostectomy
    ____ Graft

II. Septum
    ____ Septectomy
    __X__ Septoplasty
    ____ Vomer Spur Ostectomy
    __X__ Packing ____ Yes ____ No — Left ____ Right ____ Both __X__

III. Turbinates
    __X__ Inject Left ____ Right ____ Both __X__
    ____ Cauterization Left ____ Right ____ Both ____
    ____ Clamping/Excis. Left ____ Right ____ Both ____
    __X__ S.M. Resections Left __X__ Right ____ Both ____

IV. Dorsum/Bridge
    ____ Ostectomies
    ____ Rasp
    __X__ Osteotomy
    ____ Graft
        ____ Septum
        ____ Auricular
        ____ Cranial
        ____ Other

V. Columella
    ____ No Change
    __X__ Raise To _open_ Angle

Additional Comments/Procedures: _____

_____

_____

VI. Tip
    ___No Change
    <u>X</u> Reduce Alar Cartilages
        Approach: ___Cartilage Splitting Incisions
                      <u>X</u> Rim Incisions
                      ___Open Technique

    <u>X</u> Tip Grafting: Yes <u>X</u>   No ___
    ___Septum
    <u>X</u> Auricular
    ___Other:_____

VII. Base
    ___No Change
    ___Reduce Spine
    ___Augment Spine
    <u>X</u> Augment Maxilla

VIII. Alae
    ___No Change
    <u>X</u> Reduce
        ___Small
        <u>X</u> Medium
        ___Large

Additional Comments/Procedures: _____
                                            _____
                                            _____

tonide) were sprayed into the wound. The wound was closed with sutures of 4-0 Dexon.

17. A .25" Penrose drain was used to drain the area through a small postauricular inferior stab incision.

18. Compressive petroleum jelly gauze was utilized to form-fit the ear.

19. A triamcinolone acetonide 10 mg/ml (Kenalog)–bupivacaine hydrochloride (Marcaine) mixture was sprayed into all wounds.

20. A "pea-pod" graft was constructed by incising matching canoe-shaped concave cartilage grafts measuring 3.5 cm × 1 cm and placing them together similar to hands praying, with wrapped interrupted 5-0 Dexon mattress sutures. Pull-out sutures were placed through the apex and base.

21. A double-hook was then placed in the right alar-columellar wound and the base of the graft suture-passed and then placed 2–3 mm above the nasal spine. The tip of the graft was placed at the apex. This was previously measured and viewed in frontal and profile views to assure correct positioning.

22. The external nasal wounds were then closed at the columella with 6-0 nylon. The intranasal area was closed with 5-0 plain catgut. 5 mg/cc Kenalog (10 mg/ml suspension triamcinolone acetonide) was then injected into both turbinates and tip area.

23. Form-fitting tape and a form-fitting aluminum splint were then placed.

24. Ice compresses were placed on the eyes.

25. The patient was then returned to the recovery area.

Postoperative Comments

Postoperatively, the patient has a thinner, more defined nose. The airway is now satisfactory. The nasal profile was significantly improved. The major improvement was from the large "pea-pod" tip graft.

10

Recommended Instruments

The art and science of rhinoplasty is greatly facilitated with proper instrumentation. Three invaluable principles are (1) good lighting, (2) good exposure, and (3) easy, nontraumatic handling of tissue.

I find the use of a headlight and loop magnification greatly facilitates my ability to see.

It is also surprising to me that many surgeons overlook pinpoint Bovie cauterization. I find appropriate lighting, exposure, suctioning, and the use of a pinpoint cautery extremely useful in clearing the operative field of any bleeding.

Numerous and varied headlights are available. All one needs to do is to attend a large Plastic and Reconstructive Surgery meeting and progress slowly through the exhibit booths to find out which light(s) are most comfortable and personally workable. Additionally, small fiber-optic retractors are very helpful. A recommend a range be tried and available in your operating room. There are numerous unique special "retraction," "grasping," "holding," and "delivery" instruments which may suit a surgeon's particular needs.

Part of the beauty of a rhinoplastic surgeon's life is the ability to personally develop one's own instrument ideas. I highly recommend that modification of a current instrument or ideas about a new one be shared with colleagues.

The following list of instruments is a basic rhinoplasty set-up. Many surgeons collect their own favorites and have them manufactured. We should continue to investigate and try new instruments so we can provide ourselves and our patients with improvements in both the art and science of our rhinoplastic endeavors.

Useful Instruments

Instruments are the tools of the trade. The following is a list of basic instruments I have found to be useful in performing rhinoplasty:

1. Long metal suction tip
2. Packing forceps
3. 2 small double-hooks
4. Long double-hook
5. #15 blade and handle
6. Straight large clamp
7. Single-hook

8. Closed retractor, right angle
9. Open retractor, right angle
10. Medium Ragnell scissors
11. Dorsal scissors
12. Turbinate scissors
13. Small dissection scissors
14. Long Brown-Adsen forceps
15. Double-guarded osteotome
16. Hammer
17. Triple dorsal osteotome set-up (Padgett)
18. Small Brown-Adsen forceps
19. Small cobblestone rasp
20. Large cobblestone rasp
21. Double-ended rasp
22. 2-mm dissection osteotome
23. 2-mm thumb-held osteotome
24. Small needle holder
25. Large needle holder

If a septum procedure is to be performed, the following instruments will also be useful:

a. Small nasal speculum
b. Freer elevator
c. Ballenger knife

Special Instruments

Handling cartilage is much easier with proper instrumentation. Maintenance of cartilage viability is particularly important in ethnic rhinoplasty, where cartilage grafts are often critical (Fig. 10-1, 10-2). Standard crushing techniques can destroy the graft and increase the likelihood of future resorption.

Headlights are very personal. Recent advances in electronics will assure future state-of-the-art models which incorporate a self-contained portable battery pack, as well as 2.5 magnification capability.

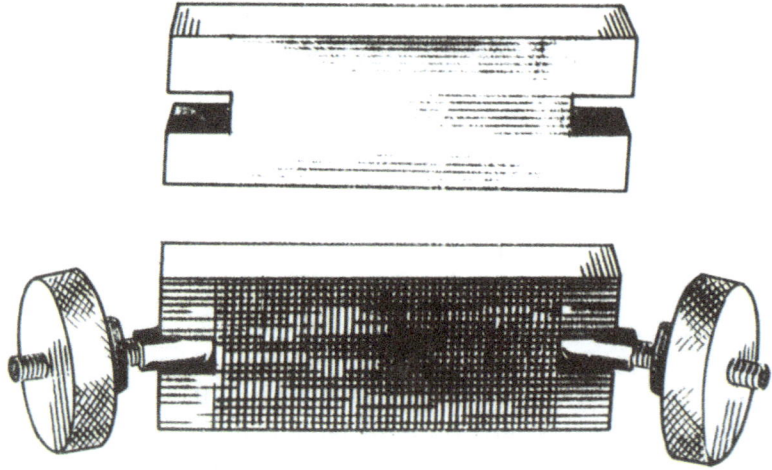

Figure 10-1
The JOST Crusher (above) has interstices, which allow only partial crushing of tissues. The turn-knobs also allow very fine adjustments in the amount of pressure being applied. The JOST cartilage crusher is utilized to crush cartilage, which is sutured with 4-0 or 5-0 Dexon.

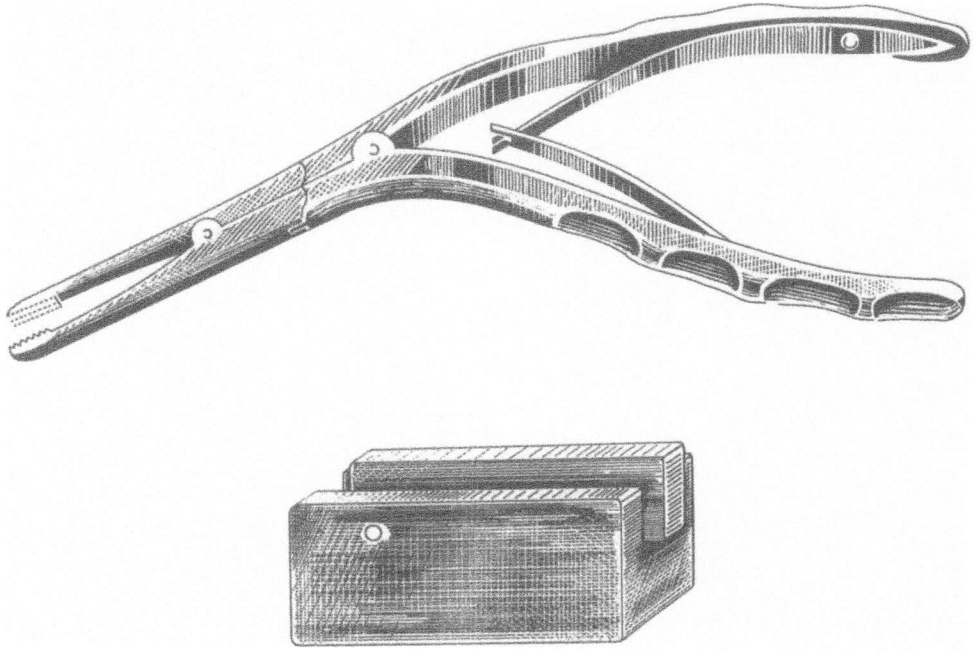

The JOST crusher and a good, comfortable fiber-optic headlight have proven to be my most useful and important pieces of "special" equipment for ethnic rhinoplasty (as well as many other procedures). The JOST crusher's different surfaces have made it indispensable to cartilage graft procedures. Its contribution with cartilage and fascia has been significant. I have enjoyed gifting colleagues with a JOST crusher over the years (including Jack Sheen, MD). Once the recipients have used the device, they don't "turn back."

Suggested Reading

Anderson, J.: On the selection of patients for rhinoplasty. *Otolaryngol. Clin. North Am.* 8:685, 1960.

Anderson, J.R.: The dynamics of rhinoplasty. Proceedings of the Ninth International Congress in Otorhinolaryngology. *Excerpta Medica, International Congress Series.* Amsterdam: Excerpta Medica, 1969, p. 206.

Ashley, F.C.: Primary and secondary correction of the nasal tip. In Millard, D.R., editor: *Symposium on Corrective Rhinoplasty*, Vol. 13., St. Louis, 1976.

Aufricht, G.: A few hints and surgical details in rhinoplasty. *Laryngoscope* 53:317, 1958.

Aufricht, G.: Rhinoplasty and the face. *Plast. Reconstr. Surg.* 43:219, 1969.

Baker, D.C.: Rhinoplasty: physiology. In Rees, T.D., Editor: *Aesthetic Plastic Surgery.* Philadelphia, 1980, W.B. Saunders Co.

Baker, D.C.: Treatment of obstructing inferior turbinates with intranasal corticosteroids. *Ann. Plast. Surg.* 3:253, 1979.

Baker, D.C., and Strauss, R.B.: Intranasal injections of long acting corticoids. *Ann. Otol. Rhinol.* 71:525, 1962.

Baker, D.C., and Strauss, R.B.: The physiologic treatment of nasal obstruction. *Clin. Plast. Surg.* 4:121, Jan. 1977.

Baker, T.J.: Patient selection and psychological evaluation. *Plast. Surg.* 5:3, 1978.

Barton, F.E., Jr.: Aesthetic aspects of partial nasal reconstructions. *Clin. Plast. Surg.* 8:77, 1981.

Beekhuis, G.J.: Surgical correction of saddle nose deformity. *Trans. Am. Acad. Ophthalmol. Otolaryngol.* 80:596, 1975.

Berman, W.E.: *Rhinoplastic Surgery.* St. Louis, 1989, The C.V. Mosby Co.

Berman, W.E.: Second rhinoplasties and composite grafts. *Trans Am. Acad. Ophthalmol. Otolaryngol.* 84: 952, 1977.

Bernstein, L.: Surgical anatomy in rhinoplasty. *Otolaryngol. Clin. North Am.* 8:549, 1975.

Bernstein, L.A.: Basic technique for surgery of the nasal lobule. *Otolaryngol. Clin. North Am.* 8:599, 1975.

Boo-Chai, K.: Augmentation rhinoplasty in the Oriental. *Plast. Reconstr. Surg.* 34:81, 1964.

Brenna, H.G., and Parkes, M.L.: Septal surgery: the high septal transfixion. *Int. Surg.* 58: 732, 1973.

Brent, B.: The versatile cartilage autograft: Current trends in clinical transplantation. *Clin. Plast. Surg.* 6:163, 1979.

Broadbent, T.R., and Matthews, V.L.: Artistic relationships in surface anatomy of the face: applications to reconstructive surgery. *Plast. Reconstr. Surg.* 20:1, 1957.

Broadbent, T.R., and Woolf, R.M.: Correction of cleft lip nasal deformity. In Georgiade, N.G., and Hagert, R.F., editors: *Symposium on Management of Cleft Lip and Palate and Associated Deformities.* St. Louis, 1974, The C.V. Mosby Co.

Brown, J.B., and McDowell, F.: *Plastic Surgery of the Nose.* St. Louis, 1965, The C.V. Mosby Co.

Bruck, H.G.: Corrective rhinoplasty: a study of 5,000 personal cases. *Arch. Orolaryngol.* 97:441–1973.

Cash, T.F., and Horton, E.E.: Aesthetic surgery: effects of rhinoplasty on the social perception of patients by others. *Plast. Reconstr. Surg.* 72:543, 1983.

Cinelli, J.A.: Lengthening of the nose by a septal flap. *Plast. Reconstr. Surg.* 43:99, 1969.

Cinelli, J.A.: Physiologic rhinoplasty principles. In Maloney, W.H., editor: *Otolaryngology.* New York, 1971, Harper & Row, Inc.

Conley, J.: Intranasal composite grafts for dorsal support. *Arch. Otolaryngol.* 111:241, 1985.

Constantian, M.B.: Grafting the projecting nasal tip. *Ann. Plast. Surg.* 14:391, May 1985.

Converse, J.M.: The cartilaginous structures of the nose. *Ann. Otol. Rhinol. Laryngol.* 64:220, 1955.

Converse, J.M.: Corrective plastic surgery of the nose. In Paparella, Shumrick, editors: *Otolaryngology*, Philadelphia, 1973, W.B. Saunders Co.

Converse, J.M.: Corrective rhinoplasty. In Converse, J.M., editor: *Reconstructive Plastic Surgery*, Vol. 2. Philadelphia, 1977, W.B. Saunders Co.

Converse, J.M.: Deformities of the nose. *Reconstructive Plastic Surgery*, Vol. 2. Philadelphia and London, 1964, W.B. Saunders Co., p. 695.

Cottle, M.H., and Loring, R.M.: Surgery of the nasal septum: new operative procedures and indications. *Ann. Otolaryngol.* 57:707, 1948.

Courtiss, E.H.: Septorhinoplasty of the traumatically deformed nose. *Ann. Plast. Surg.* 1:434, 1978.

Courtiss, E.H., Gargan, T.J., and Courtiss, G.B.: Nasal physiology. *Ann. Plast. Surg.* 13:214, 1984.

Courtiss, E.H., and Goldwyn, R.M.: The effects of nasal surgery on airflow. *Plast. Reconstr. Surg.* 72:9, 1983(a).

Courtiss, E.H., and Goldwyn, R.M.: Uptake resection of obstructing inferior turbinates: A 6-year follow-up. *Plast. Reconstr. Surg.* 72:913, 1983(b).

Courtiss, E.H., Goldwyn, R.M., and O'Brien, J.J.: Resection of obstructing inferior nasal turbinates. *Plast. Reconstr. Surg.* 62:249, 1978.

Daniel, R.K., and Lessard, M.L.: Rhinoplasty: a graded aesthetic-anatomical approach. *Ann. Plast. Surg.* 13:4361, 1984.

Dingman, R.O., and Walter, C.: Use of composite ear graft in correction of the short nose. *Plast. Reconstr. Surg.* 43:117, 1969.

Eisenberg, I.: A history of rhinoplasty. *S. Afr. Med. J.* 62:286, 1982.

Ellis, D.A., and McDonald, G.A.: Narrowing of the wide nasal tip. *J. Otolaryngol.* 13:55, Feb. 1984.

Falces, E.: Cosmetic surgery of the non-Caucasian nose. *Plast. Reconstr. Surg.* 45:317, 1970.

Falces, E., and Gorney, M.: Use of ear cartilage grafts for nasal tip reconstruction. *Plast. Reconstr. Surg.* 50:147, 1972.

Falces, E., Wesser, D., and Gorney, M.: Cosmetic surgery of the non-caucasian nose. *Plast. Reconstr. Surg.* 45:317, 1970.

Flowers, R.S.: Rhinoplasty in Oriental patients: Repair of the East Asian nose. In Daniel, R., editor: *Aesthetic Rhinoplasty.* St. Louis, 1993, The C.V. Mosby Co.

Flowers, R.S.: The surgical correction of the non-caucasian nose. *Clin. Plast. Surg.* 4:69, 1977.

Foman, S., and Bell, J.W.: Rhinoplasty—a fine art. *Arch. Otolaryngol.* 85:685, 1967.

Fredericks, S.: Tripod resection for "Pinocchio" nose deformity. *Plast. Reconstr. Surg.* 53:531, 1972.

Fry, H.J.: Cartilage and cartilage grafts. *Plast. Reconstr. Surg.* 40:426, 1967.

Fry, H.J.: Judicious turbinectomy for nasal obstruction. *Aust. N.Z. J. Surg.* 42:291, 1973.

Gerow, F.J., Stal, S., and Spira, M.: The totem pole rib graft reconstruction of the nose. *Ann. Plast. Surg.* 11:273, Oct. 1983.

Giammance, O.F.: Aesthetics and aesthetic surgery of the nasal base: Subtle indications. *Am. J. Cosm. Surg.* 2:16, 1985.

Gibson, T., and Davis, W.B.: The distortion of autogenous cartilage grafts: its causes and prevention. *Br. J. Plast. Surg.* 10:257, 1958.

Goin, M.K.: Psychological understanding and management of rhinoplasty patients. *Clin. Plast. Surg.* 43:3, 1977.

Goin, M.K., and Goin, J.: Dissatisfaction, in Kaye, B, and Gradinger, G.P., editors: *Symposium on Problems and Complications in Aesthetic Plastic Surgery of the Face* (1980), St. Louis, 1984, The C.V. Mosby Co.

Goldman, I.B.: The importance of the medial crura in nasal-tip reconstruction. *Arch. Otolaryngol.* 65:143, 1957.

Goldman, I.B.: Principles in rhinoplasty. *Minn. Med.* 50:833, 1967.

Goldman, I.B.: Rhinoplasty: its surgical complications and how to avoid them. *J. Int. Coll. Surg.* 13:285, 1950.

Goldman, I.B.: Surgical tips on the nasal tip. *Eye Ear Nose Throat Mouth.* 33:583, 1954.

Goldwyn, R.M., editor: *The Unfavorable Result in Plastic Surgery: Avoidance and Treatment.* Boston, 1972, Little, Brown, and Co.

Goldwyn, R.M.: *Long-Term Results in Plastic and Reconstructive Surgery,* Boston, 1980, Little, Brown & Co.

Goldwyn, R.M., and Shore, S.: The effects of submucous resection and rhinoplasty on the sense of smell. *Plast. Reconstr. Surg.* 41:427, 1968.

Gonzales-Ulloa, M.: The fat nose. *Aesthetic Plast. Surg.* 8:135, 1984.

Gonzales-Ulloa, M.: Planning the integral correction of the human profile. *Plast. Reconstr. Surg.* 36:364, 1966.

Gorney, M.: Correction of the deviated nose: an annotated surgical report. *Clin. Plast. Surg.* 8:201, April 1981.

Gorney, M.: Patient selection criteria: an ounce of prevention. In Kaye, B.L., and Gradinger, G.P., editors: *Symposium on Problems and Complications in Aesthetic Plastic Surgery of the Face,* Vol. 23. A.S.P.R.S., St. Louis, 1984, The C.V. Mosby Co.

Gorney, M.: The septum in rhinoplasty: form and function. In Millard, D., Jr, editor: *Symposium on Corrective Rhinoplasty.* St. Louis, 1984, The C.V. Mosby Co.

Gorney, M.D., and Falces, E.: Repair of post cleft nasal deformities with gullwing cartilage graft. In *International Congress on Cleft Palate,* Aug. 1973.

Guerrerosantos, J.: Cosmetic repair of the acute columellar-lip angle. *Plast. Reconstr. Surg.* 52:246, 1973.

Guerrerosantos, J.: Temporoparietal free fascia grafts in rhinoplasty. *Plast. Reconstr. Surg.* 74:465, 1984.

Gunter, J.P.: Anatomical observations of the lower lateral cartilages. *Arch. Otolaryngol.* 89:61, 1969.

Guyuron, B.: Precision rhinoplasty, Part I: The role of life-size photographs and soft-tissue cephalometric analysis. *Plast. Reconstr. Surg.* 81:489, 1988.

Guyuron, B.: Precision rhinoplasty, Part II: Prediction. *Plast. Reconstr. Surg.* 81:500, 1988.

Hardin, J.C., Jr.: Alar rim reconstruction by a dorsal nasal flap. *Plast. Reconstr. Surg.* 66:293, Aug. 1980.

Hinderer, K.H.: Correction of deformities of the base of the nose. Plastic and Reconstructive Surgery of the Head and Neck, in *Proceedings Second International Symposium*, Vol. 1. New York, 1977, Grune & Stratton.

Hinderer, K.H.: *Fundamentals of Anatomy and Surgery of the Nose*. Birmingham, Al., 1971, Aesculapius Publishing Co.

Hinderer, K.H.: Surgery of the nasal valve. *Int. Rhinol.* 8:60, March 1970.

Hinderer, U.T.: Relationship between the protrusion of the nasal tip and the dorsum in rhinoplasty. *Aesthet. Plast. Surg.* 8:201, 1984.

Hirshowitz, B., Kaufman, T., and Ullman, J.: Reconstruction of the tip of the nose and ala by load cycling to the nasal skin and harnessing of extra skin. *Plast. Reconstr. Surg.* 77:316, Feb. 1986.

Hoefflin, S.M.: Cartilage crusher. *Plast. Reconstr. Surg.* 81:1, 1988.

Hoefflin, S.M.: Decadron and Benadryl, in *Technical Forum: Bulletin of the International Society of Clinical Plastic Surgeons*, 1988.

Hoefflin, S.M.: Postoperative nighttime nasal taping to decrease swelling. *Plast. Reconstr. Surg.* 84:2, 1989.

Horowitz, J.H.: Persing, J.A., Nichter, L.S., et al.: Galeal-pericranial flaps in head and neck reconstruction: anatomy and application. *Am. J. Surg.* 148:489, 1984.

Horton, C.E.: Combined septoplasty and rhinoplasty. In Masters, F.W., and Lewis, J.R., Jr., editors: *Symposium on Aesthetic Surgery of the Nose, Ears, and Chin*. St. Louis, 1973, The C.V. Mosby Co.

Jackson, I.T., Smith, J., and Mixter, R.C.: Nasal bone grafting using split skull grafts. *Ann. Plast. Surg.* 11:533, Dec. 1983.

Janeke, J.B., and Wright, W.K.: Studies on the support of the nasal tip. *Arch. Otolaryngol.* 93:458, 1971.

Joseph, J.: *Nasenplastik und sonstige Gesichtplastik Nebst einem Anbang ueber Mammaplastic*, Leipzig, 1931, Kabitzsch.

Juri, J.: Secondary rhinoplasty. *Transactions of the XI International Congress of Plastic Surgery*, Montreal, Canada, 1983, p 731.

Juri, J., and Juri, C.: Secondary rhinodeformity. *Transactions of the VII International Congress of Plastic and Reconstructive Surgery*, Rio de Janeiro, 1979, p 482.

Juri, J., Juri, C., Belmont, J.A., et al.: Neighboring flaps and cartilage grafts for correction of serious secondary nasal deformities. *Plast. Reconstr. Surg.* 76:876, Dec. 1985.

Juri, J., Juri C., and Elias, J.C.: Ear cartilage grafts to the nose. *Plast. Reconstr. Surg.* 63:377, 1979.

Juri, J., Jri, C., Grilli, D.A., et al: Corrections of the secondary nasal tip. *Ann. Plast. Surg.* 15:4, 1984.

Juri, J., Juri, C., Grilli, D.A., et al.: Correction of the secondary nasal tip. *Ann. Plast. Surg.* 16:322, April 1986.

Kabaker, S.S.: An approach to aesthetic rhinoplasty in the non-Caucasian nose. *Arch. Otolaryngol.* 103:461, Aug. 1977.

Kamer, F.M., and Churukian, M.M.: Shield graft for the nasal tip. *Arch. Otolaryngol.* 110:608, 1984.

Kamer, F.M., and Cohen, A.: Median horizontal split tip. *Otolaryngol. Head Neck Surg.* 93:35, Feb. 1985.

Kamer, F.M., and Parkes, M.L.: The conservative management of the Negro nose. *Laryngoscope* 85:551, March 1975.

Kazanjian, V.H., and Converse, J.M.: *The Surgical Treatment of Facial Injuries*. Baltimore, 1972, The Williams & Wilkins Co.

Kerth, J.D., and Bytell, D.E.: Revision in unsuccessful rhinoplasty. *Otolaryngol. Clin. North Am.* 7:65, 1974.

Klatsky, S.A., and Manson, P.N.: Aesthetic rhinoplasty in patients with thick skin. *Ann. Plast. Surg.* 11:10, July 1983.

Krugman, M.E.: Photoanalysis of the rhinoplasty patient. *J. Ear, Nose & Throat* 60:56, 1981.

Man, A.: Surgical reduction of the broad nose. *Am. J. Otolaryngol.* 11:446, Nov. 1980.

Matory, W.E., Jr., and Falces, E.: Non-Caucasian rhinoplasty: A 16-year experience. *Plast. Reconstr. Surg.* 77:239, 1986.

McCarthy, J.G., and Wood-Smith, D.: Rhinoplasty. In McCarthy, J.G., editor: *Plastic Surgery*, Vol. 2, Part 2 Philadelphia: W.B. Saunders, 1990, pp 1785–1923.

McCarthy, J.G., and Zide, B.M.: The spectrum of calvaria bone grafting: introduction of the vascularized calvarial bone flap. *Plast. Reconstr. Surg.* 74:10, July 1984

McCollough, E.G., and English, J.L.: A new twist in nasa tip surgery: an alternative to the Goldman tip for the wide or bulbous lobule. *Arch. Otolaryngol.* 111:524 Aug. 1985.

McCurdy, J.A., Jr.: Surgery of the nasal tip: current concepts. *Ear Nose Throat J.* 56:238, 1977.

McDowell, F.: History of rhinoplasty. *Aesthetic Plast. Surg* 1:321, 1978.

McKinney, P.: Teaching model for rhinoplasty. *Plast. Reconstr. Surg.* 74:846, 1984.

McKinney, P., and Cook, J.Q.: A critical evaluation of 20(rhinoplasties. *Ann. Plast. Surg.* 7:357, 1981.

McKinney, P., and Cunningham, B.L.: *Rhinoplasty.* New York, 1989, Churchhill Livingstone.

McKinney, P., Johnson, P., and Wallock, J.: Anatomy of the nasal hump. *Plast. Reconstr. Surg.* 77:404, 1986.

McKinney, P., and Shively, R.: Straightening the twisted nose. *Plast. Reconstr. Surg.* 64:176, 1978.

McKinney, P., and Stainecker, M.L.: Surgery for the bulbous nasal tip. *Ann. Plast. Surg.* 11:106, 1983.

McKinney, P.W., Mossie, R.D., and Bailey, M.H.: Calibrated alar base excision: A 20-year experience. *Aesthetic Plast. Surg.* 12:71, 1988.

Meyer, R.: Total nasal reconstruction. In Conley, J., and Dickinson, J.T., editors: *Plast. and Reconstructive Surgery of the Face and Neck.* New York, 1972, Grune and Stratton.

Meyer, R., and Kesselring, U.K.: The unusually short nose. *Aesthetic Plast. Surg.* 1:271, 1977.

Meyer, R., and Kesselring, U.K.: Sculpturing and reconstructive procedures in aesthetic and functional rhinoplasty. *Clin. Plast. Surg.* 4:1, 1977.

Meyer, R.: Secondary rhinoplasty in secondary nose. *Transactions of the Seventh International Congress of Plastic and Reconstructive Surgery,* Rio de Janeiro, 1979.

Meyer, R., and Kesselring, U.K.: Reconstructive surgery of the nose. *Clin. Plast. Surg.* 8:435, 1981(c).

Meyer, R., and Kesselring, U.K.: Secondary rhinoplasty. In Regnault, P., and Daniel, R.K., editors: *Aesthetic Plastic Surgery.* Boston, 1984, Little, Brown and Co., p 201.

Meyer, R. *Secondary and Functional Rhinoplasty.* Orlando, Florida, 1988, Grune and Stratton.

Millard, D.R.: Alar cinch in the flat, flaring nose. *Plast. Reconstr. Surg.* 65:669, 1980(a).

Millard, D.R.: Alar margin sculpturing. *Plast. Reconstr. Surg.* 44:545, 1969(a).

Millard, D.R.: Problem cases in rhinoplasty. *Symposium on Aesthetic Surgery of the Nose, Ears, and Chin.* Master & Lewis Ed., St. Louis, 1973, The C.V. Mosby Co.

Millard, D.R.: Secondary corrective rhinoplasty. *Plast. Reconstr. Surg.* 44:545, 1969(b).

Millard, D.R.: Secondary rhinoplasty surgery. *Symposium on Corrective Rhinoplasty.* St. Louis, 1976, The C.V. Mosby Co.

Millard, D.R., Jr.: Adjuncts in augmentation mentoplasty and rhinoplasty. *Plast. Reconstr. Surg.* 36:48, 1965.

Millard, D.R., Jr. Adjuncts in primary rhinoplasty. In Millard, D.R., Jr., editor: *Symposium on corrective rhinoplasty.* St. Louis, 1976, The C.V. Mosby Co.

Millard, D.R., Jr.; The alar cinch in the flat, flaring nose. *Plast. Reconstr. Surg.* 65:669, 1980.

Millard, D.R., Jr.: Alar marginal resection. *Plast. Reconstr. Surg.* 40:4, 1976(b).

Millard, D.R., Jr.: Alar marginal sculpturing. *Plast. Reconstr. Surg.* 40:337, 1967(a).

Millard, D.R., Jr.: External excisions in rhinoplasty. *Br. J. Plas. Surg.* 12:340, 1960.

Millard, D.R., Jr.: Lengthening the columella. In Georgiade, N.G., and Hagert, R.F., editors: *Symposium on Management of Cleft Lip and Palate and Associated Deformities.* St. Louis, 1974, The C.V. Mosby Co.

Millard, D.R., Jr.: *Symposium on Corrective Rhinoplasty,* Vol. 13. St. Louis, 1976, The C.V. Mosby Co., p 312.

Millard, D.R., Jr.: Three very short noses and how they were lengthened. *Plst. Reconstr. Surg.* 65:10, 1979.

Millard, D.R., Jr.: The versatility of a chondromucosal flap in the nasal vestibule. *Plast. Reconstr. Surg.* 50:580, 1972b.

Monasterio, F., and Olmedo, A.: Corrective rhinoplasty before puberty: A long-term follow-up. *Plast. Reconstr. Surg.* 68:381, 1981.

Monasterio, F., and Michelena, J.: The use of augmentational rhinoplasty techniques for the correction of the non-Caucasian nose. *Clin. Plast. Surg.* Jan., 1988, p 57.

Moore, G.F., Freeman, T.J., Ogren, F.P., and Yonkers, A.J.: Extended follow-up of total inferior turbinate resection for relief of chronic nasal obstruction. *Laryngoscope* 11:1095, 1985.

Moraes de Avelar, J.: Personal contribution for the surgical treatment of Negroid noses. *Aesthetic Plast. Surg.* 1:81, 1976.

Natvig, P.: *Jacques Joseph: Surgical Sculptor.* Philadelphia, 1982, W.B. Saunders Co.

Nicolle, F.V.: Secondary rhinoplasty of the nasal tip and columella. *Scand. J. Plast. Rec. Surg.* 20:67, 1986(b).

O'Conner, G.B., McGreggor, M.W., Chapiro, L., and Tolleth, H.: The bulbous nose. *Plast. Reconstr. Surg.* 39:278, 1967.

Ofodile, F.A.: Rhinoplasty in Blacks: the Michael Jackson factor (letter). *Plast. Reconstr. Surg.* 74:846, Dec. 1984.

Ofodile, F.A., Bokhari, F.J., and Ellis, C.: The Black American nose. *Ann. Plast. Surg.* 31:209, 1993.

Ogura, J.H.: Physiologic relationships of the upper and lower airways. *Ann. Otol.* 79:495, 1970.

Orticochea, M.: A new method for total reconstruction of the nose: the ears as donor areas. *Br. J. Plast. Surg.* 24:225, 1971.

Orticochea, M.: Refined technique for reconstructing the whole nose with the conchas of the ears. *Br. J. Plast. Surg.* 33:68, 1980.

Ortiz-Monasterio, F.: Rhinoplasty in the Mestizo nose. *PSEF Teleplast,* 1993.

Ortiz-Monasterior, F., Lopez-Mas, J., and Araico, J.: Rhinoplasty in the thick-skinned nose. *Br. J. Plast. Surg.* 27:19, 1974.

Ortiz-Monasterior, F., and Olmedo, A.: Corrective rhinoplasty before puberty: A long term follow-up. *Plast. Reconstr. Surg.* 68:381, 1981.

Ortiz-Monasterio, F., and Olmedo, A.: Reconstruction of major nasal defects. *Clin. Plast. Surg.* 8:535, July 1981.

Ortiz-Monasterior, F., and Olmedo, A.: Rhinoplasty on the Mestizo nose. *Clin. Plast. Surg.* 4:89, 1977.

Ortiz-Monasterio, F., Olmedo, A., and Oscoy, L.: The use of cartilage grafts in primary aesthetic rhinoplasty. *Plast. Reconstr. Surg.* 67:597, 1981.

Ortiz-Monasterior, S.: Rhinoplasty in the thick skin nose. Abstract book first in the National Congress ISAPS, Rio de Janeiro, 1972, p 14.

Ortiz-Monasterior, F., and Olmedo, A.: Reconstruction of major nasal defects. *Clin. Plast. Surg.* 8:535, July 1981.

Ortiz-Monasterio, F., and Olmedo, A.: Secondary rhinoplasty principles of reoperation. *Transactions Seventh International Congress of Plastic and Reconstructive Surgery*, Rio de Janeiro, May 1979. Sao Paulo: Sociedade Brasileira de Cirugia Plastica, 1980.

Parkes, M.L., and Kanodia, R.: Avulsion of the upper lateral cartilage: etiology, diagnosis, surgical anatomy and management. *Laryngoscope* 91:758, May 1981.

Pearson, B.W., and Goodman, W.S.: S.M.R., septoplasty and the surgical relief of nasal obstruction. *Can. J. Otolaryngol.* 2:238, 1973.

Peck, G.C.: Aesthetic rhinoplasty. In Grabb, W.C., and Smith, J.W., editors: *Plastic Surgery*, 3rd. ed, Boston, 1979, Little, Brown and Co., p 427.

Peck, G.C.: Aesthetic rhinoplasty, II, In Barron, J.N., and Saad, M.N., editors: *Operative Plastic and Reconstructive Surgery*. Edinburgh, 1980, Churchill Livingstone.

Peck, G.C.: Aesthetic rhinoplasty of the nasal tip. In Regnault, P., and Daniel, R.K., editors: *Aesthetic Plastic Surgery*. Boston, 1984, Little, Brown & Co.

Peck, G.C.: The difficult nasal tip. *Clin. Plast. Surg.* 4:1, 1977.

Peck, G.C.: Onlay graft for nasal tip projection. *Plast. Reconstr. Surg.* 71:27, 1983.

Peck, G.C.: Rhinoplasty surgery. In Millard, D.R., Jr., editor: *Symposium on Corrective Rhinoplasty*. St. Louis, 1976, The C.V. Mosby Co.

Peck, G.C.: Surgery of the nasal tip. In Grabb, W.C., and Smith, J.W., editors: *Symposium on Aesthetic Surgery of the Nose, Ears and Chin*. St. Louis, 1973, The C.V. Mosby Co.

Peck, G.C.: *Techniques in Aesthetic Rhinoplasty*. New York, 1984, Gower Medical Publishing Ltd.

Pellicicari, D.D.: Columella and nasal tip reconstruction using multiple composite free grafts. *Plast. Reconstr. Surg.* 4:98, 1949.

Peterson, R.A.: Open-flap rhinoplasty. In Millard, D.R., Jr., editor: *Symposium on Corrective Rhinoplasty*. St. Louis, 1976, The C.V. Mosby Co.

Peterson, R.A.: Preoperative evaluation for rhinoplasty. In Millard, D.R., Jr., editor: *Symposium on Corrective Rhinoplasty*, St. Louis, 1976, The C.V. Mosby Co.

Pitanguy, I.: Surgical importance of a dermocartilaginous ligament in bulbous noses. *Plast. Reconstr. Surg.* 36:247, 1965.

Pitanguy, I., and Ceravolo, M.P.: Secondary rhinoplasty. *Aesthet. Plastic. Surg.* 6:47, 1982.

Planas, H.: The twisted nose. *Clin. Plast. Surg.* 4:55, 1977.

Pollet, J.: Three autogenous struts for nasal tip support. *Plast. Reconstr. Surg.* 49:527, 1972.

Pollet, J.: Use of osteocartilaginous fragments removed during rhinoplasty. *Yearbook of Plastic and Reconstructive Surgery*. Chicago, 1974, Yearbook, p 73.

Rees, T.D.: *Aesthetic Plastic Surgery*. Philadelphia, 1980, W.B. Saunders Co.

Rees, T.D.: An aid to the treatment of supratip swelling after rhinoplasty. *Laryngoscope* 81:308, 1971.

Rees, T.D.: *Cosmetic Facial Surgery*. Philadelphia, 1973, W.B. Saunders Co.

Rees, T.D.: Nasal plastic surgery in the Negro. *Plast. Reconstr. Surg.* 43:13, 1969.

Rees, T.D.: Secondary rhinoplasty: *Symposium on Aesthetic Surgery of the Nose, Ears and Chin*. St. Louis, 1973, The C.V. Mosby Co.

Rees, T.D.: *Secondary Rhinoplasty in Aesthetic Plastic Surgery*. Philadelphia, 1980, W.B. Saunders Co., p 388.

Rees, T.D., et al.: Composite grafts. *Third International Congress of Plastic and Reconstructive Surgery*, Amsterdam, 1963, Excerpta Medica.

Regnault, P., and Alfaro, A.: The Skoog Rhinoplasty: a modified technique. *Plast. Reconstr. Surg.* 66:578, 1980b.

Regnault, P., and Daniel, R.K.: Septorhinoplasty. In Regnault, P., and Daniel, R.K., editors: *Aesthetic Plastic Surgery*. Boston, 1984, Little Brown & Co.

Rees, T.D.: Rhinoplasty in the older adult. *Ann. Plast. Surg.* 1:27, 1978.

Rogers, B.O.: History of the development of aesthetic surgery. In Regnault, P., and Daniel, R.K., editors: *Aesthetic Plastic Surgery*. Boston 1984, Little, Brown & Co.

Rogers, B.O.: The importance of delay in timing secondary and tertiary corrections of post-rhinoplastic deformities. In *Transactions of the Fourth International Congress of Plastic and Reconstructive Surgeons*. Amsterdam, 1967, Excerpta Medica.

Rogers, B.O.: Rhinoplasty. In Goldwyn, R.M., editor: *The Unfavorable Result in Plastic Surgery*. Boston, 1972, Little, Brown & Co.

Rogers, B.O.: The role of physical anthropology in plastic surgery today. *Clin. Plast. Surg.* 1:439, 1974.

Rogers, B.O.: Secondary and tertiary correction of postrhinoplastic deformities: some dos and don'ts. In Millard, D.R., Jr., editor: *Symposium on Corrective Rhinoplasty*. St. Louis, 1976, The C.V. Mosby Co.

Rogers, B.O.: Secondary and tertiary rhinoplasty. In *Transactions of the Fourth International Congress of Plastic and Reconstructive Surgery*, Amsterdam, 1969, Excerpta Medica.

Rohrich, R.J.: Rhinoplasty in the Black patient. In R. Daniel, editor: *Aesthetic Rhinoplasty*. St. Louis, 1993, The C.V. Mosby Co.

Safian, J.: *Corrective Rhinoplastic Surgery*. New York, 1935, Hoeber Co.

Safian, J.: Deceptive concepts of rhinoplasty. *Plast. Reconstr. Surg.* 18:127, 1956.

Safian, J. Personal recollections of professor Jacques Joseph. *Plast. Reconstr. Surg.* 37:446, 1965.

Safian, L.S.: Cosmetic rhinoplasty: radiological features. *Head Neck Surg.* 7:139, 1984.

Sheen, J.H.: Absorption of small bone graft in nasal tip (letter). *Plast. Reconstr. Surg.* 56:332, 1975a.

Sheen, J.H.: Achieving more nasal tip projection by the use of a small autogenous vomer or septal cartilage grafts. *Plast. Reconstr. Surg.* 56:35, 1975a.

Sheen, J.H.: Achieving more nasal tip projection by the use of a small atuogenous vomer or septal cartilage grafts. *Plast. Reconstr. Surg.* 56:211, 1975b (Discussion by Horton, C.E.).

Sheen, J.H.: Aesthetic aspects of post-traumatic nasal reconstruction: a case study. *Clin. Plast. Surg.* 8:193, April 1981.

Sheen, J.H.: *Aesthetic Rhinoplasty*. St. Louis, 1978, The C.V. Mosby Co.

Sheen, J.H.: Finesse in rhinoplasty. In Millard, D.R., Jr., editor: *Symposium on Corrective Rhinoplasty*, St. Louis, 1976, The C.V. Mosby Co.

Sheen, J.H.: Finesse in Rhinoplasty. *Aesthetic Rhinoplasty*. St. Louis, 1978, The C.V. Mosby Co., p 267.

Sheen, J.H.: Limited turbinectomy: an adjunct to rhinoplasty. Presented at the American Society of Plastic and Reconstructive Surgeons meeting, Toronto, Unpublished, 1975c.

Sheen, J.H.: Low radix disproportion: a pitfall in rhinoplasty. Presented at the American Society of Plastic and Reconstructive Surgery, Kansas City, 1985.

Sheen, J.H.: A new look at supratip deformity. *Ann. Plast. Surg.* 3:498, Dec. 1979.

Sheen, J.H.: Secondary rhinoplasty. *Plast. Reconstr. Surg.* 56:137, 1975.

Sheen, J.H.: Secondary rhinoplasty. *Plast. Reconstr. Surg.* 56:211, 1975.

Sheen, J.H.: Secondary rhinoplasty. In Grabb, W.C., and Smith, J.N., editors: *Plastic Surgery: A Concise Guide to Clinical Practice*, 4th edition. Boston, 1991, Little, Brown, and Co., p 663.

Sheen, J.H.: Secondary rhinoplasty surgery. In Millard, D.R., editor: *Symposium on Corrective Rhinoplasty*. St. Louis, 1976, The C.V. Mosby Co, p 133.

Sheen, J.H.: The small dorsal hump. In *Transactions of the Sixth International Congress of Plastic and Reconstructive Surgery*, Paris, 1975, Masson Co.

Sheen, J.H.: Spreader grafts: a method of reconstructing the roof of the middle vault following rhinoplasty. *Plast. Reconstr. Surg.* 73:230, Feb. 1984.

Sheen, J.H., and Constantian, M.B.: Primary Rhinoplasty. In Aston, S., Smith, J.N., and Grabb, W.C., editors: *Plastic Surgery: A Concise Guide to Clinical Practice*, 4th edition. Boston, 1991, Little, Brown & Company.

Shehadi, S.I.: The nasal tip: cartilage repositioning. *Plast. Reconstr. Surg.* 74:771, Dec. 1984.

Ship, A.G.: Alar base resection for wide nostrils. *Br. J. Plast. Surg.* 28:77, 1975.

Shirakabe, Y., Shirakabe, T., and Kishimoto, T.: The classification of complications after augmentation rhinoplasty. *Aesthet. Plast. Surg.* 9:185, 1985.

Skoog, T.: A method of hump reduction in rhinoplasty. *Arch. Otolaryngol.* 83;283, 1966.

Skoog, T.: *Plastic Surgery*. Philadelphia, 1975, W.B. Saunders Co.

Smith, T.W.: Osteotomy and infraction in rhinoplasty. *Arch. Otolaryngol.* 100:266, 1974.

Snyder, G.B.: Rhinoplasty in the Negro. *Plast. Reconstr. Surg.* 47:572, 1971.

Spina, V., Kamakura, L., and Psilakis, J.: A new method for correction of the prominent nasal tip. *Plast. Reconstr. Surg.* 51:416, 1973.

Stark, R.B., and Frileck, S.F.: Conchal cartilage grafts in augmentation rhinoplasty and orbital floor fractures. *Plast. Reconstr. Surg.* 43:591, 1969.

Stevens, M.H.: General anesthesia in nasal septal surgery. *Ear Nose Throat J.* 56:22, 1977.

Stoksted, P.: The physiological cycle of the nose under normal and pathological conditions. *Acta Otolaryngol.* (Stockholm) 42:175, 1952.

Stucker, F.J., Jr.: Profile contouring including cheiloplasty. *Arch. Otolaryngol.* 105:680, 1979.

Stuzin, J.M., and Kawamoto, H.K.: Saddle nasal deformity. *Clin. Plast. Surg.* Jan., 1988, p 83.

Tessier, P.: Autogenous bone grafts taken from the calvarium for facial and cranial applications. *Clin. Plast. Surg.* 9:531, 1982.

Thomas, J.R., and McKinney, J.: Rhinoplasty: clinical categorization as a practical preoperative guide. *South. Med. J.* 78:1470, 1985.

Tobin, H.A., and Webster, R.C.: The less-than-satisfactory rhinoplasty: comparison of patient and surgeon satisfaction. *Otolaryngol. Head Neck Surg.* 94:86, Jan. 1986.

Vecchione, T.R.: Repair of the unilateral cleft lip nose using contralateral crease grafts. *Ann. Plast. Surg.* 14:148, Feb. 1985.

Vogt, T.: Tip rhinoplastic operations using a transverse columellar incision. *Aesthetic Plast. Surg.* 7:13, 1983.

Walter, C.: Composite grafts in nasal surgery. *Arch. Otolaryngol.* 90:622, 1969.

Webster, R.C.: Advances in surgery of the tip: intact rim cartilage techniques and the tip-columella-lip aesthetic complex. *Otolaryngol. Clin. North Am.* 8:615, 1975.

Webster, R.C.: Revisional rhinoplasty. *Otolaryngol. Clin. North Am.* 8:753, Oct. 1975.

Webster, R.C., and Smith, R.C.: Rhinoplasty. In Goldwyn, R.M., editor: *Long-term Results in Plastic and Reconstructive Surgery.* Boston, 1980, Little, Brown and Co.

Wheeler, E.S., Kawamoto, H.K., and Zarem, H.: Bone grafts for nasal reconstruction. *Plast. Reconstr. Surg.* 69:134, Jan. 1982.

Willemot, J.: Correction of old nasal deviation. *Plast. Reconstr. Surg.* 43:430, 1969.

Wright, W.K., Symposium: the supratip in rhinoplasty: a dilemma, II: Influence of surrounding structure and prevention. *Laryngoscope* 186:50, 1975.

Wright, W.K., and Bloom, S.M.: Rhinoplasty in adolescence. *Arch. Otolaryngol.* 92:99, July 1970.

Zarem, H.: Standards of photography. *Plast. Reconstr. Surg.* 74:137, 1984.

Zide, B.M.: Nasal anatomy: the muscles and tip sensation. *Aesthetic Plast. Surg.* 9:193, 1985.

Index

Italic page numbers indicate illustrations.

The manufacturer's authorised representative in the EU is Springer
Nature Customer Service Centre GmbH, Europaplatz 3, 69115 Heidelberg,
Germany. If you have any concerns regarding our products, please
contact ProductSafety@springernature.com

Printed and bound by CPI Group (UK) Ltd, Croydon, CR0 4YY

23/04/2026
02095658-0003